SYNTHETIC AND INTEGRATIVE BIOLOGY: PARTS AND SYSTEMS, DESIGN THEORY AND APPLICATIONS

BIOTECHNOLOGY IN AGRICULTURE, INDUSTRY AND MEDICINE

Additional books in this series can be found on Nova's website at:

https://www.novapublishers.com/catalog/index.php?cPath=23_29&seriesp=
Biotechnology+in+Agriculture%2C+Industry+and+Medicine

Additional e-books in this series can be found on Nova's website at:

https://www.novapublishers.com/catalog/index.php?cPath=23_29&seriespe=
Biotechnology+in+Agriculture%2C+Industry+and+Medicine

BIOTECHNOLOGY IN AGRICULTURE, INDUSTRY AND MEDICINE

SYNTHETIC AND INTEGRATIVE BIOLOGY: PARTS AND SYSTEMS, DESIGN THEORY AND APPLICATIONS

JAMES T. GEVONA

EDITOR

Nova Biomedical
Nova Science Publishers, Inc.
New York

LIBRARY OF CONGRESS CATALOGING-IN-PUBLICATION DATA
Available upon request.

ISBN 978-1-60876-678-9

Published by Nova Science Publishers, Inc. ✦ New York

CONTENTS

PREFACE

This new book examines the latest research in the synthetic biology which refers to both: the design and fabrication of biological components and systems that do not already exist in the natural world the re-design and fabrication of existing biological systems. It also deals with Integrative biology is the study and research of biological systems. It does not simply involve one discipline, but integrates a wide variety of disciplines that work together to find answers to scientific questions.

As explained in Chapter 1, synthetic biology involves the design and construction of new biological components and systems, not already existing in nature, as well as the re-design of existing, natural biological molecules, structures and organisms for useful purposes.

Genetic and protein engineering tools, as fast and cheap DNA sequencing and synthesis, and protein evolution in vitro, would allow for rapid design, fabrication, and testing of systems.

"Chemical synthetic biology" is concerned with the synthesis of chemical structures such as proteins, nucleic acids, and other which do not exist in nature. An example deals with the so called "never born proteins" (NBPs), whose design and construction is aimed to understand why and how the protein structures existing in nature have been selected out, with the underlying question whether they have something very particular from the structural or thermodynamic point of view. Moreover, the NBPs may also have bio-technological importance, displaying, for example, novel catalytic and structural features not observed in natural proteins.

Synthetic biology could provide the tools and understanding needed both to develop and to expand "nano-biotechnology". Proteins can be rationally modified to bind to new, non-natural substrates, being adapted for nano-technological uses. There is no need to rely on the complexity of the immune system in order to conduct combinatorial searches for new peptides of this sort. The NBPs can be produced in laboratory by modern molecular biology techniques. The principle to produce NBPs is simple: if one makes a long string of DNA purely randomly, the probability of hitting an existing sequence in nature is lowest. Then this DNA is processed by standard recombinant DNA and in vivo expression techniques, thus obtaining a polypeptide that does not exist in nature, and when this polypeptide is globularly folded, a NBP is already obtained.

The phage display technique has been used to produce very large libraries of proteins having no homology with known proteins, and being selected for binding to specific targets. The peptides are expressed in the protein coats of bacteriophage, which provided both a vector for the recognition sequences and a marker that signalled binding to the respective target.

Phage display can be considered as a practical realization of an artificial chemical evolution. As such, it is an useful tool for in vitro protein evolution, aimed to identifying new receptors and natural ligands for "orphan receptors", drug discovery (peptides might act as enzyme inhibitors and receptor agonists or antagonists, or otherwise modulate the enzyme/receptor's biological effect), "epitope discovery" (a new approach to disease diagnosis and vaccine development), design of DNA-binding proteins, source of new materials.

All this can be regarded as a kind of synthetic biology in that it involves the reshaping and redirecting of natural molecular systems, phage, typically using the tools of protein and genetic engineering.

Aquaporins (AQPs) play important roles in maintaining the water homeostasis. The anuran AQP family is known to consist of at least AQP0-AQP5, AQP7-AQP10, and two anuran-specific types, designated AQPa1 and AQPa2. In *Hyla japonica*, AQP2 (AQP-h2K) and two forms of AQPa2 (AQP-h2 and AQP-h3) reside in the tight epithelial cells of three major osmoregulatory organs: AQP-h2K in the kidney, AQP-h2 in the urinary bladder, and both AQP-h2 and AQP-h3 in the ventral pelvic skin. These AQPs are antidiuretic hormone-dependent AQPs. In Chapter 2, the authors describe in detail the anuran AQPs that have been identified to data and describe the molecular and cellular mechanisms underlying the terrestrial adaptation of anurans in terms of AQPs.

The ability to coordinate cellular responses in a population is critical to achieving certain behaviors in both natural and artificial systems. In bacteria, the coordination of cellular activity at the population level is implemented through quorum sensing. At their most basic, quorum-sensing systems are composed of three main components, making them amenable to genetic manipulation. In Chapter 3 the authors review the work researchers have done to isolate the components of these systems into well-characterized modules for use in the construction of genetic circuits that program complex cellular behaviors. Such modules have not only allowed for the incorporation of traditional quorum-sensing responses in host organisms, but have also allowed for the creation of a diverse array of novel responses based on cell-cell communication.

Synthetic morphology is a coupling of synthetic gene networks to output modules that change the shape or the morphogenetic behaviour of cells. In other words, it is the engineering of biological form. It differs from traditional surgical and tissue engineering approaches in that it is not restricted to forms that exist in nature and it works by making cells organize themselves into the desired form, rather than by manual manipulation of tissues. Synthetic biology has uses in basic science (eg testing hypotheses in developmental biology), industry (eg altering microbial associations and behaviours to improve the efficiency of fermentation, drug production and remediation of polluted soils) and medicine (engineering cell collectives for ex-corporo organ substitutes, engineering novel cell arrangements for repair of tissues or interfacing with artificial devices). Chapter 4 introduces morphogenetic 'primitives' that can be used, in different combinations and sequences, to produce engineered forms and that can be invoked by the expression of single molecules. Both bacterial and mammalian systems are described.

In Chapter 5, the study of the shell wall of Antarctic species *C. antarctica* Saidova, 1975 in SEM was carried on for the first time. The character and disposition of sand particles, pseudopore openings and inner and outer organic linings and thin structure of the apertural collar was revealed. The character and position of the aperture of this species and of the genus *Conotrochammina* on which there were some contradictory data in the previous literature was clarified. The taxonomic position of the genus was changed: it was moved from the subclass Textulariana to the subclass Hormosinana according to the terminal position of its aperture beginning from the initial stage of its shell.

As discussed in Chapter 6, characteristics of feedback loops, i.e. closed interaction chains, can often be used as indicators of the kinds of dynamics a biological system can exhibit. However, published definitions of feedback vary widely, especially in their verbal descriptions of feedback. In particular, opinions differ as to whether the sign of links in a causal chain are given by the direction of the *processes themselves*, or *how process rates respond* to changes in system state. In the latter case, a self-effect (the direct effect of a state variable on itself) may appear qualitatively different depending on whether one considers the state-dependency of the *relative* or the *absolute* rate-of-change of the variable. A fourth definition uses "feedback" as a summary measure of all disjunct loops of action in the system.

For a system of ordinary differential equations, the authors' evaluation favors a definition of "the action of state variable x on y" as being positive if an increase in x causes an increase in the rate-of-change of y. Thus, the sign of an action is given by the corresponding element in the Jacobian matrix, evaluated at the current state of the system. No predictive power seems to be lost by abandoning the competing definitions of feedback, because all authors base their mathematical treatment on the Jacobian matrix.

Although many useful quantities can be derived from a dynamical model, not all of them should be called feedback. In the authors' opinion, a positive or negative term in the rate-of-change should be called just that. Similarly, per capita growth rates may often be adequately characterized as positively or negatively density-dependent. Lumping disjunct causal loops in a single feedback term seems misleading, because disjunct loops are not causally interconnected.

The state-dependence of process rates is a fundamental feature of natural dynamical systems, which makes this notion of feedback widely applicable. This suggests that verbal and conceptual explanations focussing on how process depends on state will be heuristically useful.

Advances in biotechnology have and are providing -for the analysis of events occurring at the molecular genome-wide level- innovative tools which change deeply the scientific and medical landscape of this century. These tools in fact are not only offering more detailed and abundant data, but, also a different -systemic- vision on how molecular mechanisms operate, with direct impact on our way to perceive the chemo-physical mechanisms that underlie drug discovery, therapy delivery, and ultimately medicine and health care. To effectively take advantage of the novel technologies, biology and medicine cannot be any longer two separate and distinct fields, they need to interact in order to bring the discoveries of the fundamental mechanisms of activity of the cells into applicative actions at the patients bedside. This is carried on by the so called *translational research*. Chapter 7 will present an introduction on the technologies that are promoting these profound changes, an overview on some of the most striking changes occurring in biology, pharmacology and medicine, the areas most closely related to health care. All these concepts will be used as the rationale to deepen and promote the use of the scientific approach to complementary and alternative medicine, an area too poorly explored and yet bearing the promise to offer alternatives in the authors' way to approach diseases. This chapter aims at providing the background necessary to understand the scientific bases and current evidence that allow to perceive this area as a promising area of development, along with the limitations and issues that need to be solved.

Tissue engineering has emerged as a response to the problems associated with the substitution of tissues lost due to diseases or trauma. Nowadays, xenografts, allografts or autografts are commonly used to replace the damaged tissue. However, these options involve numerous drawbacks such as rejection, chronic inflammation and severe organ donor shortages. Tissue engineering keeps the promise to overcome these limitations by creating biological substitutes capable of replacing the injured tissue.

Cells, temporary 3D constructs and biochemical signals that trigger tissue regeneration cascades are the three major components for engineering tissues. The adequate combination of these components leads to the successful repair of damaged tissues. In addition to these three main elements, the use and development of bioreactors has come out as an essential tool for the study and achievement of engineered tissues under *in vitro* conditions while mimicking the *in vivo* environment.

Thus, tissue engineering is an interdisciplinary field that applies the principles of engineering and life sciences to develop biological substitutes that restore, maintain, or improve the tissue functions.

Chapter 8 discusses the challenge of creating engineered bone tissues by combining biological and engineering skills. In particular, it will review the issue of stem cell biology, the fabrication methods and artificial materials used for 3D constructs, the principal growth factors used in bone applications and the key role played by bioreactors. More importantly, it will highlight the interdependence of all these parameters and the need for interdisciplinary research for a successful approach.

Three examples of this "chemical synthetic biology" approach are given in Chapter 9. The first example deals with the synthesis of proteins that do not exist in nature, and dubbed as "the never born proteins" (NBPs). This research is related to the question why and how the protein structures existing in our world have been selected out, with the underlying question whether they have something very particular from the structural or thermodynamic point of view (for example, folding). The NBPs are produced in the laboratory by the modern molecular biology technique, the phage display, so as to produce a very large library of proteins having no homology with known proteins.

The second example of chemical synthetic biology has also to do with the laboratory synthesis of proteins, but, this time, adopting a prebiotic synthetic procedure, i.e., the fragment condensation of short peptides, where short means that they have a length that can be obtained by prebiotic methods.

The scheme is illustrated and discussed, being based on the fragment condensation catalyzed by peptides endowed with proteolitic activity. Selection during chain growth is determined by solubility under the contingent environmental conditions, i.e., the peptides which result insoluble are eliminated from further growth. The scheme is tested preliminarily with a synthetic chemical fragment-condensation method and brings to the synthesis of a 44-residueslong protein, which has no homology with known proteins, and which has a stable tertiary folding.

Finally, the third example, dubbed as "the minimal cell project". Here, the aim is to synthesize a cell model having the minimal and sufficient number of components to be defined as living. For this purpose, liposomes are used as shell membranes, and attempts are made to introduce in the interior a minimal genome. Several groups all around the world are active in this field, and significant results have been obtained, which are reviewed in this article. For example, protein expression has been obtained inside liposomes, generally with the green fluorescent protein. The authors' last attempts are with a minimal genome consisting of 37 enzymes, a set which is able to express proteins using the ribosomal machinery.

These minimal cells are not yet capable of self-reproduction, and this and other shortcomings within the project are critically reviewed.

In: Synthetic and Integrative Biology
Editor: James T. Gevona, pp. 1-39

ISBN: 978-1-60876-678-9
© 2010 Nova Science Publishers, Inc.

Chapter 1

PHAGE DISPLAY AS A TOOL FOR SYNTHETIC BIOLOGY: NEW PERSPECTIVES IN NANO-BIOTECHNOLOGY

Santina Carnazza[*] *and Salvatore Guglielmino*

Dept. Life Sciences, University of Messina, sal. Sperone 31,
Vill. S. Agata 98166 Messina

Abstract

Synthetic biology involves the design and construction of new biological components and systems, not already existing in nature, as well as the re-design of existing, natural biological molecules, structures and organisms for useful purposes.

Genetic and protein engineering tools, as fast and cheap DNA sequencing and synthesis, and protein evolution in vitro, would allow for rapid design, fabrication, and testing of systems.

"Chemical synthetic biology" is concerned with the synthesis of chemical structures such as proteins, nucleic acids, and other which do not exist in nature. An example deals with the so called "never born proteins" (NBPs), whose design and construction is aimed to understand why and how the protein structures existing in nature have been selected out, with the underlying question whether they have something very particular from the structural or thermodynamic point of view. Moreover, the NBPs may also have bio-technological importance, displaying, for example, novel catalytic and structural features not observed in natural proteins.

Synthetic biology could provide the tools and understanding needed both to develop and to expand "nano-biotechnology". Proteins can be rationally modified to bind to new, non-natural substrates, being adapted for nano-technological uses. There is no need to rely on the complexity of the immune system in order to conduct combinatorial searches for new peptides of this sort. The NBPs can be produced in laboratory by modern molecular biology techniques. The principle to produce NBPs is simple: if one makes a long string of DNA purely randomly, the probability of hitting an existing sequence in nature is lowest. Then this DNA is processed by standard recombinant DNA and in vivo expression techniques, thus obtaining a polypeptide that does not exist in nature, and when this polypeptide is globularly folded, a NBP is already obtained.

---

[*] E-mail address: santina.carnazza@unime.it

The phage display technique has been used to produce very large libraries of proteins having no homology with known proteins, and being selected for binding to specific targets. The peptides are expressed in the protein coats of bacteriophage, which provided both a vector for the recognition sequences and a marker that signalled binding to the respective target.

Phage display can be considered as a practical realization of an artificial chemical evolution. As such, it is an useful tool for in vitro protein evolution, aimed to identifying new receptors and natural ligands for "orphan receptors", drug discovery (peptides might act as enzyme inhibitors and receptor agonists or antagonists, or otherwise modulate the enzyme/receptor's biological effect), "epitope discovery" (a new approach to disease diagnosis and vaccine development), design of DNA-binding proteins, source of new materials.

All this can be regarded as a kind of synthetic biology in that it involves the reshaping and redirecting of natural molecular systems, phage, typically using the tools of protein and genetic engineering.

Introduction

Synthetic biology studies how to build artificial biological systems for engineering applications, using advanced tools of system design, modeling and simulation, as well as the most recent experimental techniques.

Synthetic biology involves both i) the design and construction of new biological components and systems, not already existing in nature, and ii) the re-design of existing, natural biological molecules, structures and organisms for useful purposes.

The work is fundamentally an engineering application of biological science: the focus is often on ways of taking parts of natural biological systems, characterizing and simplifying them, and using them as components of novel, engineered, highly unnatural life forms.

Biologists are interested in synthetic biology because it provides a complementary perspective from which to consider, analyze, and ultimately understand the living world. Being able to design and build a system is also one very practical measure of understanding. Physicists, chemists and others are interested in synthetic biology as an approach with which to probe the behavior of molecules and their activity inside living cells. Engineers view biology as a technology; they are interested in synthetic biology because the living world provides an apparently rich yet largely unexplored way for controlling and processing information, materials, and energy.

In this field, the experimental work has a philosophical counterpart, as it bears with fundamental questions in the origin of life. This interface between science and philosophy is arising in a special way when chemistry, physics and engineering move towards biology, and, of course, synthetic biology is the most proper medium for this merging.

Genetic and protein engineering tools, as fast and cheap DNA sequencing and synthesis, and protein evolution in vitro, would allow for rapid design, fabrication, and testing of systems. Studies of cellular function, discovery of new therapeutic targets, and detailed mechanistic and structural analyses of proteins rely on specific binding reagents. Display techniques are powerful tools to generate, select, and evolve such binding reagents completely in vitro. Novel applications include maturation of protein affinity and stability, selection for enzymatic activity, and the display of cDNA and random polypeptide libraries.

Taken together, these display techniques have great potential for biotechnological, medical and proteomic applications.

In particular, the use of phage display in screening for novel high-affinity ligands and their receptors has become crucial in functional genomics and proteomics. Since it was first reported, intensive efforts from many researchers have made phage display an invaluable component of biotechnology. Highly diverse peptide libraries can be used to isolate specific ligands for virtually any target of interest, and these ligands successfully used in various research fields. Improved library construction approaches —in combination with innovated vector design, display formats and screening methods— have further extended the technology. It seems probable that extremely diverse phage-display libraries contain multiple solutions to most binding problems, and perhaps the most effective applications are those that exhaustively explore these solutions by combining phage-display selections with high-throughput screening and DNA sequencing. These technologies will generate vast databases that explore the links between protein structure and function, and this information will in turn expedite the process of directed molecular evolution. Moreover, phage display technology extends to the synthesis of artificial proteins with random sequences.

During the past ten years, antibody phage display has evolved into a well-accepted technology, and in a short time has delivered fully human, high-quality antibodies. Phage antibodies have proven their safety and efficacy in clinical trials and are likely to play a great role in the generation of analytical reagents and therapeutic drugs. They offer major advantages in terms of speed and throughput for research and target identification/validation. The greatest challenge for the future will be to translate our ability to create binding sites with tailored size, affinity, valency and sequence, into antibody molecules with improved clinical benefit.

Recombinant phage selected by phage-display may find application also as biosorbent and diagnostic probe in micro- and nano-devices in which antibodies have been used to date. For their properties, phage probes may be exploited for development of bioaffinity sensors, whose essential elements are probes that specifically recognize and selectively bind target structures and, as parts of the analytical platform, generate a measurable signal. For example, they may be used for separation and purification of bacteria prior to their identification with polymerase chain reaction, immunoassays, flow cytometry, or other methods. Otherwise, they can be used to develop rapid real-time diagnostic arrays, by themselves recognizing and binding selectively and specifically the target, with no need of further characterization. The development of highly sensitive and accurate field-usable devices for detection of multiple biological agents could have a number of applications in biomedical field as well as in monitoring of agro-food pathogens and detection of biological warfare agents.

Tailored selection processes, in combination with easy-to-engineer phage, open the door wide for sophisticated applications in synthetic biology.

The "Never Born Proteins" (NBPs)

The chemical approach to synthetic biology is concerned with the synthesis of molecular structures and/or multi-molecular organized systems - proteins, nucleic acids, vesicular forms, and other - that do not exist in nature.

An example deals with the synthesis of proteins non-extant in nature, termed as the "never born proteins" (NBPs) [Luisi 2007].

The proteins existing in nature make only an infinitesimal fraction of the theoretically possible structures, and our life is based on a very limited number of structures. This elicits the question why and how the protein structures existing in our world have been selected out, with the underlying question whether they have something very particular from the structural or thermodynamic point of view that made the selection possible. For example, the few structures selected might be the only ones to be stable (i.e., with the correct folding); or water soluble; or those which have very particular viscosity and/or rheological properties. A second point of view is that "our" proteins have no extraordinary physical properties at all; they have been selected by "chance" among an enormous number of possibilities of quite similar compounds, and it happened that they were capable of fostering cellular life. This last belongs to the so-called "contingency" theory.

The NBPs can be produced in laboratory either by chemical synthesis – e.g. fragment condensation of short peptides with selection governed by the contingency of the environmental conditions – or the modern molecular biology techniques – such as the phage display method.

The principle to produce NBPs is simple: if one makes a long string of DNA purely randomly, the probability of hitting an existing sequence in nature is practically zero. If then this DNA is processed by standard recombinant DNA and in vivo expression techniques, a non-existing polypeptide will be obtained, which, when globularly folded, is already a NBP.

In practice, the aim is to produce a very large library of totally random, de novo proteins having no homology with known proteins, and to investigate whether these synthetic biology products are really so different with respect to natural proteins, in terms of stability, solubility, or folding.

Luisi's group [Chiarabelli et al. 2006a, 2006b; De Lucrezia et al. 2006a, 2006b] tackled the question by investigating folding ability of NBPs, considering it a particularly important and stringent criterion, as the prerequisite for the biological activity of proteins determined by their primary structure. The strategy adopted was based on the well-accepted observation that folded proteins are not easily digestible by proteases. It involved the insertion of the tripeptide PRG (proline-arginine-glycine), substrate for the proteolytic enzyme thrombin, in the otherwise totally random protein sequence. In this way, each of the new proteins had the potentiality of being digested by the enzyme, with the expectation, however, that globularly folded NBPs would be protected from digestion. The larger part of the population was rapidly hydrolyzed, but ~ 20% of the NBPs were highly resistant to the action of thrombin, suggesting that folding is indeed a general property, something that arises naturally, even for proteins of medium length. A significant percentage of periodic structure, α-helix in particular, was present, and, furthermore, the globular folding was thermoreversible, indicating to be under thermodynamic control.

It appears possible at this point to state that folding and thermodynamic stability are not properties that are restricted to extant proteins, and that, on the contrary, they appear to be rather common features of randomly created polypeptides. On the basis of this, one is tempted to propose that "our" natural proteins do not belong to a class of polypeptides with privileged physical properties. And, by inference, one could say that this kind of data permit to brake a lance in favour of the scenario of contingency.

Synthetic Biology Applications in Nanobiotechnology

Synthetic biology includes the broad redefinition and expansion of biotechnology, with the ultimate goals of being able to design and build engineered biological systems that process information, manipulate chemicals, fabricate materials and structures, produce energy, provide food, and maintain and enhance human health and our environment [Chopra and Kamma 2006].

Of course, also the NBPs may have bio-technological importance, and may be also very interesting from the structural point of view: they could, for example, display novel catalytic and structural features that have not been observed in natural proteins.

Synthetic biology, in particular, could provide the tools and understanding needed both to develop "nanobiotechnology" in a more systematic manner and to expand the scope of what it might achieve [Ball 2005].

One of the aims of protein engineering is to design proteins from scratch — for example, artificial enzymes and new protein-based materials. Some peptide materials have been successfully designed [McGrath et al. 1992; Urry et al. 1995; Deming 1997], as well as de novo peptides with specified folds [Bryson et al. 1995]. But a more difficult challenge is achieving novel catalytic function in artificial proteins with an efficacy and specificity similar to that of natural enzymes — most efforts so far have tended to use the natural combinatorial mechanism of the immune system to develop antibodies with catalytic functions [Tramontano et al. 1986]. Recently, however, advances in computational methods have been exploited to transform a non-catalytic protein receptor into a mimic of a natural enzyme by rationally mutating several residues in the binding site [Dwyer et al. 2004]. Thus, rational protein design does not necessarily have to be conducted wholly de novo: existing protein folds can be used for the "scaffolding", and one can focus simply on retooling the active site. Moreover, proteins can be rationally modified to bind to new, non-natural substrates.

These developments in protein design have been adapted for nanotechnological uses. For example, the versatility of the immune system has been used to generate antibodies that will recognize and bind to fullerenes [Chen et al. 1998], carbon nanotubes [Erlanger et al. 2001], and a variety of crystal surfaces [Izhaky and Addadi 1998].

Nature shows how soluble molecules capable of recognizing and binding to specific materials can be used to shape and control the growth of crystals and other nanostructures. There is no need to rely on the complexity of the immune system in order to conduct combinatorial searches for new peptides of this sort. Whaley et al. [2000] used an in vitro evolutionary approach to screen a combinatorial library of 12-residue peptide molecules and identify sequences that would selectively bind to a range of inorganic semiconductor surfaces. The peptides were expressed in the protein coats of bacteriophage, which provided both a vector for the recognition sequences and a marker that signalled binding to the respective surfaces.

In this way, 12-mer peptides could be identified that bind to specific crystal faces of GaAs, as well as to the surfaces of GaN, ZnS, CdS, Fe_3O_4 and $CaCO_3$. These recognition peptides might provide selective "glues" for assembling inorganic nanocrystals into complex arrangements, or for attaching them to other biomolecules for labelling or transport.

Brown's work on polypeptides that will bind to specific metals [Brown 1997] has been extended by Sarikaya and coworkers [2003] to make so-called GEPIs (genetically engineered polypeptides for inorganics) that bind a host of materials. Again, the peptides are prepared by combinatorial shuffling of sequences, coupled to a phage-display screening process. Some of these GEPIs exhibit the ability to modify crystal growth, for example switching the morphology of gold nanocrystals from cubo-octahedral (the equilibrium form) to flat triangular or pseudo-hexagonal forms [Brown S. et al. 2000].

One of the encouraging messages emerging from such efforts to use essentially biological structures for nanotechnology is that the potential hurdle of interfacing seems not to be a problem: that is to say, biology is clearly "plastic" enough to accommodate unfamiliar materials from the inorganic world.

Viruses as New Materials

Viruses are highly organized supramolecular arrays put together by a combination of non-covalent self-assembly and genetic programming. One of the attractions of viruses as nanostructured materials is that their surface chemistry is highly amenable to fine, site-specific and inheritable modification: the proteins that constitute the coat can be altered by introducing the appropriate sequence into the gene that encodes them.

Viral capsids offer the advantages of being robust and monodisperse, and can exhibit various sizes and shapes. Filamentous bacteriophage [Wilson and Finlay 1998] is a flexible rod, of 6 nm diameter and 800-2000 nm length, depending on the genome length. The capsid is mainly constituted by a protein (pVIII) arranged in a helical array with a 5-fold symmetry axis around a single-stranded DNA molecule. A series of aspartate and glutamate residues ensure a negative potential on the surface, and one tryptophan residue is buried in the hydrophobic region responsible for packing of the capsid.

Given that filamentous phages are resistant to harsh conditions such as high salt concentration, acidic pH, chaotropic agents, and prolonged storage, they are suitable candidate building blocks to meet the challenges of bottom-up nano-fabrication. Moreover, the pIII minor capsid protein of the phage can be easily engineered genetically to display ligand peptides that will bind to and modify the behaviour of target cells in selected tissues. Thus, the tactic of integrating phage display technology with tailored nanoparticle assembly processes offers opportunities for reaching specific nano-engineering and biomedical goals [Giordano et al. 2001; Trepel et al. 2002; Arap et al. 2002; Langer and Tirrell 2004; LaVan et al. 2002].

Recently an approach for fabrication of spontaneous, biologically active molecular networks consisting of phage directly assembled with gold (Au) nanoparticles has been reported [Souza et al. 2006]. In this work, it was shown that such networks are biocompatible and preserve the cell-targeting and internalization attributes mediated by a displayed peptide and that spontaneous organization (without genetic manipulation of the pVIII major capsid protein), and optical properties can be manipulated by changing assembly conditions. By taking advantage of Au optical properties, Au–phage networks were generated that, in addition to targeting cells, could function as signal reporters for fluorescence and dark-field microscopy and near-infrared (NIR) surface-enhanced Raman scattering (SERS) spectroscopy. Notably, this strategy maintains the low-cost, high-yield production of complex polymer units (phage) in host bacteria and bypasses many of the challenges in developing cell-peptide detection tools, such as complex synthesis and coupling chemistry, poor solubility of peptides, the presence of organic solvents, and weak detection signals. These networks can effectively integrate the unique signal reporting properties of Au nanoparticles while preserving the biological properties of phage. Together, the physical and biological features within these targeted networks offer convenient multifunctional integration within a single entity with potential for nanotechnology-based biomedical applications.

Furthermore, the bacteriophage MS2 was used as a potential vector for transporting the anti-tumour drug taxol, by linking it covalently to the acid-labile chemical linker groups attached to the inside of the spherical virion [Kooker et al. 2004].

On the other hand, M13 bacteriophage surfaces have been engineered with recognition peptides [Whaley et al. 2000] so that they bound ZnS or CdS, acting as templates for the synthesis of polynanocrystalline nanowires [Mao et al. 2003, 2004]. Lee *et al* [2002] combined recognition peptides with the self-organizing property of rod-shaped M13 bacteriophage to arrange inorganic nanocrystals into an ordered superstructure. The viruses spontaneously packed in concentrated solution into a layered, tilted liquid-crystalline phase. When their coats were tipped with a peptide 9-mer that bound to ZnS, the viruses act as "handles" for arranging ZnS nanocrystals into composite layers with a roughly 700 nm periodicity.

Similar modifications were made to the tubular protein sheath of the tobacco mosaic virus (TMV) so that it can bind metal ions such as cobalt, potentially enabling the virus to template magnetic nanowires and nanotubes [Schlick et al. 2005]. Each TMV tube is 300 nm long, made up of 2100 identical protein subunits. Interestingly, the wedge-shaped proteins were also able to form a variety of other potential template structures, such as shorter tubes and disks, depending on parameters such as pH and ionic strength. Functionalization of these structures with chromophores could provide mimics of the disk-shaped light harvesting complexes of photosynthetic bacteria.

More recently, a new memory effect function was reported in the hybrid system composed of TMV conjugated with platinum nanoparticles (TMV–Pt) [Tseng et al. 2006]. The augmentation of electrical conductivity in this TMV–Pt nanocomposite modifies its properties and makes it a suitable candidate for electronic applications. The function of the TMV is not just to provide a backbone for the organization of discrete nanoparticles (NP). Indeed, the TMV consists of an RNA core with rich aromatic rings, such as guanine, which can behave as charge donors, and of coat proteins, which separate the RNA and Pt NP and act as the energy barrier. These interactions between the RNA and proteins in the TMV with the Pt-NPs are responsible for charge trapping for data storage and tunnelling process in high conductance state, thus creating a conductance switching behaviour and a repeatable memory effect in the TMV–Pt devices.

Ring-shaped viruses from genetically modified M13 with two different binding peptides at each end were created [Nam et al. 2004]. When a bifunctional linker molecule binding to the two peptides was added, it secured the flexible rod-shaped viruses into rings about 200 nm in diameter. These were proposed to be used as templates for making nanoscale magnetic rings for magnetic data storage [Ball 2005].

Landscape phage obtained by phage-display technology might be looked on as a new kind of submicroscopic "fiber" [Smith and Petrenko 1997]. Each phage clone is a type of fiber with unique surface properties. These fibers are not synthesized one by one with some use in mind. Instead, billions of fibers are constructed, propagated all at once in a single vessel and portions of this enormous population are distributed to multiple end-users with many different goals. Each user must devise a method of selecting from this population those fibers that might be suitable for his or her particular applications by affinity selection or whatever other selection principle can be conceived. The phage-display approach provides a physical linkage between the peptide-substrate interaction and the DNA that encodes that interaction.

Localizable or global emergent properties cannot be transferred from the virion surface to another medium; any application that depends on such properties must therefore use phages themselves as the new material.

Of particular value would be methods that could be applied to materials with interesting electronic or optical properties. Organizing ordered inorganic nanoparticles by using biological structures as templates is essential for constructing nano-devices with new functionalities. Although natural evolution has not selected for interactions between biomolecules and such materials, phage-display libraries can be successfully used to identify, develop and amplify binding between organic peptide sequences and inorganic semiconductor substrates, as introduced at the end of the previous section. Peptides with limited selectivity for binding to metal surfaces and metal oxide surfaces have been successfully selected [Brown 1992; Brown 1997]; other researchers have used phage display to select peptides against synthetic polymers such as polystyrene [Adey et al. 1995] and yohimbine-imprinted methacrylate polymer for molecular-imprinted receptors [Berglund et al. 1998]. This approach was then extended and it was shown that combinatorial phage-display libraries can be used to evolve peptides that bind to a range of semiconductor surfaces with high specificity, depending on the crystallographic orientation and composition of the materials used [Whaley et al. 2000]. Phage-display libraries, based on a combinatorial library of random peptides-each containing 12 amino acids-fused to the pIII coat protein of M13, provided 10^9 different peptides that were reacted with crystalline semiconductor structures. Five copies of the pIII coat protein are located on one end of the phage particle, accounting for 10-16 nm of the particle. The experiments utilized different single-crystal semiconductors for a systematic evaluation of the peptide-substrate interactions. Peptide binding selective for the crystal composition (for example, binding to GaAs but not to Si) and crystalline face (for example, binding to GaAs(100), but not to GaAs(111)B) was demonstrated. In addition the preferential attachment of phage to a zinc-blended surface in close proximity to a surface of differing chemical and structural composition was reported, demonstrating the high degree of binding specificity for chemical composition.

Subsequently, phage display has been used again in selecting unique peptides against inorganic semiconductor materials [Flynn et al. 2003; Sano and Shiba 2003]. Reviews [Sarikaya et al. 2003; Sarikaya et al. 2004] have highlighted the application of phage display in selecting peptides to functionalize biomaterials such as titanium. More recently, a unique strategy for surface functionalization of an electrically conductive polymer, chlorine-doped polypyrrole (PPyCl), which has been widely researched for various electronic and biomedical applications, has been developed [Sanghvi et al. 2005]. A M13 bacteriophage library was used to screen 10^9 different 12-mer peptide inserts against PPyCl, a binding phage was isolated, and the stability and specificity, strength and mechanism of its binding to PPyCl were assessed. In these studies, phage display was used to select for peptides that specifically bound to an existing biomaterial, PPy, and were subsequently used to modify the surface of PPy. PPy is a conductive synthetic polymer that has numerous applications in fields such as drug delivery [Konturri et al. 1998] and nerve regeneration [Schmidt 1997; Valentini et al. 1992], and has been used in biosensors and coatings for neural probes [Vidal et al. 1999; Cui et al. 2001]. Different dopant ions such as chloride, perchlorate, iodine and poly(styrene sulphonate) can be used during electrochemical synthesis to provide the material with varying properties (for example, conductivity, film thickness and surface topography). PPyCl does not contain a functional group for biomolecule immobilization, making it a suitable model polymer for functionalization using a peptide selected with phage display. Further, the specific peptide selectively binding PPyCl was joined to a cell adhesive sequence and used to promote cell attachment on PPyCl, to serve as a bi-functional linker. The use of the selected peptide for PPyCl by phage display can be extended to encompass a variety of therapies and devices such as PPy-based drug delivery vehicles [Konturri et al. 1998], nerve guidance channel conduits [Schmidt et al. 1997; Valentini et al. 1992], and coatings for neural probes [Cui et al. 2001]. Furthermore, this strategy for surface functionalization can be extended to immobilize a variety of molecules to PPyCl for numerous other applications. In addition, phage display can be applied to other existing polymers (including those that are already approved and/or those polymers that lack functional chemical groups for coupling reactions like PPyCl) to develop bioactive hybrid-materials without altering their bulk properties.

Selection of peptides using phage display thus represents a simple and versatile alternative to methods based on electrostatic and hydrophobic interactions between two moieties to achieve functionalization of surfaces. It is theoretically possible to design bivalent recombinant phage with two-component recognition: such phages have the potential to bind to specific locations on a semiconductor structure by peptides displayed on pIII protein and simultaneously to specific target (molecules or cells to be captured) by peptides displayed on pVIII coat protein.

Overall, this can be regarded as a kind of synthetic biology in that it involves the reshaping and redirecting of natural molecular systems, typically using the tools of protein and genetic engineering.

Protein Engineering and Directed Evolution

Protein engineering is a relatively young discipline, aimed to develop novel useful or valuable proteins with new and uniquely functional attributes [Graff et al. 2004]. Much research is currently taking place into the understanding of the fundamental rules linking a protein's structure to its function, and it involves the application of science, mathematics and economics.

There are two main strategies for protein engineering. The first is known as rational design, in which detailed knowledge of the structure and function of the protein is used to make desired changes. This has the advantage of being generally inexpensive and easy, since site-directed mutagenesis techniques are well-developed. However, there is a major drawback in that detailed structural knowledge of a protein is often unavailable, and even when it is available, it can be extremely difficult to predict the effects of various mutations.

Computational protein design algorithms seek to identify amino acid sequences that have low energies for target structures. While the sequence-conformation space that needs to be searched is large, the most challenging requirement for computational protein design is a fast, yet accurate, energy function that can distinguish optimal sequences from similar suboptimal ones. Using computational methods, a protein with a novel fold has been designed [Yuan et al. 2005], as well as sensors for unnatural molecules [Arnold 1998].

The second strategy is known as directed evolution. This method mimics natural evolution to evolve proteins with desirable properties not found in nature, and generally produces superior results to rational design. Random mutagenesis is applied to a protein, and a selection regime is used to pick out variants that have the desired qualities. Further rounds of mutation and selection are then applied, in order to allow an increase in functional density of the protein of interest, identifying interesting mutants. It is thus possible to use this method to optimize properties that were not selected for in the original organism, including catalytic specificity, thermostability and many others.

A typical directed evolution experiment involves two steps:

1. Library creation: The gene encoding the protein of interest is mutated and/or recombined at random to create a large library of gene variants.
2. Library screening: The library is screened by the researcher using a high-throughput screen to identify mutants or variants that possess the desired properties. "Winner" mutants identified in this way then have their DNA sequenced to understand what mutations have occurred.

The evolved protein is then characterized using biochemical methods

The great advantage of directed evolution techniques is that they require no prior structural knowledge of a protein, nor it is necessary to be able to predict what effect a given mutation will have. Indeed, the results of directed evolution experiments are often surprising in that desired changes are often caused by mutations that no one would have expected. The drawback is that they require high-throughput, which is not feasible for all proteins. Large amounts of recombinant DNA must be mutated and the products screened for desired qualities. The sheer number of variants often requires expensive robotic equipment to automate the process. Furthermore, not all desired activities can be easily screened for. New advancements in high-throughput technology will greatly expand the capabilities of directed evolution.

An additional technique known as *DNA shuffling*, or *sexual Polymerase Chain Reaction* (PCR) [Stemmer 1994], mixes and matches pieces of successful variants in order to rapidly propagate beneficial mutations, thus producing better results in a directed evolution experiment. This process mimics recombination that occurs naturally during sexual reproduction and is used to rapidly increase DNA library size.

DNA shuffling is a PCR without synthetic primers. In this process, a family of related genes are first cut with enzymes. The gene fragments then are heated up to separate them into single-stranded templates. Some of these fragments will bind to other fragments that share complementary DNA regions, which in some cases will be from other family members. Regions of DNA that are non-complementary hang over the ends of the templates, and the PCR reaction then treats the complementary regions as primers and builds the new double-helical DNA. But PCR also adds bases to the overhanging piece of the primer, forming a double helix there, too. This ultimately creates a mixed structure or "chimera". In the final step, PCR reassembles these chimeras into full-length, shuffled genes.

Application of these methods to engineer protein cores, active sites and macromolecular interfaces will contribute greatly to our ability to both understand and rationally manipulate the physicochemical properties that drive protein function.

In Vitro and Biological Display Technologies

One of the most powerful strategies to improve the properties of proteins or even create new ones is to imitate the strategy of evolution in the test tube, through an in vitro iteration between diversification and selection, by means of display technologies. The directed evolution of proteins using display methods can be engineered for specific properties and selectivity. A variety of display approaches are employed for the engineering of optimized human antibodies, as well as protein ligands, for such diverse applications as protein arrays, separations, and drug development.

In vitro display technologies, namely ribosome and mRNA display [for a review, Amstutz et al. 2001; Lipovsek and Plückthun 2004], combine two important advantages for identifying and optimizing ligands by evolutionary strategies. First, by obviating the need to transform cells in order to generate and select libraries, they allow much higher library diversity. Second, by including PCR as an integral step in the procedure, they make PCR-based mutagenesis strategies convenient. The resulting iteration between diversification and selection allows true Darwinian protein evolution to occur in vitro. Successful examples of high-affinity, specific target-binding molecules selected by in-vitro display methods include peptides, antibodies, enzymes, and engineered scaffolds, such as fibronectin type III domains [Koide et al. 1998; Xu et al. 2002] and synthetic ankyrins, which can mimic antibody function [Binz et al. 2003, 2004].

Ribosome Display is a technique used to perform in vitro protein evolution to create proteins that can bind to a desired ligand. It was first developed by Mattheakis et al. [1994] for the selection of peptides and further improved for folded proteins [Hanes and Plückthun 1997; He and Taussig 1997, 2007]. A fusion protein is constructed in which the domain of interest is fused to a C-terminal tether, such that this domain can fold while the tether is still in the ribosomal tunnel. This fusion construct lacks a stop codon at the mRNA level, thus preventing release of the mRNA and the polypeptide from the ribosome. The process results in translated proteins that remain associated with ribosome and their mRNA progenitor, which is used, as a non-covalent ternary complex, to bind to an immobilized ligand in a selection step. The mRNA-protein hybrids that bind well are then reverse transcribed to cDNA and their sequence amplified via PCR. The result is a nucleotide sequence that can be used to create tightly binding proteins.

The complex of mRNA, ribosome, and protein is stabilized with the lowering of temperature and the addition of cations such as Mg^{2+}. During the subsequent panning stages, the complex is introduced to surface-bound ligand in several ways: using an affinity chromatography column with a resin bed containing ligand, a 96-well plate with immobilized surface-bound ligand, or magnetic beads that have been coated with ligand. The complexes that bind well are immobilized. Subsequent elution of the binders, via high salt concentrations, chelating agents, or mobile ligands which complex with the binding motif of the protein, allows dissociation of the mRNA. The mRNA can then be reverse transcribed back into cDNA, and thus, the genetic information of the binding polypeptides is available for analysis, then it can undergo mutagenesis, and iteratively feed into the process with greater selective pressure to isolate even better binders.

By having the protein progenitor attached to the complex, the process of ribosome display skips the microarray/peptide bead/multiple-well sequence separation that is common in assays involving nucleotide hybridization and provides a ready way to amplify the proteins that do bind without decrypting the sequence until necessary. At the same time, this method relies on generating large, concentrated pools of sequence diversity without gaps and keeping these sequences from degrading, hybridizing, and reacting with each other in ways that would create sequence-space gaps.

In addition, as ribosome display is the first method for screening and selection of functional proteins performed completely in vitro, it circumvents many drawbacks of in vivo selection technologies. First, the diversity of the library is not limited by the transformation efficiency of bacterial cells, but only by the number of ribosomes and different mRNA molecules present in the test tube. Second, random mutations can be introduced easily after each selection round, as no library must be transformed after any diversification step. This allows simple directed evolution of binding proteins over several generations.

In ribosome display, the physical link between genotype and phenotype is accomplished by an mRNA–ribosome–protein complex that is used for selection. As this complex is stable for several days under appropriate conditions, several selections can be performed. Ribosome display allows protein evolution through a built-in diversification of the initial library during selection cycles. Thus, the initial library size no longer limits the sequence space sampled.

This technology of directed evolution over many generations is currently being exploited to address fundamental questions of protein structure and stability [Jermutus et al. 2001; Hanes et al. 2000a], catalysis [Amstutz et al. 2002; Cesaro-Tadic et al. 2003], as well as interesting biomedical applications. Recently, the potential of ribosome display for directed molecular evolution was recognised and developed into a rapid and simple affinity selection strategy to obtain scFv fragments of antibodies with affinities in the low picomolar range [Schaffitzel et al. 1999; Hanes et al. 2000b]. The authors selected a range of different scFvs with picomolar affinity from a fully synthetic naïve antibody scFv library using ribosome display. All of the selected antibodies accumulated beneficial mutations throughout the selection cycles. This display method can apply also to other members of the immunoglobulin superfamily; for example single V-domains which have an important application in providing specific targeting to either novel or refractory cancer markers [Irving et al. 2001]. These works demonstrated that ribosome display not only allows the selection of library members but also further evolves them, thereby mimicking the strategy of the immune system.

It was also demonstrated that even those proteins can be selected that cannot be expressed at all in vivo [Schimmele and Plückthun 2005; Schimmele et al. 2005].

Ribosome display systems that are well proven, by the evolution of high affinity antibodies and the optimisation of defined protein characteristics, generally use an *Escherichia coli* cell extract for in vitro translation and display of an mRNA library. More recently, a cell-free translation system has been produced by combining recombinant *E. coli* protein factors with purified 70S ribosomes [Villemagne et al. 2006]. Higher cDNA yields are recovered from ribosome display selections when using a reconstituted translation system and the degree of improvement seen is selection specific. These effects are likely to reflect higher mRNA and protein stability and potentially other advantages that may include protein specific improvements in expression. Reconstituted translation systems therefore enable a highly efficient, robust and accessible prokaryotic ribosome display technology.

Competing methods for protein evolution in vitro are mRNA display, yeast display, bacterial display and phage display.

Like other biological display technologies, *mRNA display technology* provides easily accessible coding information for each peptide/protein displayed [Roberts and Szostak 1997; Nemoto et al. 1997]. In mRNA display, mRNA is first translated and then covalently bonded to the nascent polypeptide it encodes, using puromycin as an adaptor molecule. The covalent mRNA–protein adduct is purified from the ribosome and used for selection. Puromycin is an analogue of the 3' end of a tyrosyl-tRNA with a part of its structure mimics a molecule of adenosine, and the other part mimics a molecule of tyrosine. Compared to the cleavable ester bond in a tyrosyl-tRNA, puromycin has a non-hydrolysable amide bond. As a result, puromycin interferes with translation, and causes premature release of translation products. The protein and the mRNA are thus coupled and are subsequently isolated from the ribosome and purified. In the current protocol, a cDNA strand is then synthesized to form a less sticky RNA–DNA hybrid and these complexes are finally used for selection.

mRNA display technology has many advantages over the other display methods. The biological display libraries (phage, yeast and bacterial) have polypeptides or proteins expressed on the respective microorganism's cell surface, and the accompanying coding information for each polypeptide or protein is retrievable from the microorganism's genome. However, the library size for the in vivo display systems is limited by the transformation efficiency of each organism. For example, the library size for phage and bacterial display is limited to $1\text{-}10 \times 10^9$ different members. The library size for yeast display is even smaller. Moreover, these cell-based display systems only allow the screening and enrichment of peptides/proteins containing natural amino acids. In contrast, mRNA display and ribosome display are totally in vitro selection methods [Roberts 1999]. They allow a library size as large as 10^{14} different members. The large library size increases the probability to select very rare sequences, and also improves the diversity of the selected sequences. In addition, in vitro selection methods remove unwanted selection pressure, such as poor protein expression, and rapid protein degradation, which may reduce the diversity of the selected sequences. Finally, in vitro selection methods allow the application of in vitro mutagenesis and recombination techniques throughout the selection process. Moreover, although both ribosome display and mRNA display are both in vitro selection methods, mRNA display has some advantage over the former. mRNA display utilizes covalent mRNA-polypeptide complexes linked through puromycin; whereas, ribosome display utilizes stalled, noncovalent ribosome-mRNA-polypeptide complexes and selection stringency is limited. This may cause difficulties in reducing background binding during the selection cycle. In addition, the polypeptides under selection in a ribosome display system are attached to an enormous rRNA-protein complex, the ribosome itself, and there might be some unpredictable interaction between the selection target and the ribosome, thus leading to a loss of potential binders during the selection cycle. In contrast, the puromycin DNA spacer linker used in mRNA display technology is much smaller comparing to a ribosome, so having less chance to interact with an immobilized selection target. Thus, mRNA display technology is more likely to give less biased results [Gold 2001].

mRNA display has been used to select high affinity reagents from engineered libraries of linear peptides [Barrick and Roberts 2002; Barrick et al. 2001; Wilson et al. 2001; Baggio et al. 2002], constrained peptides [Baggio et al., 2002], single-domain antibody mimics [Xu et al.,2002], variable heavy domains of antibodies and single-chain antibodies [Chen 2003]. In addition, mRNA-display selections from proteomic libraries have identified cellular polypeptides that bind specific signaling proteins [Hammond et al., 2001] and small-molecule drugs, as well as polypeptide substrates of v-abl kinase [Cujec et al., 2002].

In general, in vitro display technologies prove to be valuable tools for many applications other than merely selecting polypeptide binders. They have great potential for directed evolution of protein stability and affinity, the generation of high-quality libraries by in vitro preselection, the selection of enzymatic activities, and the display of cDNA and random-peptide libraries [Amstutz et al. 2001; Lipovsek and Plückthun 2004].

In *Yeast display* (or *yeast surface display*) a protein of interest is displayed as a fusion to the Aga2p protein on the surface of yeast [Boder and Wittrup 1997, 1998]. The Aga2p protein is naturally used by yeast to mediate cell-cell contacts during yeast cell mating. As such, display of a protein via Aga2p projects the protein away from the cell surface, minimizing potential interactions with other molecules on the yeast cell wall. The use of magnetic separation and flow cytometry in conjunction with a yeast display library is a highly effective method to isolate high affinity protein ligands against nearly any receptor through directed evolution.

Advantages of yeast display over other in vitro evolution methods include eukaryotic expression and processing, quality control mechanisms of the eukaryotic secretory pathway, minimal avidity effects, and quantitative library screening through fluorescent-activated cell sorting (FACS) [Feldhaus and Siegel 2004a, 2004b].

Disadvantages include smaller mutagenic library sizes compared to alternative methods and differential glycosylation in yeast compared to mammalian cells. It should be noted that these disadvantages have not limited the success of yeast display for a number of applications, including engineering the highest monovalent ligand-binding affinity reported to date for an engineered protein [Boder et al. 2000].

Similarly, in *Bacterial Display* (or *bacterial surface display*) libraries of polypeptides displayed on the surface of bacteria can be screened using iterative selection procedures (biopanning), flow cytometry or cell sorting techniques [Francisco et al. 1993], thus simplifying the isolation of proteins with high affinity for ligands. Expression of antigens on the surface of non-virulent microorganisms is an attractive approach to the development of high-efficacy recombinant live vaccines [Georgiou et al. 1997]. Finally, cells displaying protein receptors or antibodies are of use for analytical applications and bioseparations.

Phage Display for Directed Molecular Evolution

Phage display is a fundamental tool in protein engineering as well as a method for studying protein-protein, protein-peptide, and protein-DNA interactions that utilizes bacteriophage to connect proteins with the genetic information that encodes them [Smith 1985]. This connection between genotype and phenotype enables large libraries of proteins to be screened and amplified in a process of in vitro selection that imitates the strategy of natural evolution in the test tube. Phage display technology involves the expression of random peptides on the surface of a bacteriophage, displayed as a fusion with one of the viral structural protein. The most common bacteriophages used in phage display are M13 and fd filamentous phage [Smith and Petrenko 1997; Kehoe and Kay 2005], though T4 [Ren and Black 1998], T7 [Rosenberg et al. 1996], and λ phage [Santini et al. 1998] have also been used.

Filamentous phages [Marvin 1998] are flexible, thread-like particles approximately 1 μm long and 6 nm in diameter. The bulk of their tubular capsid consists of 2700 identical subunits of the 50-residue major coat protein pVIII arranged in a helical array with a five-fold rotational axis and a coincident two-fold screw axis with a pitch of 3.2 nm. The major coat protein constitutes 87% of total virion mass. Each pVIII subunit is largely αhelical and rod-shaped; about half of its 50 amino acids are exposed to the solvent, the other half being buried in the capsid. At one tip of the particle, the capsid is capped with five copies each of minor coat proteins pVII and pIX; five copies each of minor coat proteins pIII and pVI cap the other end. The capsid encloses a single-stranded DNA. Longer or shorter plus strands —including recombinant genomes with foreign DNA inserts— can be accommodated in a capsid whose length matches the length of the enclosed DNA by including proportionally fewer or more pVIII subunits.

In 1985, recombinant DNA techniques were applied to phage to fashion a new type of molecular chimera that underlies today's phage display technology [Smith 1985]. A foreign coding sequence is spliced in-frame into a phage coat protein gene, so that the ''guest'' peptide encoded by that sequence is fused to a coat protein, and thereby displayed on the exposed surface of the virion.

In early examples of M13 filamentous phage display, polypeptides were fused to the amino-terminus of either pIII or pVIII in the viral genome [Scott and Smith 1990; Greenwood et al. 1991]. These systems were severely limited because large polypeptides (>10 residues for pVIII display) compromised coat protein function and so could not be efficiently displayed. The development of phagemid display systems solved this problem because, in such systems, polypeptides were fused to an additional coat protein gene encoded by a phagemid vector [Bass et al. 1990]. Multiple cloning sites are sometimes used to ensure that the fragments are inserted in all three possible frames so that the cDNA fragment is translated in the proper frame. The phagemid is then transformed into *E. coli* bacterial cells such as TG1 or XL1-Blue *E. coli*. The phage particles will not be released from the *E. coli* cells until these are infected with helper phage, which enables packaging of the phagemid DNA in a coat composed mainly of wild-type coat proteins from the helper phage but also containing some fusion coat proteins from the phagemid. In phagemid systems, functional polypeptide display has now been demonstrated with all five M13 coat proteins.

By cloning large numbers of DNA sequences into the phage, display libraries are produced with a repertoire of many billions of unique displayed proteins. A phage display library is, in fact, an ensemble of up to about 10 billion recombinant phage clones, each harboring a different foreign coding sequence, and therefore displaying a different guest peptide on the virion surface.

The foreign coding sequence can derive from a natural source, or it can be deliberately designed and synthesized chemically. For instance, phage libraries displaying billions of random peptides can be readily constructed by splicing degenerate synthetic oligonucleotides, obtained by combinatorial approach into the coat protein gene. Displayed peptides can be linear or disulfide-constrained [McLafferty et al. 1993; Ladner 1995; Saggio and Laufer 1993; Luzzago and Felici 1998], aimed to mimic in minute detail similar natural ligands and epitopes.

Recombinant peptides specifically binding a target of interest can be selected from random peptidic libraries (usually from 8- to 20-mer), by a process of affinity selection known as "biopanning".

By immobilizing the target protein to a solid support of some sort (e.g., on the polystyrene surface of an ELISA well or on a magnetic bead), a phage that displays a protein binding to one of those targets on its surface will be captured on the support and remain there while others are removed by washing. Those that remain —generally a minuscule fraction of the initial phage population— can then be eluted in a solution that loosens target-peptide bonds without destroying phage infectivity, propagated simply by infecting fresh bacterial host cells and so produce a phage mixture that is enriched with relevant binding phage and that can serve as input to another round of affinity selection. Phage eluted in the final step (typically after 2-4 rounds of selection) can be used to infect a suitable bacterial host, from which the phagemids can be collected and the relevant DNA sequenced to identify the interacting proteins or protein fragments.

Recent work published by Chasteen et al. [2006] shows that use of the helper phage can be eliminated by using a novel "bacterial packaging cell line" technology.

In addition, phage selection is not limited to solid support biopanning as described above but has been used also against intact cells for selection of tissue and cell targeting proteins [Samoylova et al. 2003; Spear et al. 2001]. In particular, this technology represents a powerful tool for the selection of peptides binding to specific motifs on whole cells since it is a non-targeted strategy, which also enables the identification of surface structures that may not have been considered as targets or have not yet been identified [Bishop-Hurley et al. 2005].

More recently, in vivo phage display has been used extensively to screen for novel targets of tumor therapy [Schluesener and Xianglin 2004; Li et al. 2006, Lee et al. 2002; Brown C. K. et al. 2000; Zhang et al. 2005].

Phage display is a practical realization of an artificial chemical evolution [Smith and Petrenko 1997]. Using standard recombinant DNA technology, peptides are associated with replicating viral DNAs that include their coding sequences. This confers on them the key properties of evolving organisms: replicability and mutability. Affinity for the target is an artificial analogue to the ''fitness'' that governs an individual's survival in the next generation. Because selection parameters can be designed and controlled, the phage display is an ideal instrument for directed molecular evolution.

The peptide populations so created are managed by simple microbiological methods that are familiar to all molecular biologists, and they are replicable and therefore nearly cost-free after their initial construction or selection. Therefore, phage display has the overwhelming advantage to be cheap and easy.

The proteins displayed range from short amino acid sequences to fragments of proteins [Wang et al. 1995; vanZonneveld et al. 1995], enzymes [Wang et al. 1996], receptors [Gu et al. 1995; Onda et al. 1995; Sche et al. 1999; Fakok et al. 2000], DNA and RNA binding proteins [Wu et al. 1995; Wolfe et al. 1999; Segal et al. 1999; Isalan and Choo et al. 2000; Cheng et al. 1996] and hormones [Cabibbo et al. 1995; Wrighton et al. 1996; Livnah et al. 1996].

Geysen and his colleagues introduced the term "mimotope" to refer to small peptides that specifically bind a receptor's binding site (and in that sense mimic the epitope on the natural ligand) without matching the natural epitope at the amino acid sequence level [Geysen et al.

1986a, 1986b]; the definition includes cases where the natural ligand is non-proteinaceous. Mimotopes are usually of little value in mapping natural epitopes, but may have other important uses, as identifying new receptors and natural ligands for an "orphan receptor" [Houimel et al. 2002; El-Mousawi et al. 2003], peptides that might act as enzyme inhibitors [Hyde-DeRuyscher et al. 2000; Dennis et al. 2000; Maun et al. 2003; Huang et al. 2003; Lunder et al. 2005a, 2005b; Bratkovic et al. 2005; Nakamura et al. 2001] and receptor agonists or antagonists [Skelton et al. 2002; McConnell et al. 1998; Nakamura et al. 2002; Hessling et al. 2003], "epitope discovery" [Wang and Yu 2004; Petit et al. 2003; Leinonen et al. 2002; Coley et al. 2001; Myers et al. 2000; Rowley et al. 2000], design of DNA-binding proteins [Wu et al. 1995; Wolfe et al. 1999; Segal et al. 1999; Isalan and Choo et al. 2000; Cheng et al. 1996], source of new materials [Smith and Petrenko 1997; Souza et al. 2006; Nam et al. 2004]. The proteins so synthesized can indeed be considered as non-extant, and artificial proteins with random sequence can be displayed [Nakashima et al. 2000], which permits the terminology of "never born proteins" (NBPs).

Phage display is an exponentially growing research area, and numerous reviews covering different aspects of it have been published [Felici et al. 1995; Cortese et al. 1995; Smith and Petrenko 1997]. In conclusion, then, it is a useful tool in protein engineering as well as in functional genomics and proteomics, in drug discovery and, we can say, in synthetic biology.

Antibody Phage

Over the past decade, phage-displayed antibody fragments have been the subject of intensive research [reviewed in Dall'Acqua and Carter 1998; Griffiths and Duncan 1998]. As a result, antibody phage libraries have become practical tools for drug discovery and several phage-derived antibodies are in advanced clinical trials. Phage display has provided approximately 30% of all human antibodies now in clinical development [Kretzschmar and von Ruden 2002].

Large collection of antibody fragments have been displayed on phage particles, and successfully screened with different antigens [Hust and Dubel 2004]. Since the first demonstration that it was possible to display functional antibody fragments on the surface of filamentous phage [McCafferty et al. 1990; Hoogenboom et al. 1991; Barbas et al. 1991; Breitling et al. 1991; Garrard et al. 1991], the development of this technique has led to the construction of recombinant antibody libraries displayed on the bacteriophage surface. The selection of antibodies by phage display basically relies on several factors: first, the ability to isolate or synthesize antibody gene pools to construct large, highly diverse libraries; second, the possibility to express functional antibody fragments in the periplasmic space of *Escherichia coli* [Better et al. 1988; Skerra and Plückthun 1988]; and third, the efficient coupling of expression and display of the antibody protein with the antibody's genetic information being packaged in the *E. coli* bacteriophage [Smith 1985; McCafferty et al. 1990].

Filamentous bacteriophage such as M13 and its coat protein pIII are most often used for antibody display, although T7 bacteriophage also reportedly allows antibody display [Rosenberg et al. 1996].

Both scFv (single chain Fv fragments, where the heavy and light chain V regions are linked by a linker peptide) [McCafferty et al. 1990] and Fab (Fragment antigen binding dimers) [Hoogenboom et al. 1991; Garrard et al. 1991; Chang et al. 1991] formats have been used successfully in antibody libraries displayed on phage, with the former representing the more popular choice [Carmen and Jermutus 2002]. Large repertoires of heavy and light chain V regions can be obtained through amplification by the polymerase chain reaction from the B cells of an immunized animal (usually extracted from the spleen) [Clackson et al. 1991], or hybridoma cells generated from such an animal [Orlandi et al. 1989; Chiang et al. 1989], or even immunized humans ("immunized libraries") [Persson et al. 1991; Burton et al. 1991; Graus et al. 1997; Cai and Garen 1995]; these repertoires will contain antibodies that are biased towards the immunogen, based on the host's immune response.

Alternative approaches are constituted by the "semi-synthetic libraries", where germ-line heavy and light chain V regions, cloned from human B cells, are assembled and synthetic randomization is used to introduce additional diversity at the CDR3 region to increase the repertoire [Barbas et al. 1992], and the "naïve libraries" heavy and light chain variable regions are amplified from the naïve Ig repertoire of a healthy human donor and randomly combined to produce the phage-displayed library [Carmen and Jermutus 2002; Marks et al. 1991].

An important advance has been the development of high-quality libraries with completely synthetic complementarity-determining regions. Knappik *et al* [2000] have constructed a library in which a limited number of human frameworks are used and diversity is introduced by means of synthetic cassettes. Such a system is very amenable to the generation of therapeutic antibodies because preferred frameworks can be used and affinity maturation is aided by the use of defined mutagenic cassettes.

The construction of large, high-quality antibody phage libraries has also been aided by the introduction of improved in vivo recombination systems [Sblattero and Bradbury 2000].

The selection of antibodies from phage libraries consists of two main steps: panning and screening. During panning, library phage preparations are incubated with the antigen of choice, unbound phage are discarded and remaining phage recovered after several washing steps by disrupting the phage–antigen interaction without compromising the phage infectivity (e.g. by applying pH-gradients, competitive elution conditions or proteolytic reactions). Recovered phage subsequently are amplified by infecting *E. coli* and further round(s) of panning are applied, yielding a polyclonal mixture of phage antibodies enriched for antigen-specific binders. The purified antigen can be attached to a solid support (to plastic, by adsorption, or to beads or a column matrix), the phage library run over the support, and antigen-bound phages retrieved after rinsing the support by elution; alternatively, the binding event can take place with antigen in solution, for example, using biotinylated antigen or unlabelled antigen, and the antigen-bound phages might be retrieved by incubation with streptavidin-coated magnetic beads or other ligands that capture the antigen.

The in vitro selection procedure can be performed for function, besides for binding capabilities. Selections can be performed under conditions that mediate the selection of phage antibodies with a particular characteristic, for example, under reducing conditions to retrieve disulfide-free yet stable antibodies [Proba and Wörn 1998], or in the presence of proteases to select for well-folded molecules [Kristensen and Winter 1998]. Antibodies might also be selected with or for a particular functional activity, for example, for receptor cross-linking, signalling, gene transfer or catalysis [Hoogenboom et al. 1998].

The screening process involves subsequently converting the polyclonal mixture obtained by panning into monoclonal antibodies. To this end, *E. coli* cells are infected with the phage pool, plated on selective agar dishes, and single colonies are picked. Thus, highly specific, monoclonal antibody clones are obtained, from which the antibody genes can be readily isolated for further analyses and/or engineering [Rader and Barbas 1997; Griffiths and Duncan 1998; Hoogenboom and Chames 2000; Siegel 2002].

A single phage antibody library can be distributed to thousands of users and serve as the source of cloned antibodies against an unlimited array of antigens. Because selection is based solely on affinity, many toxic and biological threat agents that could not be used to immunize animals without their prior inactivation can nevertheless serve as "native antigens" in this artificial immune system. Furthermore, phage display allows selecting of antibodies recognizing unique epitopes on biological agents that may be missed in hybridoma screening [Emanuel et al. 1996]. Another advantage of phage display contrasting it to the hybridoma technique is that the quantity of antigens required for selection of phage antibodies may be surprisingly small [Liu and Marks 2000], and the properties of selected probes can be further improved by affinity maturation and molecular evolution [Chowdhury 2002; Deng et al.1994; Worn and Plückthun 2001]. Thus, for many purposes, this system may well come to replace natural immunity in animals [Liu and Marks 2000]. With phage display, as in the in vivo immune system, antibodies can be affinity-matured in a stepwise fashion, by incorporating mutations and selecting variant cells with decreasing amounts of antigen [reviewed in Hoogenboom 1997]. Various procedures for introducing diversity in the antibody genes have been described, ranging from more-or-less random strategies (e.g. V-gene chain shuffling, error-prone PCR, mutator strains or DNA shuffling), to strategies targeting the CDR regions of the antibody for mutagenesis (e.g. oligonucleotide-directed mutagenesis, PCR). One possible disadvantage of this in vitro process is that the affinity improvement can be accompanied by the appearance of a modified fine-specificity or unwanted cross-reactivity [Ohlin et al. 1996], which the natural immune system might quickly remove. Extensive screening of the in vitro affinity-matured antibodies for changes in specificity is thus required.

There are several examples where phage antibodies selected against various biological threats have been used beneficially in various detection platforms [reviewed in Iqbal et al. 2000] and for therapeutic applications [reviewed in Kretzschmar and von Ruden 2002].

Phage as Probes in Nanobiotechnology

Development of systems for monitoring the environment and food for biological threat agents is a challenge because it requires environmentally stable, long lasting, sensitive and specific diagnostic probes capable of tight selective binding of pathogens in unfavorable conditions. To respond to the challenge, large financial investments and extensive collaborative efforts of specialists in different areas of science and technology are required. In the last years, probe technology is being revolutionized by utilizing methods of combinatorial chemistry and directed molecular evolution. In particular, phage display is recently identified [Brigati et al. 2004; Petrenko and Smith 2000; Petrenko and Sorokulova 2004; Petrenko and Vodyanoy 2003] as a new technique for development of diagnostic probes which may meet the strong criteria —fastness, sensitiveness, accuracy, and inexpensiveness— for biological monitoring [Al-Khaldi et al. 2008, 2009].

Recombinant phage probes have been selected from phage display libraries with high specificity and selectivity for a wide range of targets [Kouzmitcheva et al. 2001; Petrenko et al. 1996; Petrenko and Smith 2000; Romanov et al. 2001; Samoylova et al. 2003], including small molecules [Saggio and Laufer 1993], receptors [Balass et al. 1993; Legendre and Fastrez 2002], virus [Gough et al. 1999], bacterial spores [Knurr et al. 2003; Steichen et al. 2003; Turnbough 2003; Brigati et al. 2004], and whole-cell epitopes [Carnazza et al. 2007, 2008; Cwirla et al. 1990; Olsen et al. 2006; Petrenko and Sorokulova 2004; Sorokulova et al. 2005; Stratmann et al. 2002; Yu and Smith 1996].

Affinity-selected landscape phage probes for *Salmonella typhimurium* were demonstrated to possess the specificity, selectivity, and affinity of monoclonal antibodies and used as probes for the detection of *S. typhimurium* [Sorokulova et al. 2005].

Petrenko and Vodyanoy [2003] have discussed the potential of phage-based electronic-based (QCM) biodetectors for threat agents.

Proof-in-concept biosensors were prepared for the rapid detection of *S. typhimurium* in solution, based on affinity-selected filamentous phage prepared as probes physically adsorbed to acoustic wave piezoelectric transducers [Olsen et al. 2006].

At the same time, phage antibody chip strategy proved its efficacy in preliminary diagnostics of cancer or other diseases applications [Hong et al. 2004]; phage arrays were constructed by using five clones, displaying respectively four scFv from mouse and one humanized scFv. The targets were Cy3 fluorescence labeled protein extracts from normal lymphocytes and tumorous HeLa cells. Fluorescence intensity of phage was exploited to indicate overexpression of some proteins in the tumor cell line when compared to normal lymphocytes.

Another similar proof-of-principle experiment for phage antibody chips was also reported from the same research group [Bi et al. 2007]: a protein microarray spotted directly with ninety-six phage-displayed antibody clones, half of them deriving from cell panning with leukocytes from healthy donors, and half from panning with acute myeloid leukemia leukocytes, was created to discriminate between recognition profiles of samples from healthy donors and leukemia patients. The signals of nine of those probes showed significant difference between normal and leukemia samples.

In general, fusion of a peptide to the pIII minor coat protein, located on the tip of the phage capsid, is probably not optimal for obtaining phage probes because this expression format does not take advantage of the avidity effect gained when the binding peptides are displayed multi-valently on the major coat protein pVIII [Liao et al. 2005]. This is because pIII is the minor protein of wild phage and there are only five copies of pIII on the tip of the phage. In the pIII display system, scFv is always expressed mono-valently, and most probably, scFv will be either orientated parallel to or in contact with the surface that may restrict the freedom of scFv recognition. On the contrary, the result is surprising in pVIII display system, with a ratio of the positive signal to the negative of 3000:1. This is attributed to the amount and status of pVIII of phage, which forms the tube of phage with about 2700 copies. Using pVIII display system, not only the number of fused scFv is increased, but also the orientation is improved because there is always half of the displayed scFv stretching freely out into solution. Thus, phage antibody chip by pVIII display system seems to be very promising.

The overall data strongly suggest that new generation of selective and inexpensive phage-derived probes will serve as efficient substitutes for antibodies in separation, concentration and detection systems employed for clinical and environmental monitoring, for example by developing rapid diagnostic arrays.

The main advantages of phage probes include: the simplicity of manipulation of the phage libraries, their great variability, high binding affinity, great stability and the possibility to select probes to targets of different nature, also to small molecules or toxic compounds or immunosupressants against which it is difficult to raise natural antibodies.

In fact, while sensitive and selective, antibodies have numerous disadvantages for use as diagnostic biodetectors in biological monitoring, including high cost of production, low availability, great susceptibility to environmental conditions [Shone et al. 1985] and the need for laborious immobilization methods to sensor substrates [Petrenko and Vodyanoy 2003]. The phage probes affinity-selected from random libraries for specific and selective binding to biological targets can be an effective alternative to antibodies [Sorokulova et al. 2005].

They can act as antibody surrogates, possessing distinct advantages including durability, stability, standardization and low-cost production, while achieving equivalent specificity and sensitivity [Petrenko et al. 1996; Petrenko and Vodyanoy 2003]. A selected phage itself can be used as a probe in a detection device, without chemical synthesis of the displayed peptide or fusion to a carrier protein. For example, to be used in an automated fluorescence based sensing assay [Goldman et al. 2000] or FACS [Turnbough 2003], phage, exposing thousands of reactive amino-groups, can be conjugated with fluorescent labels and, in this format, successfully compete with antibody-derived probes.

The use of antibodies as diagnostic probes outside of a laboratory may be problematic because they are often unstable in severe environmental conditions. Environmental monitoring requires stable probes, such as landscape phage, that carry thousands of foreign peptides on their surfaces, are as specific and selective as antibodies, and can operate in non-controlled conditions. Filamentous phages are probably the most stable natural nucleoproteins capable of withstanding high temperatures (up to 80°C), denaturing agents (6–8 mol/L urea), organic solvents [e.g., 50% alcohol or acetonitrile], mild acids (pH 2), and alkaline solutions. The thermostability of a landscape phage probe was recently examined in comparison with a monoclonal antibody specific for the same target [Brigati and Petrenko 2005]. They were both stable for greater than six months at room temperature, but at higher temperatures the antibody degraded more rapidly than the phage probe. Phage retained detectable binding ability for more than 6 weeks at 63°C, and 3 days at 76°C. These results confirm that phage probes are highly thermostable and can function even after exposure to high temperatures during shipping, storage and operation.

Phage-derived probes inherit the extreme robustness of the wild-type phage and, in addition, allow fabrication of bioselective materials by self-assemblage of phages or their composites on metal, mineral, or plastic surfaces [Petrenko and Vodyanoy 2003]. The recombinant phage probes appear to be highly amenable to simple immobilization through physical adsorption directly to the sensor surface, thus providing another engineering advantage while maintaining biological functionality [Carnazza et al. 2007, 2008; Olsen et al. 2006; Sorokulova et al. 2005]. This property allows phage to be used as a recognition element in biosensors, like an inexpensive standard construction material that allows fabrication of bioselective layers by self-assembly of virions or their composites on solid surfaces [Nanduri et al. 2007b].

Protocols for immobilizing bacteriophage particles on solid surfaces have been described since the inception of phage display technology [Smith 1992]. Purified phage particles can be either directly coated to plastic surfaces, or anti-phage monoclonal antibodies can be used to tether phage particles onto the surface of multiwell plates directly from crude supernatants of infected bacteria, without any previous purification step [Dente et al. 1994].

With respect to methods relevant for phage probes used in protein chip and biosensor applications, many different technical approaches of immobilization have been exploited, such as physical adsorption, covalent bonding, and molecular recognition. For examples, phage has been immobilized by direct physical adsorption to the gold surface [Nanduri et al. 2007b], by peptide bond between amino residue on phage and carboxyl terminal on surface [Ploug et al 2001], by disulfide bond between one thiol group on phage and another on surface [Dultsev et al. 2001], and by specific recognition between hexahistidine tag on phage and nickel coated surface [Finucane et al. 1999].

In addition, phage probes can functionalize surface with less steric hindrance than antibodies, thus allowing a higher binding avidity for the target per surface unit. In fact, on the same surface unit, a greater number of phage and with a more correct orientation can be patterned in comparison to antibodies.

Therefore, different phage clones could be selected specifically binding to isolated proteins, enzyme or inorganic material, as well as to different microbial species, thus with a single array different targets might be detected at once, by performing in parallel several different assays in real-time, within the same miniaturized substrate. In this way, standardizing data from multiple separate experiments will be unnecessary, and truly meaningful comparisons may be derived. This could ultimately translate to a much lower cost per test. Much of the promise of these microarrays relies in their small dimensions, which reduce sample and reagent requirements and reaction times, while increasing the amount of data available from a single assay.

Furthermore, phage probes may find application as bio-recognition elements of real-time biosensor devices. Recombinant phage selected by phage-display selectively recognize and specifically bind complex target structures, such as bacterial cells, thus they can be used to develop rapid diagnostic arrays. In fact, traditional diagnostic systems usually involve a multi-step detection method with the use of labeled secondary antibody. Phage-displayed detection microsystems could be considered one-step, simultaneously bind and identify the target microorganism, with no need of further characterization steps.

On the other hand, in nanobiotechnology, acquisition of abundant probes and label-free, high sensitive detection now become the important issues. Generally, labeling tends to cause the deactivation of protein, owing to protein complex three-dimensional structure. The combination of phage-displayed probes and the label-free, real-time detection method based on surface plasmon resonance (SPR) technique has been proved to be fit for proteomics research. Lytic phage was used as probes on an SPR platform, SPREETATM (Texas Instrument, US), for detection of *Staphylococcus aureus* [Balasubramanian et al. 2007], and scFv antibody displayed on Lm P4:A8 phage pIII protein was used to detect *Listeria monocytogenes* and its virulence factor ActA [Nanduri et al. 2007a]. More recently, phage display technique and SPR detection method were combined to acquire abundant specific capture molecules and realize a label-free and high-sensitive protein chip [Liu et al. 2008]. A 12-amino acid peptide displayed on phage M13 coat protein pIII was selected as the probe, and it was immobilized on 11-mercapto-undecanoic acid sensor chip to fabricate a reusable phage-displayed protein chip. The interaction between the peptide and the specific ligand protein was detected on the BIAcore3000 (BIAcore AB, Sweden). Experimental results showed that the phage-displayed protein chip could act as a useful tool in proteomics research.

All of this would allow development of analytical methods for detecting and monitoring quantitative changes of agents under any conditions that warrant their recognition, including clinical based diagnostics and biological warfare applications, spanning several potential markets including biomedical and industrial use, monitoring and proteomics research.

Phage Perspectives in Synthetic Biology

In recent years it has been recognized that recombinant bacteriophages have several potential applications in the modern biotechnology industry: they have been proposed, beside for the above described sophisticated design of antibody drugs and detection of pathogenic bacteria, as alternatives to antibiotics (phage-therapy); as delivery vehicles for protein and DNA vaccines; as gene therapy delivery vehicles; and as tools for screening libraries of proteins, peptides or antibodies. This diversity, with the ease of their manipulation and production, means that they have potential uses in research, therapeutics and manufacturing in both the biotechnology and medical fields [for a review, Clark and March 2006].

Phage-display libraries can be screened in several ways to isolate displayed peptides or proteins with practical applications [Benhar 2001; Willats 2002; Wang and Yu 2004]. For example, it is possible to isolate displayed peptides binding target proteins with affinities similar to those of antibodies, which can then be used as therapeutics that act either as agonists or through the inhibition of receptor–ligand interactions [Ladner et al. 2004].

Furthermore, phage-displayed peptides may be used as signal peptides able to trigger complex cell responses. Overall, phage-display selection of peptides mimicking ligands of cell receptors involved in modulating cell processes such as proliferation, apoptosis and differentiation, opens the door for their potential applications, respectively, in regenerative medicine, anti-tumoral development and stem cell differentiation.

Phages have been used as potential vaccine delivery vehicles in two different ways: by directly vaccinating with phages carrying vaccine antigens on their surface or by using the phage particle to deliver a DNA vaccine expression cassette that has been incorporated into the phage genome [Clark and March 2004a, 2004b]. In phage-display vaccination, phage can be designed to display a specific antigenic peptide or protein on their surface. Alternatively, phage displaying peptide libraries can be screened with a specific antiserum to isolate novel protective antigens or mimotopes – peptides that mimic the secondary structure and antigenic properties of a protective carbohydrate, protein or lipid, despite having a different primary structure [Folgori et al. 1994; Phalipon et al. 1997]. The serum of convalescents can also be used to screen phage-display libraries to identify potential vaccines against a specific disease, without prior knowledge of protective antigens [Meola et al. 1995]. Rather than generating a transcriptional fusion to a coat protein, substances can also be artificially conjugated to the surface of phages after growth, which further increases the range of antigens that can be displayed [Molenaar et al. 2002]. More recently, it has also been shown that unmodified phages can be used to deliver DNA vaccines more efficiently than standard plasmid DNA vaccination [Clark and March 2004a, 2004b; March et al. 2004; Jepson and March 2004]. The vaccine gene, under the control of a eukaryotic expression cassette, is cloned into a standard lambda bacteriophage, and purified whole phage particles are injected into the host. The phage coat protects the DNA from degradation and, because it is a virus-like particle, it should target the vaccine to the antigen presenting cells.

One particularly novel use for phage-displayed peptides is in targeted therapy. One example was in the development of a nasally delivered treatment against cocaine addiction [Dickerson et al. 2005]: whole phage particles delivered nasally can enter the central nervous system where a specific phage-displayed antibody can bind to cocaine molecules and prevent their action on the brain. Theoretically it might also be possible to modify the surface of a bacteriophage by incorporating specific protein sequences to preferentially target the particle to particular cell types, e.g. galactose residues to target galactose-recognizing hepatic receptors in the liver [Molenaar et al. 2002] or peptides isolated by screening phage-display libraries to target dendritic [Curiel et al. 2004] or Langerhans cells [McGuire et al. 2004]. To screen phage for the ability to target specific tissue types, phage-display libraries have been passed through mice several times and at each stage phage were isolated from specific tissues [Rajotte et al. 1998]. A similar in vivo screening strategy was also used to isolate phage displaying peptides that showed increased cytoplasmic uptake into mammalian cells [Ivanenkov and Menon 2000]. Phage-displayed peptides so selected may be used as targeted vehicle for antibiotics or anti-tumorals, or act themselves as targeted anti-bacterials and anti-tumorals. Specific phage-displayed peptides could be used, for example, in anticancer therapy either directly inducing apoptosis processes or targeting anti-tumorals to cancer cells, or also targeting to microorganisms that in turn specifically infect tumoral cells. Recently, in vivo phage display has been used to analyze the structure and molecular diversity of tumor vasculature and to select tumor-specific antigens which have revealed stage- and type-specific markers of tumor blood vessels [Li et al. 2006; Brown C. K. et al. 2000]. Peptides identified by this approach also work as vehicles to transport cargo therapeutic reagents to tumors. These peptides and their corresponding cellular proteins and ligands may provide molecular tools to selectively target the addresses of tumors and their pathological blood vessels and might increase the efficacy of therapy while decreasing side effects.

Finally, phages have also been proposed as potential therapeutic gene delivery vectors [Barry et al. 1996; Dunn 1996]. The phage coat protects the DNA from degradation after injection, and the ability to display foreign molecules on the phage coat also enables targeting of specific cell types, a prerequisite for effective gene therapy. Both artificial covalent conjugation [Larocca et al. 1998] and phage display [Larocca et al. 1999] have been used to display targeting and/or processing molecules on the phage surface. This demonstrates, again, the versatility of phage, showing that tissue targeting can be achieved either by rational design or by the screening of random phage-display libraries.

Conclusion

Synthetic biology could provide the tools and understanding needed both to develop and to expand "nano-biotechnology". Proteins can be rationally modified to bind to new, non-natural substrates, and NBPs can be produced in laboratory by modern molecular biology techniques, being adapted for nano-technological uses. There is no need to rely on the complexity of the immune system in order to conduct combinatorial searches for new proteins of this sort.

Protein engineering and directed evolution in vitro would allow for rapid design, fabrication, and testing of novel and unique systems. Totally in vitro – ribosome and mRNA-display – and biological – yeast, bacterial and phage display – display techniques are powerful tools to generate, select, and evolve such "synthetic" proteins, and they have great potential for biotechnological, medical and proteomic applications.

In particular, phage display technology has become a fundamental tool in functional genomics and proteomics, and intensive research efforts have made it an invaluable component of biotechnology. Specific ligands can be selected for virtually any target of interest and successfully used in several research fields. Phage display is used for studying protein-protein, protein-peptide, and protein-DNA interactions; moreover, it extends to the synthesis of artificial proteins with random sequences.

During the past ten years, phage display has evolved into a well-accepted technology, and in a short time has delivered both sophisticated, high-quality antibody phage and recombinant phage probes for detection of pathogenic agents. Phage antibodies are likely to play a great role in the generation of analytical reagents and therapeutic drugs, offering major advantages in terms of speed and throughput for research and target identification/validation. Recombinant phage selected by phage-display find application also as biosorbent and diagnostic probe in micro- and nano-devices, as effective surrogates of antibodies, used to date. For their properties, phage probes may meet the strong criteria —stability, fastness, sensitiveness, accuracy, and inexpensiveness— for development of bioaffinity sensors for biological monitoring. Highly sensitive and accurate field-usable devices could have a number of applications in biomedical field as well as in environment and food monitoring, and detection of biological warfare agents.

Several other potential applications in the modern biotechnology industry have been recently recognized for recombinant phage – phage-therapy, gene delivery, phage-display vaccination, targeted therapy, next-generation nanoelectronic devices.

Tailored selection processes, in combination with improved library construction and innovated vector design and display formats, open the door wide for sophisticated applications in synthetic biology.

References

Adey, N. B., Mataragnon, A. H., Rider, J. E., Carter, J. M. & Kay, B. K. (1995). Characterization of phage that bind plastic from phage-displayed random peptide libraries. *Gene,* **156**, 27-31.

Al-Khaldi, S. F., Mossoba, M. M., Yakes, B. J., Brown, E., Sharma, D. & Carnazza, S. (2008). Recent Advances in microbial discovery using metagenomics, DNA microarray, biosensors, molecular subtyping, and phage recombinant probes. In: M. K. Moretti, & L. J. Rizzo, (Eds.), *Oligonucleotide Array Sequence Analysis* (Chapter 4, 123-147). Nova Science Publishers, Inc.

Al-Khaldi, S. F., Mossoba, M. M., Yakes, B. J., Brown, E., Sharma, D. & Carnazza, S. (2009). The biggest winners in DNA and protein sequence analysis: metagenomics, DNA microarray, biosensors, molecular subtyping, and phage recombinant probes. *International Journal of Medical and Biological Frontiers* (Nova Science Publishers), 15(3/4), 4.

Amstutz, P., Pelletier, J. N., Guggisberg, A., Jermutus, L., Cesaro-Tadic, S., Zahnd, C. & Plückthun, A. (2002). In vitro selection for catalytic activity with ribosome display. *J. Am. Chem. Soc.,* **124**, 9396-403.

Amstutz, P., Forrer, P., Zahnd, C. & Plückthun, A. (2001). In vitro display technologies: novel developments and applications. *Curr. Opin. Biotechnol.,* **12**, 400-5.

Arap, W., Kolonin, M. G., Trepel, M., Lahdenranta, J., Cardo-Vila, M., Giordano, R. J., Mintz, P. J., Ardelt, P. U., Yao, V. J., Vidal, C. I., et al. (2002). Steps toward mapping the human vasculature by phage display. *Nat. Med.,* **8**,121-7.

Arnold, F. H. (1998). Design by directed evolution. *Acc. Chem. Res.,* **31**(3), 125-31.

Baggio, R., Burgstaller, P., Hale, S. P., Putney, A. R., Lane, M., Lipovsek, D., Wright, M. C., Roberts, R. W., Liu, R., Szostak, J. W. & Wagner, R. W. (2002). Identification of epitope-like consensus motifs using mRNA display. *J. Mol. Recognit.,* **15**, 126-34.

Balass, M., Heldman, Y., Cabilly, S., Givol, D., Katchalski-Katzir, E. & Fuchs, S. (1993). Identification of a hexapeptide that mimics a conformation-dependent binding site of acetylcholine receptor by use of a phage-epitope library. *Proc. Natl. Acad. Sci. USA,* **90**, 10638-42.

Balasubramanian, S., Sorokulova, I. B., Vodyanoy, V. J. & Simonian, A. L. (2007). Lytic phage as a specific and selective probe for detection of *Staphylococcus aureus*. A surface plasmon resonance spectroscopic study. *Biosens. Bioelectr.,* **22**, 948-55.

Ball, P. (2005). Synthetic biology for nanotechnology. Tutorial. *Nanotechnology,* **16**, R1-R8.

Barbas, C. F., Bain, J. D., Hoekstra, D. M. & Lerner, R. A. (1992). Semisynthetic combinatorial libraries: a chemical solution to the diversity problem. *Proc. Natl. Acad. Sci. USA,* **89**, 4457-61.

Barbas, C. F., Kang, A. S., Lerner, R. A. & Benkovic, S. J. (1991). Assembly of combinatorial antibody libraries on phage surfaces: the gene III site. *Proc. Natl. Acad. Sci. USA,* **88**, 7978-82.

Barrick, J. E. & Roberts, R. W. (2002). Sequence analysis of an artificial family of RNA-binding peptides. *Protein Sci.,* **11**, 2688-96.

Barrick, J. E., Takahashi, T. T., Balakin, A. & Roberts, R. W. (2001). Selection of RNA-binding peptides using mRNA-peptide fusions. *Methods,* **23**, 287-93.

Barry, M. A., Dower, W. J. & Johnston, S. A. (1996). Toward cell-targeting gene therapy vectors: selection of cell-binding peptides from random peptide-presenting phage libraries. *Nat. Med.,* **2**, 299-305.

Bass, S., Green, R. & Wells, J. A. (1990). Hormone phage: an enrichment method for variant proteins with altered binding properties. *Proteins: Struct. Funct. Genet.,* **8**, 309-14.

Benhar, I. (2001). Biotechnological applications of phage and cell display. *Biotechnol. Adv.,* **19**, 1-33.

Berglund, J., Lindbladh, C., Nicholls, I. A. & Mosbach, K. (1998). Selection of phage display combinatorial library peptides with affinity for a yohimbine imprinted methacrylate polymer. *Anal. Commun.,* **35**, 3-7.

Better, M., Chang, C. P., Robinson, R. R. & Horwitz, A. H. (1988). *Escherichia coli* secretion of an active chimeric antibody fragment. *Science,* **240**, 1041-3.

Bi, Q., Cen, X., Wang, W., Zhao, X., Wang, X., Shen, T. & Zhu, S. (2007). A protein microarray prepared with phage-displayed antibody clones. *Biosens. Bioelectron.,* **22**(12), 3278-82.

Binz, H. K., Amstutz, P., Kohl, A., Stumpp, M. T., Briand, C., Forrer, P., Grütter, M. G. & Plückthun, A. (2004). High-affinity binders selected from designed ankyrin repeat protein libraries. *Nat. Biotechnol., 22,* 575-82.

Binz, H. K., Stumpp, M. T., Forrer, P., Amstutz, P. & Plückthun, A. (2003). Designing repeat proteins: well-expressed, soluble and stable proteins from combinatorial libraries of consensus ankyrin repeat proteins. *J. Mol. Biol., 332,* 489-503.

Bishop-Hurley, S. L., Schmidt, F. J., Erwin, A. L. & Smith, A. L. (2005). Peptides selected for binding to a virulent strain of *Haemophilus influenzae* by phage display are bactericidal. *Antimicrob. Agents Chemother., 49,* 2972-8.

Boder E. T., Midelfort K. S. & Wittrup K. D. (2000). Directed evolution of antibody fragments with monovalent femtomolar antigen-binding affinity. *Proc. Nat. Acad. Sci. USA,* **97**(20), 10701-5.

Boder, E. T. & Wittrup, K. D. (1997). Yeast surface display for screening combinatorial polypeptide libraries. *Nat. Biotech., 15,* 553-57.

Boder, E. T. & Wittrup, K. D. (1998). Optimal screening of surface-displayed polypeptide libraries. *Biotechnol. Prog., 14,* 55-62.

Bratkovic, T., Lunder, M., Popovic, T., Kreft, S., Turk, B., Strukelj, B. & Urleb, U. (2005). Affinity selection to papain yields potent peptide inhibitors of cathepsins L, B, H, and K. *Biochem. Biophys. Res. Commun., 332*(3), 897-903.

Breitling, F., Dübel, S., Seehaus, T., Klewinghaus, I. & Little, M. (1991). A surface expression vector for antibody screening. *Gene, 104,* 147-53.

Brigati, J. R. & Petrenko, V. A. (2005). Thermostability of landscape phage probes. *Anal. Bioanal. Chem., 382,* 1346-50.

Brigati, J., Williams, D. D., Sorokulova, I. B., Nanduri, V., Chen, I. H., Turnbough, C. L., Jr. & Petrenko, V. A. (2004). Diagnostic probes for *Bacillus anthracis* spores selected from a landscape phage library. *Clin. Chem., 50,* 1899-906.

Brown, C. K., Modzelewski, R. A., Johnson, C. S. & Wong, M. K. (2000). A novel approach for the identification of unique tumor vasculature bonding peptides using an *E. coli* peptide display library. *Ann. Surg. Oncol.* 7(10), 743-9.

Brown, S. (1992). Engineered iron oxide-adhesion mutants of the *Escherichia coli* phage 1 receptor. *Proc. Natl Acad. Sci. USA, 89,* 8651-5.

Brown, S. (1997). Metal-recognition by repeating polypeptides. *Nat. Biotechnol., 15,* 269-72.

Brown, S., Sarikaya, M. & Johnson, E. (2000). Genetic analysis of crystal growth. *J. Mol. Biol., 299,* 725-32.

Bryson, J. W., Betz, S. F., Lu, H. S., Suich, D. J., Zhou, H. X., O'Neil, K. T. & DeGrado, W. F. (1995). Protein design: a hierarchic approach. *Science, 270,* 935-41.

Burton, D. R., Barbas, C. F. 3rd, Persson, M. A., Koenig, S., Chanock, R. M. & Lerner, R. A. (1991). A large array of human monoclonal antibodies to type 1 human immunodeficiency virus from combinatorial libraries of asymptomatic individuals. *Proc. Natl. Acad. Sci. USA, 88,* 10134-7.

Cabibbo, A., Sporeno, E., Toniatti, C., Altamura, S., Savino, R., Paonessa, G. & Ciliberto, G. (1995). Monovalent phage display of human interleukin (hIL)-6: Selection of superbinder variants from a complex molecular repertoire in the hIL-6 D-helix. *Gene, 167,* 41-7.

Cai, X. & Garen, A. (1995). Anti-melanoma antibodies from melanoma patients immunised with genetically modified antilogous tumor cells: selection of specific antibodies from single-chain Fv fusion phage libraries. *Proc. Natl. Acad. Sci. USA, 92,* 6537-41.

Carmen, S. & Jermutus, L. (2002). Concepts in antibody phage display. *Brief Funct. Genomic Proteomic*, **1**(2), 189-203.

Carnazza, S., Foti, C., Gioffrè, G., Felici, F. & Guglielmino, S. (2008). Specific and selective probes for *Pseudomonas aeruginosa* from phage-displayed random peptide libraries. *Bios. Bioelectron.*, **23**, 1137-44.

Carnazza, S., Gioffrè, G., Felici, F. & Guglielmino, S. (2007). Recombinant phage probes for *Listeria monocytogenes*. *J. Phys. Condensed Matter*, **19**, 395011.

Cesaro-Tadic, S., Lagos, D., Honegger, A., Rickard, J. H., Partridge, L. J., Blackburn, G. M. & Plückthun, A. (2003). Turnover-based in vitro selection and evolution of biocatalysts from a fully synthetic antibody library. *Nat. Biotechnol.*, **21**, 679-85.

Chang, C. N., Landolfi, N. F. & Queen, C. (1991). Expression of antibody Fab domains on bacteriophage surfaces. *J. Immunology*, **147**, 3610-4.

Chasteen, L., Ayriss, J., Pavlik, P. & Bradbury, A. R. (2006). Eliminating helper phage from phage display. *Nucleic Acids Res.*, **34**(21), *e145* [Epub 2006 Nov 6].

Chen, B. X., Wilson, S. R., Das, M., Coughlin, D. J. & Erlanger, B. F. (1998). Antigenicity of fullerenes: antibodies specific for fullerenes and their characteristics. *Proc. Natl. Acad. Sci. USA*, **95**, 10809-13.

Chen, Y. (2003). *Novel approach to generate human monoclonal antibodies by PROfusion*[TM] *Technology*. Cambridge Healthtech Institute 4th Annual Conference on Recombinant Antibodies. Cambridge, MA, USA.

Cheng, X., Kay, B. K. & Juliano, R. L. (1996). Identification of a biologically significant DNA-binding peptide motif by use of a random phage display library. *Gene*, **171**, 1-8.

Chiang, Y. L., Sheng-Dong, R., Brow, M. A. & Larrick, J. W. (1989). Direct cDNA cloning of the rearranged immunoglobulin variable region. *Biotechniques*, **7**, 360-6.

Chiarabelli, C., Vrijbloed, J. W., Thomas, R. M. & Luisi, P. L. (2006a). Investigation of de novo totally random biosequences. Part I. A general method for in vitro selection of folded domains from a random polypeptide library displayed on phage. *Chem. Biodiv.*, **3**, 827-39.

Chiarabelli, C., Vrijbloed, J. W., De Lucrezia, D., Thomas, R. M., Stano, P., Polticelli, F., Ottone, T., Papa, E. & Luisi, P. L. (2006b). Investigation of de novo totally random biosequences. Part II. On the folding frequency in a totally random library of de novo proteins obtained by phage display. *Chem. Biodiv.*, **3**, 840-59.

Chopra, P. & Kamma, A. (2006). Engineering life through Synthetic Biology. *In Silico Biology*, **6**, 401-10.

Chowdhury, P. S. (2002). Targeting random mutations to hotspots in antibody variable domains for affinity improvement. In P. M. O'Brien, & R. Aitken (Eds.), *Antibody Phage Display: Methods and Protocols*. (pp. 269-86). Totowa, NJ: Humana Press.

Clackson, T., Hoogenboom, H. R., Griffiths, A. D. & Winter, G. (1991). Making antibody fragments using phage display libraries. *Nature*, **352**, 624-8.

Clark, J. R. & March, J. B. (2004a). Bacterial viruses as human vaccines? *Expert Rev. Vaccines*, **3**, 463-76.

Clark, J. R. & March, J. B. (2004b). Bacteriophage-mediated nucleic acid immunization. *FEMS Immunol. Med. Microbiol.*, **40**, 21-6.

Clark, J. R. & March, J. B. (2006). Bacteriophages and biotechnology: vaccines, gene therapy and antibacterials. *Trends Biotech.*, **24**, 212-8.

Coley, A. M., Campanale, N. V., Casey, J. L., Hodder, A. N., Crewther, P. E., Anders, R. F., Tilley, L. M. & Foley, M. (2001). Rapid and precise epitope mapping of monoclonal antibodies against *Plasmodium falciparum* AMA1 by combined phage display of fragments and random peptides. *Protein Eng.,* **14**, 691-8.

Cortese, R., Monaci, P., Nicosia, A., Luzzago, A., Felici, F., Galfre, G., Pessi, A., Tramontano, A. & Sollazzo, M. (1995). Identification of biologically active peptides using random libraries displayed on phage. *Curr. Opin. Biotechnol.,* **6**, 73-80.

Cui, X., Hetke, J. F., Wiler, J. A., Anderson, D. J. & Martin, D. C. (2001). Electrochemical deposition and characterization of conducting polymer polypyrrole/PSS on multichannel neural probes. *Sensors Actuat. A,* **93**, 8-18.

Cujec, T. P., Medeiros, P. F., Hammond, P., Rise, C. & Kreider, B. L. (2002). Selection of v-abl tyrosine kinase substrate sequences from randomized peptide and cellular proteomic libraries using mRNA display. *Chem. Biol.,* **9**, 253-264.

Curiel, T. J., Morris, C., Brumlik, M., Landry, S. J., Finstad, K., Nelson, A., Joshi, V., Hawkins, C., Alarez, X., Lackner, A. & Mohamadzadeh, M. (2004). Peptides identified through phage display direct immunogenic antigen to dendritic cells. *J. Immunol.,* **172**, 7425-31.

Cwirla, S. E., Peters, E. A., Barrett, R. W. & Dower, W. J. (1990). Peptides on phage: a vast library of peptides for identifying ligands. *Proc. Natl. Acad. Sci. USA,* **87**, 6378-82.

Dall'Acqua, W. & Carter, P. (1998). Antibody engineering. *Curr. Opin. Struct. Biol.,* **8**, 443-50.

De Lucrezia, D., Franchi, M., Chiarabelli, C., Gallori, E. & Luisi, P. L. (2006a). Investigation of de novo totally random biosequences. Part III. RNA foster: a novel assay to investigate RNA folding structural properties. *Chem. Biodiv.,* **3**, 860-8.

De Lucrezia, D., Franchi, M., Chiarabelli, C., Gallori, E. & Luisi, P. L. (2006b). Investigation of de novo totally random biosequences. Part IV. Folding properties of de novo, totally random RNAs. *Chem. Biodiv.,* **3**, 869-77.

Deming, T. J. (1997). Polypeptide materials: new synthetic methods and applications. *Adv. Mater.,* **9**, 299-311.

Deng, S. J., MacKenzie, C. R., Sadowska, J., Michniewicz, J., Young, N. M., Bundle, D. R. & Narang, S. A. (1994). Selection of antibody single-chain variable fragments with improved carbohydrate binding by phage display. *J. Biol. Chem.,* **269**, 9533-8.

Dennis, M. S., Eigenbrot, C., Skelton, N. J., Ultsch, M. H., Santell, L., Dwyer, M. A., O'Connell, M. P. & Lazarus, R. A. (2000). Peptide exosite inhibitors of factor VIIa as anticoagulants. *Nature,* **404**, 465-70.

Dente, L., Cesareni, G., Micheli, G., Felici, F., Folgori, A., Luzzago, A., Monaci, P., Nicosia, A. & Delmastro, P. (1994). Monoclonal antibodies that recognize filamentous phage: tools for phage display technology. *Gene,* **148**(1), 7-13.

Dickerson, T. J., Kaufmann, G. F. & Janda, K. D. (2005). Bacteriophage-mediated protein delivery into the central nervous system and its application in immunopharmacotherapy. *Expert Opin. Biol. Ther.,* **5**, 773-81.

Dultsev, F. N., Speight, R. E., Fiorini, M. T., Blackburn, J. M., Abell, C., Ostanin, V. P. & Klenerman, D. (2001). Direct and quantitative detection of bacteriophage by "hearing" surface detachment using a quartz crystal microbalance. *Anal. Chem.,* **73**(16), 3935-9.

Dunn, I. S. (1996). Mammalian cell binding and transfection mediated by surface-modified bacteriophage lambda. *Biochimie,* **78**, 856-61.

Dwyer, M. A., Looger, L. L. & Hellinga, H. W. (2004). Computational design of a biologically active enzyme. *Science,* **304**, 1967-71.

El-Mousawi, M., Tchistiakova, L., Yurchenko, L., Pietrzynski, G., Moreno, M., Stanimirovic, D., Ahmad, D. & Alakhov, V. (2003). A vascular endothelial growth factor high affinity receptor 1-specific peptide with antiangiogenic activity identified using a phage display peptide library. *J. Biol. Chem.,* **278**, 46681-91.

Emanuel, P., O'Brien, T., Burans, J., DasGupta, B. R., Valdes, J. J. & Eldefrawi, M. (1996). Directing antigen specificity towards botulinum neurotoxin with combinatorial phage display libraries. *J. Immunol. Methods,* **193**, 189-97.

Erlanger, B. F., Chen, B.-X., Zhu, M. & Brus, L. (2001). Binding of an anti-fullerene IgG monoclonal antibody to single wall carbon nanotubes. *Nano Lett.,* **1**, 465-7.

Fakok, V. A., Bratton, D. L., Rose, D. M., Pearson, A., Ezekewitz, R. A. B. & Henson, P. M. (2000). A receptor for phosphatidylserine-specific clearance of apoptotic cells. *Nature,* **405**, 85-90.

Feldhaus, M. J. & Siegel, R. W. (2004a). Flow cytometric screening of yeast surface display libraries. *Methods Mol. Biol.,* **263**, 311-32.

Feldhaus, M. J. & Siegel, R. W. (2004b). Yeast display of antibody fragments: A discovery and characterization platform. *J. Immunol. Methods,* **290**, 69-80.

Felici, F., Luzzago, A., Monaci, P., Nicosia, A., Sollazzo, M. & Traboni, C. (1995). Peptide and protein display on the surface of filamentous bacteriophage. In M. R. El-Gewely (Ed.), *Biotechnology Annual Review* (Volume 1, 149-83). Amsterdam, The Netherlands: Elsevier Science B.V.

Finucane, M. D., Tuna, M., Lees, J. H. & Woolfson, D. N. (1999). Core-directed protein design. I. An experimental method for selecting stable proteins from combinatorial libraries. *Biochemistry,* **38**, 11604-12.

Flynn, C. E., Mao, C., Hayhurst, A., Williams, J. L., Georgiou, G., Iversona B. & Belcher, A. M. (2003). Synthesis and organization of nanoscale semiconductor materials using evolved peptide specificity and viral capsid assembly. *J. Mater. Chem.,* **13**, 2414-21.

Folgori, A., Tafi, R., Meola, A., Felici, F., Galfré, G., Cortese, R., Monaci, P. & Nicosia, A. (1994). A general strategy to identify mimotopes of pathological antigens using only random peptide libraries and human sera. *EMBO J.,* **13**, 2236-43.

Francisco, J. A., Campbell, R., Iverson, B. L. & Georgiou, G. (1993). Production and fluorescence-activated cell sorting of *Escherichia coli* expressing a functional antibody fragment on the external surface. *Proc. Nat. Acad. Sci. USA,* **90**, 10444-8.

Garrard, L. J., Yang, M., O'Connell, M. P., Kelley, R. F. & Henner, D. J. (1991). Fab assembly and enrichment in a monovalent phage display system. *Bio/Technology,* **9**, 1373-7.

Georgiou, G., Stathopoulos, C., Daugherty, P. S., Nayak, A. R., Iverson, B. L. & Curtis, R. III. (1997). Display of heterologous proteins on the surface of microorganisms: from the screening of combinatorial libraries to live recombinant vaccines. *Nat. Biotech.,* **15**, 29-34.

Geysen, H. M., Rodda, S. J. & Mason, T. J. (1986a). A priori delineation of a peptide which mimics a discontinuous antigenic determinant. *Mol. Immunol.,* **23**, 709-15.

Geysen, H. M., Rodda, S. J. & Mason, T. J. (1986b). The delineation of peptides able to mimic assembled epitopes. *Ciba Found. Symp.,* **119**, 130-49.

Giordano, R. J., Cardo-Vila, M., Lahdenranta, J., Pasqualini, R. & Arap, W. (2001). Biopanning and rapid analysis of selective interactive ligands. *Nat. Med.,* **7**, 1249-53.

Gold, L. (2001). mRNA display: diversity matters during in vitro selection. *Proc. Natl. Acad. Sci. USA,* **98**(9), 4825-6.

Goldman, E. R., Pazirandeh, M. P., Mauro, J. M., King, K. D., Frey, J. C. & Anderson, G. P. (2000). Phage-displayed peptides as biosensor reagents. *J. Mol. Recognit.,* **13**, 382-7.

Gough, K.C., Cockburn, W. & Whitelam, G.C. (1999). Selection of phage-display peptides that bind to cucumber mosaic virus coat protein. *J. Virol. Methods,* **79**, 169-80.

Graff, C. P., Chester, K., Begent, R. & Wittrup, K. D. (2004). Protein Engineering Design and Selection. *Prot. Eng. Des. Sel.,* **17**, 293-304.

Graus, Y. F., de Baets, M. H., Parren, P. W., Berrih-Aknin, S., Wokke, J., van Breda Vriesman, P. J. & Burton, D. R. (1997). Human anti-nicotinic acetylcholine receptor recombinant Fab fragments isolated from thymus-derived phage display libraries from myasthenia gravis patients reflect predominant specificities in serum and block the action of pathogenic serum antibodies. *J. Immunol.,* **158**, 1919-29.

Greenwood, J., Willis, A.E. & Perham, R.N. (1991). Multiple display of foreign peptides on a filamentous bacteriophage. *J. Mol. Biol.,***220**, 821-7.

Griffiths, A. D. & Duncan, A. R. (1998). Strategies for selection of antibodies by phage display. *Curr. Opin. Biotechnol.,* **9**, 102-8.

Gu, H. D., Yi, Q. A., Bray, S. T., Riddle, D. S., Shiau, A. K. & Baker, D. (1995). A phage display system for studying the sequence determinants of protein-folding. *Protein Science,* **4**, 1108-17.

Hammond, P. W., Alpin, J., Rise, C. E., Wright, M. & Kreider, B. L. (2001). In vitro selection and characterization of Bcl-X(L)-binding proteins from a mix of tissue-specific mRNA display libraries. *J. Biol. Chem.,* **276**, 20898-906.

Hanes, J. & Plückthun, A. (1997). In vitro selection and evolution of functional proteins using ribosome display. *Proc. Natl. Acad. Sci. USA,* **94**, 4937-42.

Hanes, J., Jermutus, L. & Plückthun, A. (2000a). Selecting and evolving functional proteins in vitro by ribosome display. *Methods Enzymol.,* **328**, 404-30.

Hanes, J., Schaffitzel, C., Knappik, A. & Plückthun, A. (2000b). Picomolar affinity antibodies from a fully synthetic naïve library selected and evolved by ribosome display. *Nat. Biotechnol.,* **18**, 1287-92.

He, M. & Taussig, M. J. (1997). Antibody-ribosome-mRNA (ARM) complexes as efficient selection particles for in vitro display and evolution of antibody combining sites. *Nucleic Acids Res.,* **25**, 5132-4.

He, M. & Taussig, M. J. (2007). Eukaryotic Ribosome Display with in situ DNA recovery. *Nat. Methods,* **4**, 281-8.

Hessling, J., Lohse, M. J. & Klotz, K. N. (2003). Peptide G protein agonists from a phage display library. *Biochem. Pharmacol.,* **65**, 961-7.

Hong, L., Liao, W., Zhao, X. S. & Zhu, S. G. (2004). Phage antibody chip for discriminating proteomes from different cells. *Acta Phys.-Chim. Sin.,* **20**, 1182-5.

Hoogenboom, H. R. (1997). Designing and optimizing library selection strategies for generating high-affinity antibodies. *Trends Biotechnol.,* **15**, 62-70.

Hoogenboom, H. R. & Chames, P. (2000). Natural and designer binding sites made by phage display technology. *Immunol. Today,* **21**, 371-8.

Hoogenboom, H. R., de Bruïne, A. P., Hufton, S. E., Hoet, R. M., Arends, J. W. & Roovers, R. C. (1998). Antibody phage display technology and its applications. *Immunotechnology, 4*, 1-20.

Hoogenboom, H. R., Griffiths, A. D., Johnson, K. S., Chiswell, D. J., Hudson, P. & Winter, G. (1991). Multi-subunit proteins on the surface of filamentous phage: methodologies for displaying antibody (Fab) heavy and light chains. *Nucl. Acids Res., 19*, 4133-7.

Hooker, J. M., Kovacs, E. W. & Francis, M. B. (2004). Interior surface modification of bacteriophage MS2. *J. Am. Chem. Soc., 126*, 3718-9.

Houimel, M., Schneider, P., Terskikh, A., and Mach, J. P. Starovasnik, M. A. & Lowman, H. B. (2002). Stable "zeta" peptides that act as potent antagonists of the high-affinity IgE receptor. *Proc. Natl. Acad. Sci. USA, 99*, 1303-8.

Huang, L., Sexton, D. J., Skogerson, K., Devlin, M., Smith, R., Sanyal, I., Parry, T., Kent, R., Enright, J., Wu, Q. L., Conley, G., DeOliveira, D., Morganelli, L., Ducar, M., Wescott, C. R. & Ladner, R. C. (2003). Novel peptide inhibitors of angiotensin-converting enzyme 2. *J. Biol. Chem., 278*, 15532-40.

Hust, M. & Dubel, S. (2004). Mating antibody phage display with proteomics. *Trends in Biotechnology, 22*, 8-14

Hyde-DeRuyscher, R., Paige, L. A., Christensen, D. J., Hyde-DeRuyscher, N., Lim, A., Fredericks, Z. L., Kranz, J., Gallant, P., Zhang, J., Rocklage, S. M. et al. (2000). Detection of small-molecule enzyme inhibitors with peptides isolated from phage-displayed combinatorial peptide libraries. *Chem Biol, 7*, 17-25.

Iqbal, S. S., Mayo, M. W., Bruno, J. G., Bronk, B. V., Batt, C. A. & Chambers, J. P. (2000). A review of molecular recognition technologies for detection of biological threat agents. *Biosens. Bioelectron., 15*, 549-78.

Irving, R. A., Coia, G., Roberts, A., Nuttall, S. D. & Hudson, P. J. (2001). Ribosome display and affinity maturation: from antibodies to single V-domains and steps towards cancer therapeutics. *J. Immunol. Methods, 248*, 31-45.

Isalan, M. & Choo, Y. (2000). Engineered zinc finger proteins that respond to DNA modification by HaeII and HhaI methyltransferase enzymes. *J. Mol. Biol., 295*, 471-7.

Ivanenkov, V. V. & Menon, A. G. (2000). Peptide-mediated transcytosis of phage display vectors in MDCK cells. *Biochem. Biophys. Res. Commun., 276*,251-7.

Izhaky, D. & Addadi, L. (1998). Pattern recognition of antibodies for two-dimensional arrays of molecules. *Adv. Mater., 10*, 1009-13.

Jepson, C. D. & March, J. B. (2004). Bacteriophage lambda is a highly stable DNA vaccine delivery vehicle. *Vaccine, 22*, 2413-9.

Jermutus, L., Honegger, A., Schwesinger, F., Hanes, J. & Plückthun, A. (2001). Tailoring in vitro evolution for protein affinity or stability. *Proc. Natl. Acad. Sci. USA, 98*, 75-80.

Kehoe, J. W. & Kay, B. K. (2005). Filamentous phage display in the new millennium. *Chem. Rev., 105*(11), 4056-72.

Knappik, A., Ge, L., Honegger, A., Pack, P., Fischer, M., Wellnhofer, G., Hoess, A., Wolle, J., Plückthun, A. & Virnekas, B. (2000). Fully synthetic human combinatorial antibody libraries (HuCAL) based on modular consensus frameworks and CDRs randomized with trinucleotides. *J. Mol. Biol., 296*, 57-86.

Knurr, J., Benedek, O., Heslop, J., Vinson, R. B., Boydston, J. A., McAndrew, J., Kearney, J. F. & Turnbough, C. L. (2003). Peptide ligands that bind selectively to spores of *Bacillus subtilis* and closely related species. *Appl. Environ. Microbiol., 69*, 6841-7.

Koide, A., Bailey, C. W., Huang, X., Koide, S. (1998). The fibronectin type III domain as a scaffold for novel binding proteins. *J. Mol. Biol.*, **284**, 1141-51.

Konturri, K., Pentti, P. & Sundholm, G. (1998). Polypyrrole as a model membrane for drug delivery. *J. Electroanal. Chem.*, **453**, 231-8.

Kouzmitcheva, G. A., Petrenko, V. A. & Smith, G. P. (2001). Identifying diagnostic peptides for lyme disease through epitope discovery. *Clin. Diagn. Lab. Immunol.*, **8**, 150-60.

Kretzschmar, T. & von Ruden, T. (2002). Antibody discovery: phage display. *Curr. Opin. Biotechnol.*, **13**, 598-602.

Kristensen, P. & Winter, G. (1998). Proteolytic selection for protein folding using filamentous bacteriophages. *Fold. Des.*, **3**, 321-8.

Ladner, R. C. (1995). Constrained peptides as binding entities. *Trends Biotechnol.*, **13**, 426-30.

Ladner, R. C., Sato, A. K., Gorzelany, J. & de Souza, M. (2004). Phage display-derived peptides as therapeutic alternatives to antibodies. *Drug Discov. Today,* **9**, 525-9.

Langer, R. & Tirrell, D. A. (2004). Designing materials for biology and medicine. *Nature,* **428**, 487-92.

Larocca, D., Kassner, P. D., Witte, A., Ladnera, R. C., Pierce, G. F. & Baird, A. (1999). Gene transfer to mammalian cells using genetically targeted filamentous bacteriophage. *FASEB J.,* **13**, 727-34.

Larocca, D., Witte, A., Johnson, W., Pierce, G. F. & Baird, A. (1998). Targeting bacteriophage to mammalian cell surface receptors for gene delivery. *Hum. Gene Ther.,* **9**, 2393-9.

LaVan, D. A., Lynn, D. M. & Langer, R. (2002). Moving smaller in drug discovery and delivery. *Nat. Rev. Drug. Discov.,* **1**, 77-84.

Lee, L., Buckley, C., Blades, M. C., Panayi, G., George, A. J. & Pitzalis, C. (2002). Identification of synovium-specific homing peptides by in vivo phage display selection. *Arthritis Rheum.,* **48**(8), 2109-20.

Lee, S.-W., Mao, C., Flynn, C. E. & Belcher, A. M. (2002). Ordering of quantum dots using genetically engineered viruses. *Science,* **296**, 892-5.

Legendre, D. & Fastrez, J. (2002). Construction and exploitation in model experiments of functional selection of a landscape library expressed from a phagemid. *Gene,* **290**, 203-15.

Leinonen, J., Wu, P. & Stenman, U. H. (2002). Epitope mapping of antibodies against prostate-specific antigen with use of peptide libraries. *Clin. Chem.,* **48**, 2208-16.

Li, X. B., Schluesener, H. J. & Xu, S. Q. (2006). Molecular addresses of tumors: selection by in vivo phage display. *Arch. Immunol. Ther. Exp. (Warsz),* **54**(3), 177-81.

Li, X. B., Schluesener, H. J. & Xu, S. Q. (2006). Molecular addresses of tumors: selection by in vivo phage display. *Arch. Immunol. Ther. Exp. (Warsz),* **54**(3), 177-81.

Liao, W., Hong, L., Wei, F., Zhu, S. G. & Zhao, X. S. (2005). Improving phage antibody chip by pVIII display system. *Acta Physico-Chimica Sinica,* **21**, 508-11.

Lipovsek, D. & Plückthun, A. (2004). In-vitro protein evolution by ribosome display and mRNA display. *J. Imm. Methods,* **290**, 51-67.

Liu, B. & Marks, J. D. (2000). Applying phage antibodies to proteomics: selecting single chain Fv antibodies to antigens blotted on nitrocellulose. *Anal. Biochem.,* **286**, 119-28.

Liu, F., Luo, Z., Ding, X., Zhu, S. & Yu, X. (2008). Phage-displayed protein chip based on SPR sensing. *Sens. Actuators B: Chem.,* doi:10.1016/j.snb.2008. 11.031.

Livnah, O., Stura, E. A., Johnson, D. L., Middleton, S. A., Mulcahy, L. S., Wrighton, N. C., Dower, W. J., Jolliffe, L. K. & Wilson, I. A. (1996). Functional mimicry of a protein hormone by a peptide agonist: the EPO receptor complex at 2.8 Å. *Science,* **273**, 464-71.

Luisi, P. L. (2007). Chemical aspects of synthetic biology. *Chemistry and Biodiversity,* **4**, 603-21.

Lunder, M., Bratkovic, T., Doljak, B., Kreft, S., Urleb, U., Strukelj, B. & Plazar, N. (2005a). Comparison of bacterial and phage display peptide libraries in search of target-binding motif. *Appl. Biochem. Biotechnol.,* **127**(2), 125-31.

Lunder, M., Bratkovic, T., Kreft, S. & Strukelj, B. (2005b). Peptide inhibitor of pancreatic lipase selected by phage display using different elution strategies. *J. Lipid Res.,* **46**(7), 1512-6.

Luzzago, A. & Felici, F. (1998). Construction of disulfide-constrained random peptide libraries displayed on phage coat protein VIII. *Methods Mol. Biol.,* **87**, 155-64.

Mao, C., Flynn, C. E., Hayhurst, A., Sweeney, R., Qi, J., Georgiou, G., Iverson, B. & Belcher, A. M. (2003). Viral assembly of oriented quantum dot nanowires. *Proc. Natl Acad. Sci. USA,* **100**, 6946-51.

Mao, C., Solis, D. J., Reiss, B. D., Kottmann, S. T., Sweeney, R. Y., Hayhurst, A., Georgiou, G., Iverson, B., Belcher, A. M. (2004). Virus-Based toolkit for the directed synthesis of magnetic and semiconducting nanowires. *Science,* **303**, 213-7.

March, J. B., Clark, J. R. & Jepson, C. D. (2004). Genetic immunization against hepatitis B using whole bacteriophage lambda particles. *Vaccine,* **22**, 1666-71.

Marks, J. D., Hoogenboom, H. R., Bonnert, T. P., McCafferty, J., Griffiths, A. D. & Winter, G. (1991). By-passing immunization: human antibodies from V-gene libraries displayed on phage. *J. Mol. Biol.,* **222**, 581-97.

Marvin, D.A. (1998). Filamentous phage structure, infection and assembly. *Curr. Opin. Struct. Biol.,* **8**, 150-8.

Mattheakis, L. C., Bhatt, R. R. & Dower, W.J. (1994). An in vitro polysome display system for identifying ligands from very large peptide libraries. *Proc. Natl. Acad. Sci. USA,* **91**, 9022-6.

Maun, H. R., Eigenbrot, C. & Lazarus, R. A. (2003). Engineering exosite peptides for complete inhibition of factor VIIa using a protease switch with substrate phage. *J. Biol. Chem.,* **278**, 21823-30.

McCafferty, J., Griffiths, A. D., Winter, G. & Chiswell, D. J. (1990). Phage antibodies: filamentous phage displaying antibody variable domains. *Nature,* **348**, 552-4.

McConnell, S. J., Dinh, T., Le, M. H., Brown, S. J., Becherer, K., Blumeyer, K., Kautzer, C., Axelrod, F. & Spinella, D. G. (1998). Isolation of erythropoietin receptor agonist peptides using evolved phage libraries. *Biol. Chem.,* **379**, 1279-86.

McGrath, K. P., Fournier, M. J., Mason, T. L. & Tirrell, D. A. (1992). Genetically directed synthesis of new polymeric materials. Expression of artificial genes encoding proteins with repeating -(AlaGly)3ProGluGly- elements. *J. Am. Chem. Soc.,* **114**, 727-33.

McGuire, M. J., Sykes, K. F., Samli, K. N., Timares, L., Barry, M. A., Stemke-Hale, K., Tagliaferri, F., Logan, M., Jansa, K., Takashima, A., Brown, K. C. & Johnston, S. A. (2004). A library-selected, Langerhans cell targeting peptide enhances an immune response. *DNA Cell Biol.,* **23**, 742-52.

McLafferty, M. A., Kent, R. B., Ladner, R. C. & Markland, W. (1993). M13 bacteriophage displaying disulfide-constrained microproteins. *Gene,* **128**, 29-36.

Meola, A., Delmastro, P., Monaci, P., Luzzago, A., Nicosia, A., Felici, F., Cortese, R. & Galfre, G. (1995). Derivation of vaccines from mimotopes. Immunologic properties of human hepatitis B virus surface antigen mimotopes displayed on filamentous phage. *J. Immunol.*, **154**, 3162-72.

Molenaar, T. J., Michon, I., de Haas, S. A. M., van Berkel, T. J. C., Kuiper, J. & Biessen, E. A. L. (2002). Uptake and processing of modified bacteriophage M13 in mice: implications for phage display. *Virology*, **293**, 182-91.

Myers, M. A., Davies, J. M., Tong, J. C., Whisstock, J., Scealy, M., Mackay, I. R. & Rowley, M. J. (2000). Conformational epitopes on the diabetes autoantigen GAD65 identified by peptide phage display and molecular modelling. *J. Immunol.*, **165**, 3830-8.

Nakamura, G. R., Reynolds, M. E., Chen, Y. M., Starovasnik, M. A. & Lowman, H. B. (2002). Stable "zeta" peptides that act as potent antagonists of the high-affinity IgE receptor. *Proc. Natl. Acad. Sci. USA*, **99**, 1303-8.

Nakamura, G. R., Starovasnik, M. A., Reynolds, M. E. & Lowman, H. B. (2001). A novel family of hairpin peptides that inhibit IgE activity by binding to the high-affinity IgE receptor. *Biochemistry*, **40**, 9828-35.

Nakashima, T., Ishiguro, N., Yamaguchi, M., Yamauchi, A., Shima, Y., Nozaki, C., Urabe, I. & Yomo, T. (2000). Construction and characterization of phage libraries displaying artificial proteins with random sequences. *J. Biosci. Bioeng.*, **90**, 253-9.

Nam, K. T., Peelle, B. R., Lee, S..-W & Belcher, A. M. (2004). Genetically driven assembly of nanorings based on the M13 virus. *Nano Lett.*, **4**, 23-7.

Nanduri, V., Bhunia, A. K., Tu, S.-I., Paoli, G. C. & Brewster, J. D. (2007a). SPR biosensor for the detection of *L. monocytogenes* using phage-displayed antibody. *Biosens. Bioelectr.*, **23**, 248-52.

Nanduri, V., Sorokulova, I. B., Samoylov, A. M., Simonian, A. L., Petrenko, V. A. & Vodyanoy, V. (2007b). Phage as a molecular recognition element in biosensors immobilized by physical adsorption. *Biosens. Bioelectron.*, **22**, 986-92.

Nemoto, N., Miyamoto-Sato, E., Husimi, Y. & Yanagawa, H. (1997). In vitro virus: bonding of mRNA bearing puromycin at the 3'-terminal end to the C-terminal end of its encoded protein on the ribosome in vitro. *FEBS Lett.*, **414**, 405-8.

Ohlin, M., Owman, H., Mach, M. & Borrebaeck, C. A. (1996). Light chain shuffling of a high affinity antibody results in a drift in epitope recognition. *Mol. Immunol.*, **33**, 47-56.

Olsen, E. V., Sorokulova, I. B., Petrenko, V. A., Chen, I. H., Barbaree, J. M. & Vodyanoy, V. J. (2006). Affinity-selected filamentous bacteriophage as a probe for acoustic wave biodetectors of *Salmonella typhimurium*. *Biosens. Bioelectron.*, **21**, 1434-42.

Onda, T., LaFace, D., Baier, G., Brunner, T., Honma, N., Mikayama, T., Altman, A. & Green, D. R. (1995). A phage display system for detection of T cell receptor-antigen interactions. *Mol. Immunol.*, **32**, 1387-97.

Orlandi, R., Güssow, D. H., Jones, P. T. & Winter, G. (1989). Cloning immunoglobulin variable domains for expression by the polymerase chain reaction. *Proc. Natl. Acad. Sci. USA*, **86**, 3833-7.

Persson, M.A., Caothien, R. H. & Burton, D. R. (1991). Generation of diverse high-affinity human monoclonal antibodies by repertoire cloning. *Proc. Natl. Acad. Sci. USA*, **88**, 2432-6.

Petit, M. A., Jolivet-Reynaud, C., Peronnet, E., Michal, Y. & Trepo, C. (2003). Mapping of a conformational epitope shared between E1 and E2 on the serum-derived human hepatitis C virus envelope. *J. Biol. Chem.,* **278**, 44385-92.

Petrenko, V. A. & Smith, G. P. (2000). Phages from landscape libraries as substitute antibodies. *Protein. Eng.,* **13**, 589-92.

Petrenko, V. A. & Sorokulova, I. B. (2004). Detection of biological threats. A challenge for directed molecular evolution. *J. Microbiol. Methods,* **58**, 147-68.

Petrenko, V. A. & Vodyanoy, V. J. (2003). Phage display for detection of biological threat agents. *J. Microbiol. Methods,* **53**, 253-62.

Petrenko, V. A., Smith, G. P., Gong, X. & Quinn, T. (1996). A library of organic landscapes on filamentous phage. *Protein. Eng.,* **9**, 797-801.

Phalipon, A., Folgori, A., Arondel, J., Sgaramella, G., Fortugno, P., Cortese, R., Sansonetti, P. J. & Felici, F. (1997). Induction of anti-carbohydrate antibodies by phage library-selected peptide mimics. *Eur. J. Immunol.,* **27**, 2620-5.

Ploug, M., Østergaard, S., Gårdsvoll, H., Kovalski, K., Holst-Hansen, C., Holm, A., Ossowski, L. & Danø, K. (2001). Peptide-derived antagonists of the urokinase receptor. Affinity maturation by combinatorial chemistry, identification of functional epitopes, and inhibitory effect on cancer cell intravasation. *Biochemistry,* **40**(40), 12157-68.

Proba, K., Wörn, A., Honegger, A. & Plückthun, A. (1998). Antibody scFv fragments without disulfide bonds made by molecular evolution. *J. Mol. Biol.,* **275**, 245-53.

Rader, C. & Barbas, C. F. (1997). Phage display of combinatorial antibody libraries. *Curr. Opin. Biotechnol.,* **8**, 503-8.

Rajotte, D., Arap, W., Hagedorn, M., Koivunen, E., Pasqualini, R. & Ruoslahti, E. (1998). Molecular heterogeneity of the vascular endothelium revealed by in vivo phage display. *J. Clin. Invest.,* **102**, 430-7.

Ren, Z. & Black, L. W. (1998). Phage T4 SOC and HOC display of biologically active, full-length proteins on the viral capsid. *Gene,* **215**, 439-44.

Roberts, R.W. (1999). Totally in vitro protein selection using mRNA-protein fusions and ribosome display. *Curr. Opin. Chem. Biol.,* **3**(3), 268-73.

Roberts, R. W. & Szostak, J. W. (1997). RNA-peptide fusions for the in vitro selection of peptides and proteins. *Proc. Natl. Acad. Sci. USA,* **94**(23), 12297-302.

Romanov, V. I., Durand, D. B. & Petrenko, V. A. (2001). Phage display selection of peptides that affect prostate carcinoma cells attachment and invasion. *Prostate,* **47**, 239-51.

Rosenberg, A., Griffin, K., Studier, F. W., McCormick, M., Berg, J., Novy, R. & Mierendorf, R. (1996). T7Select® phage display system: a powerful new protein display system based on bacteriophage T7. *Innovations (Newsletter of Novagen, Inc.),* **6**, 1-6.

Rowley, M. J., Scealy, M., Whisstock, J. C., Jois, J. A., Wijeyewickrema, L. C. & Mackay, I. R. (2000). Prediction of the immunodominant epitope of the pyruvate dehydrogenase complex E2 in primary biliary cirrhosis using phage display. *J. Immunol.,* **164**, 3413-9.

Saggio, I. & Laufer, R. (1993). Biotin binders selected from a random peptide library expressed on phage. *Biochem. J.,* **293**(3), 613-6.

Samoylova, T. I., Petrenko, V. A., Morrison, N. E., Globa, L. P., Baker, H. J. & Cox, N. R. (2003). Phage probes for malignant glial cells. *Mol. Cancer Ther.,* **2**, 1129-37.

Sanghvi, A. B., Miller, K. P.-H., Belcher, A. M. & Schmidt, C. E. (2005). Biomaterials functionalization using a novel peptide that selectively binds to a conducting polymer. *Nature Materials,* **4**, 496-502.

Sano, K. & Shiba, K. (2003). A hexapeptide motif that electrostatically binds to the surface of titanium. *J. Am. Chem. Soc.,* **125**, 14234-5.

Santini, C., Brennan, D., Mennuni, C., Hoess, R. H., Nicosia, A., Cortese, R. & Luzzago, A. (1998). Efficient display of an HCV cDNA expression library as C-terminal fusion to the capsid protein D of bacteriophage lambda. *J. Mol. Biol.,* **282**, 125-35.

Sarikaya, M., Tamerler, C., Jen, A. K.-Y., Schulten, K. & Baneyx, F. (2003). Molecular biomimetics: nanotechnology through biology. *Nat. Mater.,* **2**, 577-85.

Sarikaya, M., Tamerler, C., Schwartz, D. T. & Baneyx, F. (2004). Materials assembly and formation using engineered polypeptides. *Annu. Rev. Mater. Res.,* **34**, 373-408.

Sblattero, D. & Bradbury, A. (2000). Exploiting recombination in single bacteria to make large phage antibody libraries. *Nat. Biotechnol.,* **18**, 75-80.

Schaffitzel, C., Hanes, J., Jermutus, L. & Plückthun, A. (1999). Ribosome display: an in vitro method for selection and evolution of antibodies from libraries. *J. Immunol. Methods,* **231**, 119-35.

Sche, P. P., McKenzie, K. M., White, J. D. & Austin, D. J. (1999). Display cloning: functional identification of natural receptors using cDNA-phage display. *Chem. Biol.,* **6**, 707-16.

Schimmele, B. & Plückthun, A. (2005). Identification of a functional epitope of the Nogo receptor by a combinatorial approach using ribosome display. *J. Mol. Biol.,* **352**, 229-41.

Schimmele, B., Gräfe N. & Plückthun, A. (2005). Ribosome display of mammalian receptor domains. *Protein Eng. Des. Sel.,* **18**, 285-94.

Schlick, T. L., Ding, Z., Kovacs, E. W. & Francis, M. B. (2005). Dual-surface modification of the tobacco mosaic virus. *J. Am. Chem. Soc.,* **127**, 3718-23.

Schluesener, H. J. & Xianglin, T. (2004). Selection of recombinant phages binding to pathological endothelial and tumor cells of rat glioblastoma by in vivo display. *J. Neurol. Sci.,* **224(1-2)**, 77-82.

Schmidt, C. E., Shastri, V. R., Vacanti, J. P. & Langer, R. (1997). Stimulation of neurite outgrowth using an electrically conducting polymer. *Proc. Natl Acad. Sci. USA,* **94**, 8948-53.

Scott, J. K. & Smith, G. P. (1990). Searching for peptide ligands with an epitope library. *Science,* **249**, 386-90.

Segal, D. J., Dreier, B., Beerli, R. R. & Barbas, C. F. III (1999). Toward controlling gene expression at will: selection and design of zinc finger domains recognizing each of the 5'-GNN-3' DNA target sequences. *Proc. Natl. Acad. USA,* **96**, 2758-63.

Shone, C., Wilton-Smith, P., Appleton, N., Hambleton, P., Modi, N., Gatley, S. & Melling, J. (1985). Monoclonal antibody-based immunoassay for type A *Clostridium botulinum* toxin is comparable to the mouse bioassay. *Appl. Environ. Microbiol.,* **50**, 63-7.

Siegel, D. L. (2002). Recombinant monoclonal antibody technology. *Transfus. Clin. Biol.,* **9**, 15-22.

Skelton, N. J., Russell, S., de Sauvage, F. & Cochran, A. G. (2002). Amino acid determinants of beta-hairpin conformation in erythropoeitin receptor agonist peptides derived from a phage display library. *J. Mol. Biol.,* **316**, 1111-25.

Skerra, A. & Plückthun, A. (1988). Assembly of a functional immunoglobulin Fv fragment in *Escherichia coli. Science,* **240**, 1038-41.

Smith, G. P. (1985). Filamentous fusion phage: novel expression vectors that display cloned antigens on the virion surface. *Science,* **228**(4705), 1315-7.

Smith, G. P. (1992). Cloning in fUSE vectors. Available from: Prof. G. P. Smith, Division of Biological Sciences, University of Missouri, URL: http://www.biosci.missouri.edu/smithgp/PhageDisplayWebsite/PhageDisplayWebsiteInd ex.html.

Smith, G. P. & Petrenko, V. A. (1997). Phage Display. *Chem. Rev., 97,* 391-410.

Sorokulova, I. B., Olsen, E. V., Chen, I. H., Fiebor, B., Barbaree, J. M., Vodyanoy, V. J., Chin, B. A. & Petrenko, V. A. (2005). Landscape phage probes for *Salmonella typhimurium. J. Microbiol. Methods, 63,* 55-72.

Souza, G. R., Christianson, D. R., Staquicini, F. I., Ozawa, M. G., Snyder, E. Y., Sidman, R. L., Miller, J. H., Arap, W. & Pasqualini, R. (2006). Networks of gold nanoparticles and bacteriophage as biological sensors and cell-targeting agents. *PNAS, 103,* 1215-20.

Spear, M. A., Breakefield, X. O., Beltzer, J., Schuback, D., Weissleder, R., Pardo, F. S. & Ladner, R. (2001). Isolation, characterization, and recovery of small peptide phage display epitopes selected against viable malignant glioma cells. *Cancer Gene Ther., 8,* 506-11.

Steichen, C., Chen, P., Kearney, J. F. & Turnbough, C. L. Jr. (2003). Identification of the immunodominant protein and other proteins of the *Bacillus anthracis* exosporium. *J. Bacteriol., 185,* 1903-10.

Stemmer, W. P. (1994). Rapid evolution of a protein in vitro by DNA shuffling. *Nature, 370*(6488), 389-91.

Stratmann, J., Strommenger, B., Stevenson, K. & Gerlach, G. F. (2002). Development of a peptide-mediated capture PCR for detection of *Mycobacterium avium* subsp. *paratuberculosis* in milk. *J. Clin. Microbiol., 40,* 4244-50.

Tramontano, A., Janda, K. D. & Lerne, R. A. (1986). Catalytic antibodies. *Science, 234,* 1566-70.

Trepel, M., Arap, W. & Pasqualini, R. (2002). In vivo phage display and vascular heterogeneity: implications for targeted medicine. *Curr. Opin. Chem. Biol., 6,* 399-404.

Tseng, R. J., Tsai, C., Ma, L., Ouyang, J., Ozkan, C. S. & Yang, Y. (2006). Digital memory device based on tobacco mosaic virus conjugated with nanoparticles. *Nature Nanotechnology, 1,* 72-7.

Turnbough, C. L. Jr. (2003). Discovery of phage display peptide ligands for species-specific detection of *Bacillus* spores. *J. Microbiol. Methods, 53,* 263-71.

Urry, D. W., McPherson, D. T., Xu, J., Gowda, D. C. & Parker, T. M. (1995). In C. Gebelein, & C. E. Carraher (Eds.), *Industrial Biotechnological Polymers* (pp. 259-281). Lancaster, PA: Technomic.

Valentini, R. F., Vargo, T. G., Gardella, J. A. Jr. & Aebischer, P. (1992). Electrically conductive polymeric substrates enhance nerve fibre outgrowth in vitro. *Biomater., 13,* 183-90.

vanZonneveld, A. J., vandenBerg, B. M. M., vanMeijer, M., and Pannekoek, H. (1995). Identification of functional interaction sites on proteins using bacteriophage-displayed random epitope libraries. *Gene, 167,* 49-52.

Vidal, J. C., Garcia, E. & Castillo, J. R. (1999). In situ preparation of a cholesterol biosensor: entrapment of cholesterol oxidase in an overoxidized polypyrrole film electrodeposited in a flow system: Determination of total cholesterol in serum. *Anal. Chim. Acta., 385,* 213-22.

Villemagne, D., Jackson, R. & Douthwaite, J. A. (2006). Highly efficient ribosome display selection by use of purified components for in vitro translation. *J. Immunol. Methods*, **313**, 140-8.

Wang, C. I., Yang, Q. & Craik, C. S. (1996). Phage display of proteases and macromolecular inhibitors. *Combinatorial Chemistry*, **267**, 52-68.

Wang, L. F. & Yu, M. (2004). Epitope identification and discovery using phage display libraries: applications in vaccine development and diagnostics. *Curr. Drug Targets*, **5**, 1-15.

Wang, L. F., Duplessis, D. H., White, J. R., Hyatt, A.D. & Eaton, B. T. (1995). Use of a gene-targeted phage display random epitope library to map an antigenic determinant on the Bluetongue Virus outer capsid protein Vp5. *J. Immunol. Methods*, **178**, 1-12

Weaver-Feldhaus, J. M., Lou, J., Coleman, J. R., Siegel, R. W., Marks, J. D. & Feldhaus, M.J. (2004). Yeast mating for combinatorial Fab library generation and surface display. *FEBS Lett.*, **564**(1-2), 24-34.

Whaley, S. R., English, D. S., Hu, E. L., Barbara, P. F. & Belcher, A. M. (2000). Selection of peptides with semiconductor binding specificity for directed nano-crystal assembly. *Nature*, **405**, 665-8.

Willats, W. G. (2002). Phage display: practicalities and prospects. *Plant Mol. Biol.*, **50**, 837-54.

Wilson, D. R. & Finlay, B. B. (1998). Phage display: application, innovations, and issues in phage and host biology. *Can. J. Microbiol.*, **44**, 313-29.

Wilson, D. S., Keefe, A. D. & Szostak, J. W. (2001). The use of mRNA display to select high-affinity protein-binding peptides. *Proc. Natl. Acad. Sci. USA*, **98**, 3750-5.

Wolfe, S. A., Greisman, H. A., Ramm, E. I. & Pabo, C.O. (1999). Analysis of zinc fingers optimized via phage display: evaluating the utility of a recognition code. *J. Mol. Biol.*, **285**, 1917-34.

Worn, A. & Plückthun, A. (2001). Stability engineering of antibody single-chain Fv fragments. *J. Mol. Biol.*, **305**, 989-1010.

Wrighton, N. C., Farrell, F. X., Chang, R., Kashyap, A. K., Barbone, F. P., Mulcahy, L. S., Johnson, D. L., Barrett, R. W., Jolliffe, L. K. & Dower, W. J. (1996). Small peptides as potent mimetics of the protein hormone erythropoietin. *Science*, **273**, 458-64.

Wu, H., Yang, W. P. & Barbas, C. F. (1995). Building zinc fingers by selection - toward a therapeutic application. *Proceedings of the National Academy of Sciences of the United States of America*, **92**, 344-8.

Xu, L., Aha, P., Gu, K., Kuimelis, R. G., Kurz, M., Lam, T., Lim, A. C., Liu, H., Lohse, P. A., Sun, L., Weng, S., Wagner, R. W. & Lipovsek, D. (2002). Directed evolution of high-affinity antibody mimics using mRNA display. *Chem. Biol.*, **9**, 933-42.

Yu, J. & Smith, G. P. (1996). Affinity maturation of phage-displayed peptide ligands. *Methods Enzymol.*, **267**, 3-27.

Yuan, L., Kurek, I., English, J. & Keenan, R. (2005). Laboratory-directed protein evolution. *Microbiol. Mol. Biol. Rev.*, **69**(3), 373-92.

Zhang, L., Hoffman, J. A. & Ruoslahti, E. (2005). Molecular profiling of heart endothelial cells. *Circulation*, **112**(11), 1601-11.

In: Synthetic and Integrative Biology
Editor: James T. Gevona, pp. 41-60

ISBN: 978-1-60876-678-9
© 2010 Nova Science Publishers, Inc.

Chapter 2

INTEGRATIVE BIOLOGY OF AQUAPORINS IN ANURAN AMPHIBANS

Shigeyasu Tanaka[1,2,*] *and Masakazu Suzuki*[2]

[1]Integrated Bioscience Section, Graduate School of Science and Technology,
Shizuoka University, Shizuoka 422-8529, Japan
[2]Department of Biology, Faculty of Science, Shizuoka University,
Shizuoka 422-8529, Japan

Abstract

Aquaporins (AQPs) play important roles in maintaining the water homeostasis. The anuran AQP family is known to consist of at least AQP0-AQP5, AQP7-AQP10, and two anuran-specific types, designated AQPa1 and AQPa2. In *Hyla japonica*, AQP2 (AQP-h2K) and two forms of AQPa2 (AQP-h2 and AQP-h3) reside in the tight epithelial cells of three major osmoregulatory organs: AQP-h2K in the kidney, AQP-h2 in the urinary bladder, and both AQP-h2 and AQP-h3 in the ventral pelvic skin. These AQPs are antidiuretic hormone-dependent AQPs. In this review, we describe in detail the anuran AQPs that have been identified to data and describe the molecular and cellular mechanisms underlying the terrestrial adaptation of anurans in terms of AQPs.

Keywords: aquaporin, anuran amphibians, antidiuretic hormone-dependent aquaporin, kidney, urinary bladder, ventral pelvic skin, metamorphosis

1. Introduction

Water is the major constituent of almost all life forms, accounting for approximately 50-95% of the body weight of all living organisms. It is essential to the continued survival of all organisms. Water has unique physical and chemical properties that have earned it the name of

---

* E-mail address: sbstana@ipc.shizuoka.ac.jp. Fax: +81-54-238-4783. Corresponding author: Shigeyasu Tanaka, Integrated Bioscience Section, Graduate School of Science and Technology, Shizuoka University, Ohya 836, Suruga-ku, Shizuoka 422-8529, Japan.

"universal solvent" due to its ability to act as a solvent for many substances. Organisms depend upon this property, which maintains life by stabilizing biomolecular structures, contributing to intra- and extracellular biochemical reactions and functioning as a transport medium of biomolecules. Organisms originated in a primitive marine environment approximately 4 billion years ago and subsequently evolved gradually to life in fresh water or on dry land. As such, the evolution of organisms is intricately linked with water and the importance of this inorganic molecule to all living processes.

Anuran amphibians, the most numerous order of the Amphibia, are widely distributed throughout and have adapted to various water environments, ranging from freshwater and seawater to forests and arid desert (Pough, 2007; Frost, 2008). Most anurans go through an aquatic stage – the tadpole stage – before they metamorphose into their adult form, which is able to adapt to life on land. Adult anurans, with the exception of some aquatic species, are terrestrial and, as such, exposed to evaporative water loss through their thin skin when on dry land (Lillywhite, 2006). It is important to understand the adaptive processes involved with this change from aquatic to a terrestrial lifestyle in terms of water adaptation. To adapt to their habitats, anurans have developed various complicated systems for maintaining water balance. For example, in general, most adult anuran amphibians do not drink water through their mouth, rather they absorb water through the ventral pelvic skin (also referred to as the pelvic patch) and reabsorb water from urine in the urinary bladder (Bently and Main, 1972; Bently and Yorio, 1979).

The plasma membrane, formed by a phospholipid bilayer, functions as an exquisitely selective barrier against the entry of ions, small neutral solutes, and water into cells. It is slightly permeable to water by simple diffusion. However, some types of cells and tissues, such as red blood cell, mammalian kidneys, and anuran skin and urinary bladder, exhibit high water permeability, giving rise to the hypothesis that specialized water transport molecules (water channels) may exist in these cells and tissues. Freeze-fracture electron microscopic studies have suggested that intramembrane particles in the amphibian urinary bladder and skin may be water channel proteins because they translocate from their cytoplasmic pools to the plasma membrane following stimulation by vasopression (Chevalier et al., 1974; Kachadorian et al., 1975; Brown et al., 1983).

2. Aquaporin Family

In 1992, a water channel was identified in the plasma membrane of red blood cells, which was subsequently named aquaporin (AQP) (Agre et al., 1995). Aquaporins are a class of integral membrane proteins that form a selective water pore in the plasma membrane of various cells of animals, plants, and microorganisms (Zardoya, 2005). There are at least 13 different members of the AQP protein family (AQP0-AQP12) that mediate bidirectional water transport across the plasma membrane in response to osmotic gradients and differences in hydrostatic pressure. A common characteristic of the AQP protein family commonly is that they contain a conserved sequence of arginine, proline, and alanine, called the NPA motif. Aquaporin proteins can be categorized into two subfamilies, orthodox AQPs and aquaglyceroporins, based on their transport function. Orthodox AQPs, such as AQP0, AQP1, AQP2, AQP4, and AQP5, conduct only water, whereas aquaglyceroporin, including AQP3, AQP7, AQP9, and AQP10, transport not only water but also small neutral solutes, such as glycerol and urea (Ishibashi et al., 2000; Takata et al., 2004). AQP6, AQP8, AQP11, and AQP12 have recently been grouped as unorthodox AQPs because their functions are not yet fully defined (Ishibashi, 2006; Rojek et al., 2008).

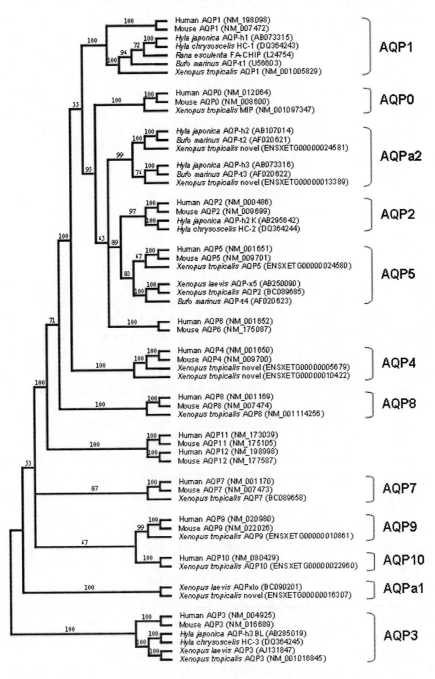

Figure 1. Phylogenetic relationships among AQP0-12, AQPa1, and AQPa2 seen in a neighbor joining (NJ) unrooted tree of AQPs from the human, mouse, and anurans. [modified from Ogushi et al. (2007)].

The phylogenetic analysis of AQP proteins from anurans and mammals presented in Figure 1 indicates that anuran AQPs can be divided into 12 clusters: types 0-5, 7-10, and two anuran-specific types designated as a1 and a2 (the letter "a" represents anuran). Types 0-5 correspond to mammalian AQP0 - AQP5, and AQP7 - AQP10, respectively. The cluster of type a1 AQPs comprises AQPxlo from *Xenopus laevis* oocytes (Virkki et al., 2002) and *X. tropicalis* novel AQP (ENSXETG00000016307), and that of type a2 AQPs contains AQP-h2 and AQP-h3 from the tree frog, *Hyla japonica*, AQP-t2 (AF02622) and AQP-t3 (AF020622) from the toad, *Bufo marinus*, and novel AQPs (ENSXETG00000013389, ENSXETG00000024581) from *X. tropicalis*. It is of interest that the AQPs of the AQP2 and type a2 clusters belong to different groups even through all of them, can be stimulated by arginine vasotocin (AVT; the non-mammalian vertebrate counterpart of vasopressin).

In the following sections, anuran AQP0 - AQPP3, AQP5, AQPa1, and AQPa2 will be described in detail in term of structure and function.

3. Amphibian Aquaporins

3.1. AQP0

AQP0 was originally identified as a major intrinsic protein of 26 kDa (MIP, also called MIP26). The cDNA of bovine MIP was cloned and sequenced by Gorin et al. (1984), who determined that the protein is composed of 263 amino acid residues containing six transmembrane regions with both C- and N-termini on the cytoplasmic side. The absence of an *N*-glycosylation site is characterstic of this AQP0. AQP0 is the most abundant membrane protein in lens fiber cells (Gorin et al., 1984), and its deficiency results in the development of cataract (Shiels et al., 2001). AQP0 facilitates the transport of water and small neutral solutes, such as glycerol, across the plasma membrane (King et al., 2004; Varadaraj et al., 2005). It also has functional roles in the adhesion, structure, and organization of lens fiber cells, thereby maintaining the transparency of the lens (Shiels et al., 2000). Several lines of evidence suggest that proteolytic cleavage induces AQP0 to form junctions. In young fiber cells of the lens cortex, AQP0 exists as a full-length protein of 26 kDa, but a portion of this AQP0 is proteolytically cleaved in an age-dependent manner as fiber cells grow older and become buried deeper in the lens core (Takemoto et al., 1986). Gonen et al. (2004) demonstrated that cleavage of the intracellular C-terminus enhances the adhesive properties of the extracellular surface of AQP0, inducing a conformational change in the molecule and thereby changing the function of AQP0 from a water pore in the cortex to an adhesion molecule in the lens core (Engel et al., 2008).

In anuran amphibians, AQP0 has been cloned only in *X. tropicallis* (NM_001097347); the protein is composed of 234 amino acid residues (Figure 2). Studies using *Xenopus* AQP0 antibody recently generated in our laboratory revealed that *Xenopus* AQP0 also resides in the plasma membrane of the lens fiber cells in *X. laevis* (unpublished data).

We have hypothesized that anuran AQP2, AQPa2, and AQP5 may have arisen through local gene duplication of a single ancestral AQP gene, probably paralog AQP0. Evidence supporting this hypothesis is provided by the clustering of anuran *AQP2*, *AQPa2*, and *AQP5* in the region of *FAIM2* and *RACGAP1*, and the lack of *AQP2*, *AQPa2*, and *AQP5* in fish, although fish *AQP0* is located between *FAIM2* and *RACGAP1* (Suzuki and Tanaka, 2009).

```
Xt-AQP0    MM------WE-FRSFAFWRAIFAEFFATMFYVFFGLGAS-LKWAAGPA--    40
AQP-h1     MASE-------FKKMAFWRAVIAEFLAMIMFVFISIGAA-LGFNFPIQEK    42
AQPxlo     MVSHLAFLKNMKLKIRTQNLYVRCGLAEF-----LGTLILI-LFGCGSV     43
AQP-h2K    MMIVR--LWE-LRSVAFTRAVFVEFFATLLFVMFGIGSS-LNWPGAPP--    44
AQP-h3BL   MGRQKEVLNSISGMLRIRNKLIRQALAEC------LGTLILV-MFGCGSV    43
AQP-h2     M------KEMCTGP-FTRAFAGELIGTSIFVFFGLGSA-MSWPSALP--   39
AQP-h3     M-----LKELCAGFNFK-AFLAELIATLVFVFVGLGST-LSWTGALP--   40
                  *                                      *

Xt-AQP0    ------N-V-LNIALA--FGFALATLVQSVGHISGAHINPAVTFAFLIG    79
AQP-h1     INETVGRTQDIVKVSLA--FGLSIATMAQSVGHISGAHINPAVTLGCLLS    90
AQPxlo     AQMELSGFAKAQFLSVNMAFGFAVTAGAYVCAGVSGAHINPAVSLAMFIL    93
AQP-h2K    ------S-V-LQVALA--FGLGIGTLVQAFGHISGAHINPAVTLAFMVG    83
AQP-h3BL   AQVVLSKGSHGLFLTVNLAFGFAVMLGILIAGQVSGGHINPAVTFALCIM    93
AQP-h2     -------T-V-LQIAFT--FGLGIGTLVQTFGHISGAHINPAVTVAFLVS    78
AQP-h3     -------T-V-LQIAFT--FGLGIGTMVQAVGHISGAHINPAVTIALLVG    79
                                              **         ** * *

Xt-AQP0    SQMSFFRAIF-YIAAQLLGAVAGAAVLYGVTPTAVRGNL-ALNTIHPGVS    127
AQP-h1     CQISILKAVM-YIIAQCLGAVVATAILSGITSNLA-GNTLGLNGLSNGVT    138
AQPxlo     KKLSW-KLFLIYCLAQFLGAFIGAALVFSLYYDALHVYSNGNWTVYGPQS    142
AQP-h2K    SQISFMRAVF-YVGAQLLGAVSGAAIIQGLTPFEVRGNL-SVNGLFNNTE    131
AQP-h3BL   AREPWIK-FPVYTLAQTLGAFLGAGIVYGLYYDAIWYFANDQLYVMGPNG    142
AQP-h2     SQISLFRAVC-YVCAQLLGAVIGAALLYQFTPEDVHGSF-GVNMPSNNAT    126
AQP-h3     ARISLIQTVF-YVIAQMLGAVIGAALLYEFSPSDIRGGF-GVNQPSNNTS    127
                *  ** ***

Xt AQP0    LGQA--------T----TV--EAFLTLQFVLCIFATFDERRNGRMGSVSL    163
AQP-h1     AGQG--------L----GV--EIMVTFQLVLCVVAVTDRRRRDVSGSVPL    174
AQPxlo     TAGIFASYPSEHLSVINGFTDQVIATAALLICILAILDEANNAAPRGLQP    192
AQP-h2K    AGKA--------F----VV--ELFLTLQLILCIFASTDDRRTDIVGSPAL    167
AQP-h3BL   TAGIFATYPTEHLTIMNGFFDQFIGTAALVVCVLAIVDPYNNPIPRGLEA    192
AQP-h2     EGQA--------V----TV--EIILTLQLVLCIYACTDDRRDDNVGSPSL    162
AQP-h3     PGQA--------V----AV--EIILTMQLVLCIFATTDSRRTDNIGSPAI    163
                          *       *  *  *

Xt AQP0    AL-GFSVALGHLFGIYYT-GASMNPARSFAPAVLTRNFVNHWVYWVGPII    211
AQP-h1     AI-GLSVALGHLIAIDYT-GGMNPARSFGSAVVAKNFQYHWIFWVGPMI    222
AQPxlo     FLIGIMVLLVGLAMG-FNCGYPINPARDLAPRFFTAIAG-----WGSEVF    236
AQP-h2K    SI-GLSVTLGHLLGIYYT-GCSMNPARSFAPAVVTGDFNAHWVFWLGPLF    215
AQP-h3BL   FTVGFVVLVIGLSMG-FNSGYAVNPARDFGPRIFTALAG-----WGTEVF    236
AQP-h2     SI-GLSVVLGHLVGIYFT-GCSMNPARSFGPALVVGNFNTHWIFWIGPFV    210
AQP-h3     SI-GLSVVLGHLLGIYYT-GCSMNPARSFGPALITGNFEYHWIFWVAPIT    211
                *   *     *           *  * *      ****

Xt AQP0    GGAVGGLVYDFILFPRMRGLNERLSILKGARPAEPEGQ-RETIRDPI-EL    259
AQP-h1     GGAAAAIIYDFILAPRTSDLTDRLKVWTNG-----QVE-----EY---EL    259
AQPxlo     SAGGHWWWVPVLG-PLVGGVVGAVIYEVFIEFHHPS-PNQKQESEEPTEG    284
AQP-h2K    GATVGSLMYNFIFIPNTKTFSERIAILRGELEPQEDWEERDMRRRQSMEL    265
AQP-h3BL   SAGGQWWWVPIVS-PLLGAFAGVLVYQLMIGCHIEPAPESTEQENVKLSN    285
AQP-h2     GAILASLIYNYVLCPQEQSFSEKLSVLLGRIPAMQEEEEDWEERQEQPRR    260
AQP-h3     GAIFACLIYDYIFAPQFISPSERLEIIRGNILQENEKEERRKQSVGLNSV    261
                *

Xt AQP0    KTQ-SL---------                                     264
AQP-h1     DGEDA--RMEMKPK-                                     271
AQPxlo     INRPHYELVQSSA--                                     297
AQP-h2K    HSTQTIPRSGMTEKV                                     280
AQP-h3BL   VKHK--E--RI----                                     292
AQP-h2     KSMEL--QTL-----                                     268
AQP-h3     YSQTNSKEKM-----                                     271
```

Figure 2. Comparison of the predicted sequences of anuran AQPs. Gaps indicated by dashed lines have been introduced to obtain maximum homology. NPA motifs are outlined. C in the solid triangle, S in solid circle, and N-circle indicate mercurial-inhibition sites, phosphorylation sites for protein kinase A, and *N*-glycosilation sites, respectively. Xt-AQP0 is from *Xenopus tropicalis* MIP (NM_001097347). The residues that match those of AQP are indicated by an asterisk. The asterisk indicates AQP-h1, AQP-h2K, AQP-h3BL, AQP-h2, ad AQP-h3 are from *Hyla japonica* (Tanii et al., 2002; Hasegawa et a., 2003; Ogushi et al., 2007; Akabane et al., 2007). AQPxlo is from *Xenopus laevis* (Virkki et al., 2002).

3.2. AQP1

The AQP1 cluster includes mouse AQP1 (Moon et al., 1995), AQP-h1 from *H. japonica* (Tanii et al., 2002), FA-CHIP from *Rana esculenta* (Abrami et al., 1994), and AQP-t1 from *B. marinus* (Ma et al., 1996). *Hyla* AQP-h1 is composed of 271 amino acid residues (Figure 2). Hydropathy analysis has predicted six transmembrane regions with an N-terminus and a C-terminus localized in the cytoplasm, similar to other aquaporins. AQP-h1 contains two NPA motifs. A series of studies on the atomic structure of rat AQP1 revealed a selective mechanism for water permeation through a channel pore (Yasui, 2004; de Groot and Grubmuller, 2005). For rat AQP1, a pair of NPA motifs is located in the pore entrance, where AQP1 builds the specific passage of water molecules. These motifs and other amino acid residues that are important for maintaining the pore selectivity of mammalian AQP1, i.e., Phe, His, Cys, and Arg (de Groot and Grubmuller, 2005), are conserved in *Hyla* AQP-h1. Therefore, it would appear that AQP-h1 also conserves the basic architecture of a water channel.

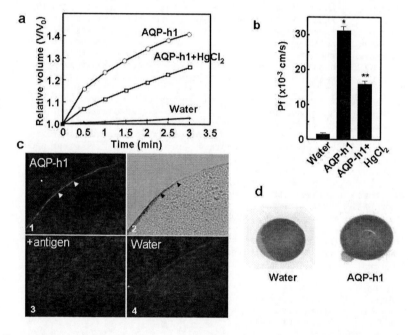

Figure 3. Expression of AQP-h1 in *Xenopus* oocytes. (a) Time course of the osmotic swelling. Oocytes were microinjected with or without cRNA encoding AQP-h1. Some AQP-h1-injected oocytes were incubated with 0.3 mM $HgCl_2$. (b) Osmotic water permeabiltity (Pf) was calculated from the initial rate of oocyte swelling. All data shown are mean ± SE of measurements from 10-11 oocytes in each experimental group. (c) Immunofluorescence images for AQP-h1 protein in AQP-h1-injected oocytes. (1) After completion of the swelling experiments, immunoreactive AQP-h1 materials (red) are visible in the plasma membrane, but not in any other parts in the oocyte. (2) The corresponding Nomarski differential interference image. (3) In the absorption test, positive immunoreactive materials obtained with anti-AQP-h1 are nearly eliminated at background levels in the AQP-h1-injected oocyte. (4) No positive immunoreactive materials were seen on the section of water-injected oocyte. (d) Photograph of water and AQP-h1-injected oocytes. In the AQP-h1-injected oocyte, the eruption of the cytoplasm from the oocyte is visible.

Tanii et al. (2002) explored the physiological properties of AQP-h1 by this AQP in *Xenopus* oocytes. Specifically, oocytes were injected with AQP-h1 cRNA and transferred to hypo-osmotic (70 mOsm) Barth's solution where they were observed to swell. The degree of swelling in the AQP-h1 cRNA-injected oocytes was significantly higher than that in water-injected oocytes, and the coefficient of osmotic water permeability, *Pf*, of the former was about 18-fold greater than the control (Tanii et al., 2002) (Figure 3a, b). This enhanced water permeability of the AQP-h1 cRNA-injected oocytes was inhibited by 48% when 0.3 mM $HgCl_2$ was administrated concomitantly with the AQP-h1 cRNA (Figure 3b). AQP-h1 protein was also expressed in the AQP-h1-injected oocytes (Figure 3c). Taken together, these results confirm that AQP-h1 functions as a water channel (Figure 3).

Tanii et al. (2002) detected AQP-h1 not only in the pelvic skin but also in other various tissues, but not in blood cells and the liver. Immunohistochemistry studies have shown that rat AQP1 exists on continuous capillaries in diverse tissues (Nielsen et al., 1993). With reference to amphibian osmoregulatory organs, AQP-h1 has been observed along the blood vessels in the skin and urinary bladder and along the mesothelium in the urinary bladder, as has another frog aquaporin, FA-CHIP, from *R. esculenta* (Abrami et al., 1997). Although the morphology of the subepithelial capillaries in the amphibian pelvic skin and urinary bladder has not been documented in detail, physiological studies indicate that the high rates of water uptake across the pelvic skin are maintained with a functional circulation (Parsons et al., 1993) and the water osmotically absorbed through the pelvic skin enters subcutaneous blood capillaries rather than the lymphatic system (Word and Hillman, 2005).

AQP1 has recently been localized to the endothelial cells of the subepidermal capillaries in *B. bufo* (Willumsen et al., 2007), as has *Rana* FA-CHIP (Abrami et al., 1997) and *Hyla* AQP-h1 (Suzuki et al., 2007). These results empirically support the possible role of AQP1 in the transport of cutaneously absorbed water into the blood flow.

3.3. AQPa1

AQPxlo has been cloned from *X. laevis* oocytes (Virkki et al., 2002). This AQP is a six transmembrane protein encoding 297 amino acids and containing the NPA motif in loops B and E and a consensus protein kinase A/G phosphorylation at Ser-97 in loop B (Figure 2). Ser-97 is also part of a consensus protein kinase C phosphorylation motif at residues 97-99. AQPxlo also contains a putative *N*-glycosylation site at Asn-134. Northern blot analysis demonstrated that this AQP is expressed in *X. laevis* fat bodies and oocytes, with a weaker signal in the kidney. AQPxlo expression increases both the *Pf* and the uptake of glycerol and urea, indicating that it can be classified as an aquaglyceroporin. However, AQPxlo excludes larger polyols and thiourea. An alkaline extracellular pH (pHo) has been shown to increase the *Pf* and to a lesser extent urea uptake, but not glycerol uptake. It is of interest that low $HgCl_2$ concentrations (0.3-10 μM) are able to reduce the *Pf* and urea uptake, whereas high concentrations (300-1000 μM) reverse this inhibition. These results indicate that AQPxlo is a unique AQP among anuran amphibians.

3.4. AQP2

We have recently identified the anuran ortholog of AQP2, AQP-h2K, from the kidney of *H. japonica* (Ogushi et al., 2007). AQP-h2K consists of 280 amino acid residues with a relative molecular mass of 30,531 Da (Figure 2). This AQP has six transmembrane regions, with the N-terminus and C-terminus in the cytoplasm. AQP-h2K contains two conserved NPA motifs found in all AQP family members as well as a cysteine just upstream from the second NPA motif. Other amino acid residues shown to be important for pore selectivity in mammalian AQP1, such as Phe-55, His-177, Cys-186, and Arg-192 (de Groot *and* Grubmuller, 2005), are also conserved in AQP-h2K (Ogushi et al., 2007). In addition, two possible *N*-linked glycosylation sites at Asn-120 and Asn-128, one protein kinase C phosphorylation site at Ser-236, and one protein kinase A phosphorylation site at Ser-262 are predicted (Figure 2). The physiological properties of AQP-h2K were assessed by expressing it in *Xenopus* oocytes, and the *Pf* of AQP-h2K was found to be approximately fourfold greater than that of the control (Ogushi et al., 2007). AQP-h2K mRNA was observed to be strongly expressed in the kidney, and immunofluorescence labeling localized AQP-h2K protein to the collecting duct. In adult anurans, AVT exerts antidiuretic effects on both the kidney and urinary bladder to aid water economy (Bentley, 2002). The renal effect of AVT is considered to be weak in aquatic species, such as *X. laevis* (Kloas and Hanke, 1992). In contrast, the kidney of most adult anurans shows significant antidiuretic responses to AVT in two modes: a decreased glomerular filtration rate and increased water reabsorption across the renal tubule (Pang, 1983; Bentley, 2002). The adult kidney is a mesonephros, and the nephrons comprise a glomerulus in the Bowman's capsule and a renal tubule; the latter is divided into morphologically distinguishable segments: a neck segment, proximal tubule, thin intermediate segment, early distal tubule, late distal tubule, and connecting tubule linked to the collecting duct (Uchiyama and Yoshizawa, 2002; Hillyard et al., 2009). The anuran renal tubule does not have an extended U-shaped medullary portion comparable to the Henle's loop in the avian and mammalian kidneys, so that hyperosmotic urine cannot be produced during antidiuretic response (Bentley, 1998).

AQP-h2K was observed in abundance in the cytoplasm and only barely in the apical plasma membrane of the principal cells under hydrated conditions (Ogushi et al., 2007). After stimulation with AVT, however, a large population of AQP-h2K appeared to be translocated from the cytoplasmic pool to the apical membrane, suggesting that this AQP is a key player in AVT-dependent water reabsorption in the anuran kidney. It seems likely that AQP-h2K controls the transport of water from the tubular fluid into the principal cells of the collecting duct through AVT-dependent translocation; in this function, it resembles mammalian AQP2 in the kidney (Sasaki and Noda, 2007).

3.5. AQPa2

Hyla AQP-h2 is a protein comprising 268 amino acids with a relative molecular mass of 29,204 Da (Figure 2). This AQP also has six transmembrane regions with an N-terminus and a C-terminus in the cytoplasm, and two conserved NPA motifs with a cysteine just upstream from the second NPA motif. Similarly, *Hyla* AQP-h3 is a six transmembrane protein composed of 271 amino acids with molecular mass of 29,204 Da (Figure 2). Both of these AQP proteins contain putative protein kinase phosphorylation sites (at Ser-262 in AQP-h2 and at Ser-255 in AQP-h3).

A critical process for AVT-dependent water absorption in the pelvic skin is carried out in the first-reacting cell layer, which is the outermost layer of the stratum granulosum of the epidermis (Voute and Ussing, 1968). During normal hydration, both AQP-h2 and AQP-h3 appear to be located in an intracellular pool and along the entire plasma membrane of principal cells in the stratum granulosum (Hasegawa et al., 2003; Akabane et al., 2007). Hasegawa et al. (2003) reported that, following AVT stimulation, most of AQP-h2 and AQP-h3 in the principal cells of the first-reacting cell layer translocated into the apical plasma membrane. AQP-h2 also translocated from the intracellular pool to the apical membrane of granular cells in the urinary bladder, followed by phosphorylation at Ser-262 (Hasegawa et al., 2005).

3.6. AQP3

The anuran ortholog of AQP3, AQP-h3BL, has been cloned from the urinary bladder of *H. japonica* (Akabane et al., 2007). The AQP-h3BL protein is composed of 292 amino acid residues with two canonical NPA motifs and one putative *N*-linked glycosylation site at Asn-141 (Figure 2). Expression assays using *Xenopus* oocytes demonstrated that AQP-h3BL transports both water and glycerol (Akabane et al., 2007).

Immunofluorescence labeling demonstrated that AQP-h3BL is localized to the collecting duct and distal tubule in the kidney and present in the basolateral plasma membrane of the principal cells (Akabane et al., 2007).

Immunohistological analysis revealed that AQP-h3BL is extensively distributed over the ventral skin and dorsal skin in *Hyla*. AQP-h3BL appears to be located along the basolateral plasma membrane of principal cells in the stratum granulosum, stratum spinosum, and stratum germinativum of the epidermis (Akabane et al., 2007). It is possible that this protein supplies water to rehydrate the epidermis suffering evaporative water loss, similar to the mammalian AQP3 that also resides along the basolateral plasma membrane of keratinocytes in the epidermis (Matsuzaki et al., 1999; Sougrat et al., 2002). As an aquaglyceroporin, AQP-h3BL transports not only water but also glycerol (Akabane et al., 2007). In mammals, glycerol exerts beneficial effects on the epidermis, including stratum corneum hydration, cutaneous elasticity, skin barrier repair, wound-healing processes, among others (Fluhr et al., 2008). AQP3-deficient mice exhibit reduced stratum corneum hydration and skin elasticity and show impaired barrier recovery after removal of the stratum corneum, they also show a remarkable reduction in the glycerol content of the stratum corneum (Hara et al., 2002). These phenotype abnormalities are, however, corrected by the oral administration of glycerol (Hara and Verkman, 2003). These lines of evidence suggest that mammalian AQP3 plays a crucial role in the transport of glycerol into the epidermis, thereby maintaining the healthy condition of the epidermis. The conserved cellular and subcellular localization of AQP3 in the *Hyla* epidermis implies that anuran AQP3 may have similar functions in the epidermis via glycerol transport.

In *Xenopus*, reverse transcriptase (RT)-PCR analysis detected a higher expression of AQP-x3BL mRNA in the ventral skin than in the dorsal skin (Mochida et al., 2008). This result was supported by immunofluorescence staining, which revealed a stark difference in labeling intensity for AQP-x3BL between the dorsal and ventral skin. Strong labels for AQP-x3BL were observed along the basolateral membrane of the principal cells in the ventral skin, while the labels were barely detectable in the dorsal skin (Mochida et al., 2008). Loveridge (1970) reported that, when placed on the land, the aquatic *Xenopus* loses water by evaporation more rapidly than other anurans and dies within less than 10 h, possibly due partially to a shortage of AQP-x3BL in the dorsal skin. One hypothesized potential function of AQP-x3BL is to protect the epidermis against rapid cutaneous desiccation by supplying water and glycerol.

3.7. AQP5

In all anuran species, cutaneous glands are basically composed of mucous glands and granular glands (also called serous glands or poison glands) (Suzuki and Tanaka, 2009). The water found in the secreted fluid, especially that from the mucous glands, is considered to be important in the maintenance of a moist skin, cutaneous gas exchange, and thermoregulation (Lillywhite and Licht, 1975; Clarke, 1997).

In *X. laevis*, the anuran AQP5 ortholog, AQP-x5, has been localized to the skin glands (Kubota et al., 2006). AQP-x5 is a recently identified anuran water channel that consists of 273 amino acid residues and contains two NPA motifs, a mercurial-sensitive Cys-181, and a putative phosphorylated motif site for protein kinase A at Ser-257 (Kubota et al., 2006) (Figure 2). The swelling assay using *Xenopus* oocytes confirmed that this AQP facilitates water permeability, and immunohistochemical and immunoelectron microscopic studies revealed the presence of AQP-x5 in the apical plasma membrane of acinar cells of the small granular glands (Fujikura et al., 1988; Kubota et al., 2006). AQP-x5 has also been found in the apical plasma membrane of flattened cells located in the intermediate region between the acinus and excretory duct of mucous glands (Kubota et al., 2006), although it is not known whether these flattened cells, like acinar cells, are able to discharge glycoproteins. Immunohistochemical labeling experiments further indicated that AQP5 may be present in the apical membrane of acinar cells of the mucous or seromucous glands in *H. japonica*, *R. japonica*, and *B. marinus* (Kubota et al., 2006); however, no immuno-positive labeling was detected in the granular glands, however. These findings suggest that anuran AQP5 may mediate the water efflux in the apical membrane of acinar cells of the mucous glands and *Xenopus* small granular glands.

4. Terrestrialism in Amphibians

4.1. Molecular Regulation of Water Balance in Anuran Amphibians

In general, those anuran species adapted to the terrestrial environment, such as *Bufo* (terrestrial) and *Hyla* (arboreal), have a ventral pelvic skin that is highly permeable to water and a bladder that has a high capacity to store urine. In contrast, aquatic anuran species, such as *X. laevis*, have a ventral pelvic skin with a low permeability to water and a urinary bladder with a low storage capacity (Bentley and Main, 1972; Bentley, 2002).

As mentioned above, we have recently identified tree distinct types of AVT-dependent AQPs in the tree frog: AQP-h2 and AQP-h3 in the ventral pelvic skin, AQP-h2 in the urinary bladder, and AQP-h2K in the kidney. Transepithelial water transport seems to be accomplished by these AQPs in concert with AQP-h3BL. AQP-h2 and AQP-h3 are specifically expressed in the ventral pelvic skins of tree frogs, where water absorption occurs (Tanii et al., 2002; Hasegawa et al., 2003). In response to stimulation by AVT, these AQP proteins are translocated to the apical plasma membrane for the purpose of absorbing water through the membrane, whereas the water that exited from the cytoplasm through the AQP-h3BL protein moves into capillaries through AQP1 in the connective tissues for rehydration of the body (Suzuki and Tanaka, 2009). In contrast to AQP-h2 and AQP-h3, the localization of AQP-h3BL does not change following AVT stimulation (Akabane et al., 2007). In addition to localizing AQP-h3BL protein in the basolateral membrane, we also demonstrated that both AQP-h2 and AQP-h3 proteins are located at the basolateral plasma membrane of the first-reacting granular cells in the non-stimulated ventral pelvic skin of tree frogs (Hasegawa et al., 2003). An interesting study to be carried out in the future would be to determine whether AQP-h3BL, AQP-h2, and AQP-h3 are colocalized on the plasma membrane and intracellular vesicles.

Although *Hyla* AQP-h2 is translocated from the cytoplasm to the apical plasma membrane of the *Hyla* urinary bladder in response to AVT stimulation (Hasegawa et al., 2005), AQP-h2 immunoreactivity in the *Xenopus* bladder remains in the cytoplasm, with little movement to the apical membrane after AVT stimulation (Mochida et al., 2008). This finding indicates that the response of *Xenopus* to AVT is considerably weaker than that of semi-terrestrial, terrestrial, and arboreal anurans (Ewer, 1952; Bentley, 2002; Hasegawa et al., 2003, 2005). Thus, it would appear that anuran species possess different osmoregulatory systems through AVT-dependent AQPs that are dependent upon the species terrestrial adaptation niche.

In *H. japonica*, AQP-x5 is located in the apical plasma membrane of the acinar cells of skin glands and AQP-h3BL in the basolateral membrane (Akabane et al., 2007). The leads to the hypothesis that water is absorbed through the AQP-x3BL protein in the secretory cells from the capillaries in the underlying connective tissues and is secreted through the AQP-x5 protein from the apical membrane onto the body surface.

In mammalian salivary glands, the driving force for water transport is considered to be derived from Cl^- and Na^+ secreted from the acinar cells to the lumen following stimulation of the α_1-adrenoreceptor, acetylcholine receptor, or substance P receptor (Edgar, 1992). In the small granular and mucous glands of *Xenopus*, the osmotic pressure gradient - the osmotic pressure of the lumen becomes higher than that of the cytoplasm in the secretory cells - is generally considered to be generated by similar mechanism, i.e., through the transport of ions. This gradient seems to be established by the transport of Cl^- via the cystic fibrosis transmembrane regulator (CFTR) Cl^- channels or via Cl^- channels from the cytoplasm when the secretory cells are stimulated with catecholeamine (Castillo and Orce, 1997; Engelhardt et al., 1994; Koefoed-Johnsen et al., 1952; Mills, 1985). In anuran mucous glands, moreover, it is likely that the depolarization induced by activating the CFTR Cl^- channels activates the co-expressed maxi K^+ channels and that this mechanism is responsible for the active K^+ efflux to the lumen, resulting in the increase of osmotic pressure in the glandular lumen (Sorensen et al., 2001). However, in the mammalian salivary gland, it is believed that the Cl^- co-transports Na^+ into the lumen through the tight junction (Edgar, 1992). If the latter is the mechanism establishing the osmotic gradient, then Na^+ may be transported in the same manner into the lumen (Nielsen, 1990). We also found mitochondria-rich (MR) cells dispersed among the secretory cells in the small granular and mucous glands. It is therefore possible that MR cells play a pivotal role in regulating the osmotic pressure of the lumen in these glands. The presence of MR cells has previously been reported in mucous glands of *H. japonica*, *R. japonica*, and *B. marinus* (Kubota et al., 2006). Because MR cells contain vacuolar type H^+-ATPase, these cells are considered to excrete H^+ into the lumen. The MR cells in the small granular glands contain carbonic anhydrase II (Suzuki and Tanaka, 2009), suggesting that MR cells produce HCO_3^-. It is possible that an electrophoretic Cl^-/HCO_3^- exchanger drives Cl^- entry via in MR cells (Jensen et al., 2002). Thus, MR cells may play a role in adjusting the osmotic gradient in the lumen. Our proposed model is shown in Figure 4. Taken together, these results lead us to suggest that the small granular or mucous glands in the frog play an important role in the secretion of water by providing the body surface with moisture and by regulating body temperature via the loss of heat by evaporation (Lillywhite, 1971).

4.2. Adaptation from the Aquatic Tadpole to the Terrestrial Adult Anuran

The skin of the aquatic tadpole undergoes a number of changes during the metamorphosis of the tadpole into a terrestrial adult frog. The ventral pelvic skin of the adult bullfrog is more permeable to water than that of its tadpole (Bentley and Greenwald, 1970).

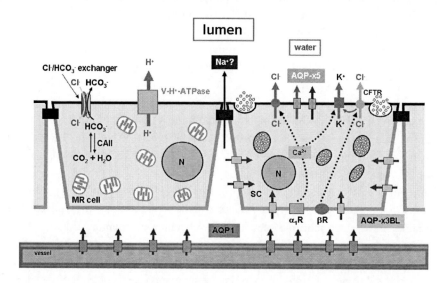

Figure 4. The hypothesis of the molecular mechanism underlying water secretion in the small granular and mucous glands. The osmotic pressure gradient is generally considered to be generated through the transport of ions from the acinar cells of skin glands. Mitochondria-rich (MR) cells play a pivotal role in the regulation of osmotic pressure of the lumen in these glands. Because MR cells contain V-ATPase, these cells are considered to excrete H^+ into the lumen. The negative apical voltage also drives Cl^- entry via an electrophoretic Cl^-/HCO_3^- exchanger in MR cells. Thus, MR cells may play a role in adjusting the osmotic gradient in the lumen. See text, for details. SC, secretory cell; N, nucleus; MR cell, mitochondria-rich cell; α_1R, α_1-adrenergic receptor; βR, β-adrenergic receptor; CAII, carbonic anhydrase II.

Consequently, the study of the spatial and temporal expression of AQP-h2 and AQP-h3 proteins in the ventral pelvic skin of the tree frog during metamorphosis is of particular interest (Hasegawa et al., 2004).

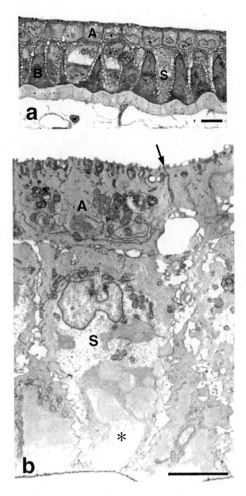

Figure 5. Light (a) and electron (b) micrographs showing sections of the ventral pelvic skin at Gosner stage 37. Larval skin is composed of a single layer of apical cell (A), with skein cells (S) and basal cells (B) in the underlayer. The arrow and asterisk in b indicate a tight junction and the figure of Eberth, respectively. Bar: 10 μm (a); 5 μm (b) [adapted from Hasegawa et al. (2004)].

The larval pelvic skin at Gosner stage 37 (Toe developmental stages) is composed of a single layer of apical cells, with skein cells and basal cells in the underlayer (Figure 5). Electron microscopic studies (Hasegawa et al., 2004) revealed the presence of tight junctions between the apical cells, and granular-like structures in the cytoplasm beneath the apical plasma membrane as well as an abundance of mitochodria and lysosomes near the nucleus. The skein cells were found to be connected to the basal lamina by means of developed hemi-desmosomes, where keratin fibers, called the figure of Eberth, were present (Figure 5). At the climactic stage, especially stage 42, the skin was organized into the same three layers as found in adulthood: the stratum corneum, the granulosum, and the germinativum (Figure 6). Mitochondria-rich cells were often observed in the epithelium. However, the apical cells and skein cells characteristic of the larval pelvic skin were not present. Several granules and keratin fibers were present in the granular cells, just as in the adult skin (Figure 6).

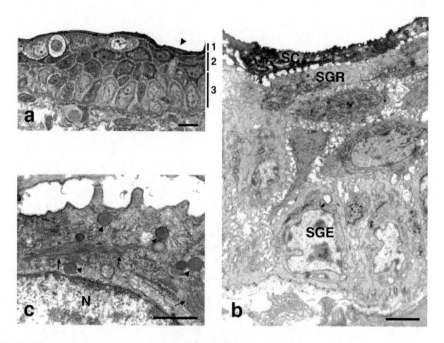

Figure 6. Light (a) and electron (b, c) micrographs showing specimens of ventral pelvic skin at Gosner 42. (a) The skin is organized into three layers: the stratum corneum (1), the granulosum (2), and the germinativum (3), composing granular cells and mitochondria-rich cells (arrowhead). (b) An electron micrograph showing the pelvic skin at low magnification. SC, stratum corneum; SGR, stratum granulosum; SGE, stratum germinativum. (c) An elctron micrograph showing part of a granular cell. Arrowheads, granules; Arrows, keratin fibers; N, nucleus. Bar: 10 μm (a), 1 μm (b). [adapted from Hasegawa et al. (2004)].

Immunofluorescence staining of the ventral pelvic skin at different metamorphic stages revealed the absence of immunopositive reactions for AQP-h2 and AQP-h3 during the premetamorphic and prometamorphic stages (Figure 7a1-c1, a2-c2). At the climactic stages, especially at stages 42 and 43, granular cells immunopositive for both AQP-h2 and AQP-h3 were detected (Figure 7a3-c3). Positive labeling was observed in the basolateral plasma membrane of the granular cells in one or two sublayers of the stratum granulose, located just before the stratum corneum. This finding suggests that both AQP-h2 and AQP-h3 are important for the land-dwelling adult frog to be able to absorb water from its ventral pelvic skin. During the transformation of the larval skin into the adult type, the apical cells and skein cells are lost as a consequence of the repeated division of the basal cells and their differentiation into granular cells (Robinson and Heintzelman, 1987). Expression of the AQP proteins is first observed during this developmental transformation of basal cells into granular cells, and this expression continues without disruption into adulthood. The V2-type AVT receptor mRNA is first expressed at stage 42, which is also the stage at which the AQP proteins are first expressed. The expression of AQP proteins establishes a mechanism for the increased ability of the frog to absorb water across the skin, which occurs in parallel with the change in the structure of the ventral pelvic skin. Thus, AQP expression in the ventral pelvic skin is consistent with the morphological changes that occur in the skin during the adaptation from life in water to that on land.

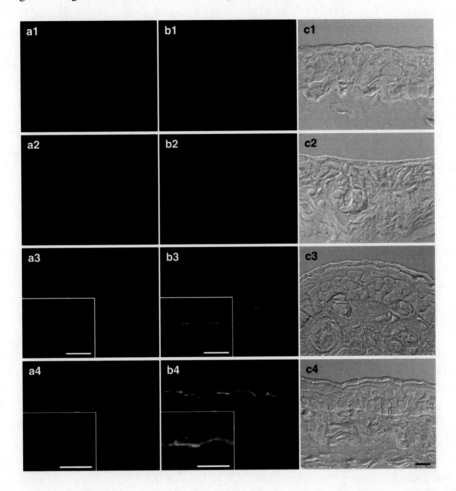

Figure 7. Double-immunofluorescence micrographs showing developmental stages of ventral pelvic skin labeled for AQP-h2 (a, red) and AQP-h3 (b, green); c, Nomarski image for a and b. a1-c1, Gosner stage 40; a2-c2, stage 41; a3-c-3, stage 42; a4-c4, stage 43. Insets in a3, b3, a4, and b4 show a higher magnification of each of the figures. Bars: 10 μm (a-c), 10 μm (inset). [adapted from Hasegawa et al. (2004)].

4.3. Water Adaptation of Anurans Depends upon Different Terrestrial Environments

Anuran amphibians are divided into four groups according to their habitats - aquatic, semi-terrestrial, terrestrial, and arboreal species. Interestingly, we found the expression of AQP-h2- and AQP-h3-like proteins/genes in the pelvic skin of the terrestrial toad, *B. japonica*, to be similar to that in the tree-adapted frog, *H. japonica*. On the other hand, expression of the AQP-h3-like protein or gene in the pelvic skin was observed in all frogs - from aquatic species to terrestrial dwellers -, but the AQP-h2-like protein was not found to be expressed in the pelvic skin of aquatic and semi-terrestrial frogs. The latter protein was, however, detected in the urinary bladder of all frogs. A general characteristic of the terrestrial environment-adapted species, such as *Hyla* (arboreal) and *Bufo* (terrestrial), is that their ventral pelvic skin is highly permeable to water and their urinary bladder has a high capacity for urine storage. The pelvic skins of these anuran species absorb water in a process involving an AQP-h2-like protein in concert with an AQP-h3-like protein (Ogushi et al., 2010). One possible explanation for this coordinated process is that as anurans evolved into the drier terrestrial environments, the urinary bladder-type AQP started to be expressed in the pelvic skin and to transport water together with the ventral pelvic-type AQP.

In conclusion, terrestrial and tree frogs that have adapted to environments with scant water absorb water through their ventral pelvic skin by the mediation of a ventral pelvic skin-type AQP working in concert with a urinary bladder-type AQP.

Acknowledgments

This work was supported in part by a grant-in aid for science research from the Ministry of Education, Science, Sports, and Culture of Japan to ST and MS.

References

Abrami, L., Simon, M., Rousselet, G., Berthonaud, V., Buhler, J. M. & Ripoche, P. (1994). Sequence and functional expression of an amphibian water channel, FA-CHIP: a new member of the MIP family. *Biochim Biophys Acta*, **1192**, 147-151.

Abrami, L., Gobin, R., Berthonaud, V., Thanh, H. L., Ripoche, P. & Verbavatz, J. M. (1997). Localization of the FA-CHIP water channel in frog urinary bladder. *Eur J Cell Biol*, **73**, 215-221.

Agre, P., Brown, D. & Nielsen, S. (1995). Aquaporin water channels: unanswered questions and unresolved controversies. *Curr Opin Cell Biol*, **7**, 472-483.

Akabane, G., Ogushi, Y., Hasegawa, T., Suzuki, M. & Tanaka, S. (2007). Gene cloning and expression of an aquaporin (AQP-h3BL) in the basolateral membrane of water-permeable epithelial cells in osmoregulatory organs of the tree frog. *Am J Physiol Regul Integr Comp Physiol*, **292**, R2340-R2351.

Bentley, P. J. & Greenwald, L. (1970). Neurohypophysial function in bullfrog (*Rana catesbeiana*) tadpoles. *Gen Comp Endocrinol*, **14**, 412-415.

Bentley, P. J. & Main, A. R (1972). Zonal differences in permeability of the skin of some anuran Amphibia. *Am J Physiol*, **223**, 361-363.

Bentley, P. J. & Yorio, T. (1979). Do frogs drink?. *J Exp Biol*, **79**, 41-46.

Bentley, P. J. (1998). Hormones and osmoregulation. In: P. J. Bentley, (Eds.), Comparative Vertebrate Endocrinology (3rd endition, 337-378). Cambridge, UK: Cambridge University.

Bentley, P. J. (2002). The Amphibia. In: S. D., Bradshw, W., H. C., Burggren, Heller, S., Ishii, H., Langer, G., Neuweiler, D. J. Randall, (Eds.), Endocrines and Osmoregulation: A Comparative Account in Vertebrates(pp. 155-18), Berlin, Germany: Springer-Verlag.

Brown, D., Grosso, A. & DeSousa, R. C. (1983). Correlation between water flow and intramembrane particle aggregates in toad epidermis. *Am J Physiol*, **245**, C334-342.

Castillo, G. A. & Orce, G. G. (1997). Response of frog and toad skin to norepinephrine. *Comp Biochem Physiol A Physiol*, **118**, 1145-1150.

Chevalier, J., Bourguet, J. & Hugon, J. S. (1974). Membrane associated particles: distribution in frog urinary bladder epithelium at rest and after oxytocin treatment. *Cell Tissue Res*, **152**, 129-140.

Clarke, B. T. (1997). The natural history of amphibian skin secretions, their normal functioning and potential medical applications. *Biol Rev Camb Philos Soc*, **72**, 365-379.

de Groot, B. L. & Grubmuller, H. (2005). The dynamics and energetics of water permeation and proton exclusion in aquaporins. *Curr Opin Struct Biol*, **15**, 176-183.

Edgar, W. M. (1992). Saliva: its secretion, composition and functions. *Br Dent J*, **172**, 305-312.

Engel, A., Fujiyoshi, Y., Gonen, T. & Walz, T. (2008). Junction-forming aquaporins. *Curr Opin Struct Biol*, **18**, 229-235.

Engelhardt, J. F., Smith, S. S., Allen, E., Yankaskas, J. R., Dawson, D. C. & Wilson, J. M. (1994). Coupled secretion of chloride and mucus in skin of *Xenopus laevis*: possible role for CFTR. *Am J Physiol*, **267**, C491-500.

Ewer, R. (1952). The Effects of posterior pituitary extracts on water balance in *Bufo carens* and *Xenopus laevis*, together with some general considerations of anuran water economy. *J Exp Biol*, **29**, 429-439.

Fluhr, J. W., Darlenski, R. & Surber, C. (2008). Glycerol and the skin: holistic approach to its origin and functions. *Br J Dermatol*, **159**, 23-34.

Frost, D. R. (2008). Amphibian Species of the World: an Online Reference. Ver. 5.2 (15 July, 2008). Electronic Database accessible at http:research.amnh.org/herpetology/ampbian/index.php. American Museum of Natural History, New York

Fujikura, K., Kurabuchi, S., Tabuchi, M. & Inoue, S. (1988). Morphological and distribution of the skin glands in *Xenopus laevis* and their response to experimental stimulations. *Zool Sci*, **5**, 415-430.

Gorin, M. B., Yancey, S. B., Cline, J., Revel, J. P. & Horwitz, J. (1984). The major intrinsic protein (MIP) of the bovine lens fiber membrane: characterization and structure based on cDNA cloning. *Cell*, **39**, 49-59.

Gonen, T., Sliz, P., Kistler, J., Cheng, Y. & Walz, T. (2004). Aquaporin-0 membrane junctions reveal the structure of a closed water pore. *Nature*, **429**, 193-197.

Hara, M., M, a T. & Verkman, A. S. (2002). Selectively reduced glycerol in skin of aquaporin-3 deficient mice may account for impaired skin hydration, elasticity and barrier recovery. *J Biol Chem*, **277**, 46616-46621.

Hara, M. & Verkman, A. S. (2003). Glycerol replacement corrects defective skin hydration, elasticity, and barrier function in aquaporin-3-deficient mice. *Proc Natl Acad Sci*, USA, **100**, 7360-7365.

Harvey, B. J. (1992). Energization of sodium absorption by the H^+-ATPase pump in mitochondria-rich cells of frog skin. *J Exp Biol*, **172**, 289-309.

Hasegawa, T., Sugawara, Y., Suzuki, M. & Tanaka, S. (2004). Spatial and temporal expression of the ventral pelvic skin aquaporins during metamorphosis of the tree frog, *Hyla japonica*. *J Membr Biol*, **199**, 119-126.

Hasegawa, T., Suzuki, M. & Tanaka, S. (2005). Immunocytochemical studies on translocation of phosphorylated AQP-h2 protein in granular cells of the frog urinary bladder before and after stimulation with vasotocin. *Cell Tissue Res*, **322**, 407-415.

Hillyard, D. S., Mobjerg, N., Tanaka, S. & Larsen, E. H. (2009). Osmotic and ion regulation in amphibians.The Amphibia. In: D. H. Evans, (Eds.), Osmotic and Ionic Regulation: Cells and Animals, (367-441), Boca Raton, FL: CRC press.

Ishibashi, K. (2006). Aquaporin subfamily with unusual NPA boxes. *Biochim Biophys Acta*, **1758**, 989-93.

Ishibashi, K., Kuwahara, M. & Sasaki, S. (2000). Molecular biology of aquaporins. *Rev Physiol Biochem Pharmacol*, **141**, 1-32.

Jensen, L. J., Willumsen, N. J. & Larsen, E. H. (2002). Proton pump activity is required for active uptake of chloride in isolated amphibian skin exposed to freshwater. *J. Comp.. Physiol*, [B], **172**, 503-511.

Kachadorian, W. A., Wade, J. B. & DiScala, V. A, (1975). Vasopressin: induced structural change in toad bladder luminal membrane. *Science*, **190**, 67-69.

King, L. S., Kozono, D. & Agre, P. (2004). From structure to disease: the evolving tale of aquaporin biology. *Nat Rev Mol Cell Biol*, **5**, 687-698.

Kloas, W. & Hanke, W. (1992). Localization and quantification of atrial natriuretic factor binding sites in the kidney of *Xenopus laevis*. *Gen Comp Endocrinol*, **85**, 26-35.

Koefoed-Johnsen, V., Ussing, H. H. & Zerahn, K. (1952). The origin of the short-circuit current in the adrenaline stimulated frog skin. *Acta Physiol Scand*, **27**, 38-48.

Kubota, M., Hasegawa, T., Nakakura, T., Tanii, H., Suzuki, M. & Tanaka, S. (2006). Molecular and cellular characterization of a new aquaporin, AQP-x5, specifically expressed in the small granular glands of *Xenopus* skin. *J Exp Biol*, **209**, 3199-3208.

Lillywhite, H. B. (1975). Physiological correlates of basking in amphibians. *Comp Biochem Physiol A*, **52**, 323-330.

Lillywhite, H. B. (2006). Water relations of tetrapod integument. *J Exp Biol*, **209**, 202-226.

Loveridge, J. (1970). Observations on nitrogenous excretion and water relations of *Chiromantis xerampelina* (Amphibia, Anura). *Arnoldia*, **5**, 1-6.

Ma, T., Yang, B. & Verkman, A. S. (1996). cDNA cloning of a functional water channel from toad urinary bladder epithelium. *Am J Physiol*, **271**, C1699-C1704.

Matsuzaki, T., Suzuki, T., Koyama, H., Tanaka, S. & Takata, K. (1999). Water channel protein AQP3 is present in epithelial exposed to the environment of possible water loss. *J Histoichem Cytochem*, **47**, 1275-1286.

Mochida, H., Nakakura, T., Suzuki, M., Hayashi, H., Kikuyama, S. & Tanaka, S. (2008). Immunolocalization of a mammalian aquaporin 3 homologue in water-transporting epithelial cells in several organs of the clawed toad *Xenopus laevis*. *Cell Tissue Res*, **333**, 297-309.

Moon, C., Williams, J. B., Preston, G. M., Copeland, N. G., Gilbert, D. J., Nathans, D., Jenkins, N. A. & Agre, P. (1995). The mouse aquaporin-1 gene. *Genomics*, **30**, 354-357.

Nielsen, S., Smith, B. L., Christensen, E. I. & Agre, P. (1993). Distribution of the aquaporin CHIP in secretory and resorptive epithelia and capillary endothelia. *Proc Natl Acad Sci*, USA, **90**, 7275-7279.

Nielsen, R. (1990). Isotonic secretion via frog skin glands in vitro. Water secretion is coupled to the secretion of sodium ions. *Acta Physiol Scand*, **139**, 211-221.

Ogushi, Y., Mochida, H., Nakakura, T., Suzuki, M. & Tanaka, S. (2007). Immunocytochemical and phylogenetic analyses of an arginine vasotocin-dependent aquaporin, AQP-h2K, specifically expressed in the kidney of the tree frog, *Hyla japonica*. *Endocrinology*, **148**, 5891-5901.

Ogushi, Y., Akabane, G., Hasegawa, T., Mochida, H., Matsuda, M., Suzuki, M. & Tanaka, S. (2010). Water adaptation strategy in anuran amphibians: molecular diversity of aquaporins. *Endovrinology*, **151**, 165-173.

Pang, P. K. (1983). Evolution of control of epithelial transport in vertebrates. *J Exp Biol*, **106**, 283-299.

Parsons, R. H., McDevitt, V., Aggerwal, V., Le Blang, T., Manley, K., Kim, N., Lopez, J. & Kenedy, A. A. (1993). Regulation of pelvic patch water flow in *Bufo marinus*: role of bladder volume and ANG II. *Am J Physiol*, **264**, R1260-1265.

Pough, F. H. (2007). Amphibian biology and husbandry. ILAR J, 48, 203-213.

Robinson, D. H. & Heintzelman, M. B. (1987). Morphology of ventral epidermis of *Rana catesbeiana* during metamorphosis. *Anat Rec*, **217**, 305-317.

Rojek, A., Praetorius, J., Frokiaer, J., Nielsen, S. & Fenton, R. A. (2008). A current view of the mammalian aquaglyceroporins. *Annu Rev Physiol*, **70**, 301-327.

Sasaki, S. & Noda, Y. (2007). Aquaporin-2 protein dynamics within the cell. *Curr Opin Nephrol Hypertens*, **16**, 348-352.

Shiels, A., Mackay, D., Bassnett, S., Al-Ghoul, K. & Kuszak, J. (2000). Disruption of lens fiber cell architecture in mice expressing a chimeric AQP0-LTR protein. *FASEB J*, **14**, 2207-2212.

Shiels, A., Bassnett, S., Varadaraj, K., Mathias, R., Al-Ghoul, K., Kuszak, J., Donoviel, D., Lilleberg, S., Friedrich, G. & Zambrowicz, B. (2001). Optical dysfunction of the crystalline lens in aquaporin-0-deficient mice. *Physiol Genomics*, **7**, 179-186.

Sorensen, J. B., Nielsen, M.S., Gudme, C. N., Larsen, E. H. & Nielsen, R. (2001). Maxi K+ channels co-localised with CFTR in the apical membrane of an exocrine gland acinus: possible involvement in secretion. *Pflugers Arch*, **442**, 1-11.

Sougrat, R., Morand, M., Gondran, C., Barre, P., Gobin, R., Bonte, F., Dumas, M. & Verbavatz, J. M, (2002). Functional expression of AQP3 in human skin epidermis and reconstructed epidermis. *J Invest Dermatol*, **118**, 678-685.

Suzuki, M., Hasegawa, T., Ogushi, Y. & Tanaka, S. (2007). Amphibian aquaporins and adaptation to terrestrial environments: a review. *Comp Biochem Physiol A Mol Integr Physiol*, **148**, 72-81.

Suzuki, M. & Tanaka, S. (2009). Molecular and cellular regulation of water homeostasis in anuran amphibians by aquaporins. *Comp Biochem Physiol A*, in press

Takata, K., Matsuzaki, T. & Tajika, Y. (2004). Aquaporins: water channel proteins of the cell membrane. *Prog Histochem Cytochem*, **39**, 1-83.

Takemoto, L., Takehana, M. & Horwitz, J. (1986). Covalent changes in MIP26K during aging of the human lens membrane. *Invest Ophthalmol Vis Sci*, **27**, 443-446.

Tanii, H., Hasegawa, T., Hirakawa, N., Suzuki, M. & Tanaka, S. (2002). Molecular and cellular characterization of a water channel protein, AQP-h3, specifically expressed in the frog ventral skin. *J Membr Biol*, **188**, 43-53.

Uchiyama, M. & Yoshizawa, H. (2002). Nephron structure and immunohistochemical localiztion of ion pumps and aquaporins in the kidney of frogs inhabiting different environments. In: N., Hazon, & G. Flik, (Eds.), Osmoregulation and Drinking in Vertebrates, (pp.109-128), Oxford, UK: BIOS Scientific Publishers.

Varadaraj, K., Kumari, S., Shiels, A. & Mathias, R. T. (2005). Regulation of aquaporin water permeability in the lens. *Invest Ophthalmol Vis Sci*, **46**, 1393-1402.

Virkki, L. V., Franke, C., Somieski, P. & Boron, W. F. (2002). Cloning and functional characterization of a novel aquaporin from *Xenopus laevis* oocytes. *J Biol Chem*, **277**, 40610-40616.

Voute, C. L. & Ussing, H. H. (1968). Some morphological aspects of active sodium transport. The epithelium of the frog skin. *J Cell Biol*, **36**, 625-638.

Willumsen, N. J., Viborg, A. L. & Hillyard, S. D. (2007). Vascular aspects of water uptake mechanisms in the toad skin: perfusion, diffusion, confusion. *Comp Biochem Physiol A Mol Integr Physiol*, **148**, 55-63.

Word, J. M. & Hillman, S. S. (2005). Osmotically absorbed water preferentially enters the cutaneous capillaries of the pelvic patch in the toad *Bufo marinus*. *Physiol Biochem Zool*, **78**, 40-47.

Yasui, M. (2004). Molecular mechanisms and drug development in aquaporin water channel diseases: structure and function of aquaporins. *J Pharmacol Sci*, **96**, 260-263.

Zardoya, R. (2005). Phylogeny and evolution of the major intrinsic protein family. *Biol Cell*, **97**, 397-414.

In: Synthetic and Integrative Biology
Editor: James T. Gevona, pp. 61-76

ISBN: 978-1-60876-678-9
© 2010 Nova Science Publishers, Inc.

Chapter 3

APPLICATIONS OF BACTERIAL QUORUM-SENSING SYSTEMS IN SYNTHETIC BIOLOGY

Daniel J. Sayut, Pavan K.R. Kambam,
William G. Herrick and Lianhong Sun[*]
Department of Chemical Engineering, University of Massachusetts,
Amherst, MA, USA

Abstract

The ability to coordinate cellular responses in a population is critical to achieving certain behaviors in both natural and artificial systems. In bacteria, the coordination of cellular activity at the population level is implemented through quorum sensing. At their most basic, quorum-sensing systems are composed of three main components, making them amenable to genetic manipulation. Here we review the work researchers have done to isolate the components of these systems into well-characterized modules for use in the construction of genetic circuits that program complex cellular behaviors. Such modules have not only allowed for the incorporation of traditional quorum-sensing responses in host organisms, but have also allowed for the creation of a diverse array of novel responses based on cell-cell communication.

Introduction

Cellular engineering has traditionally been a top-down process in which biological systems are altered using environmental conditions or by discrete changes to cellular networks through gene mutations. The field of synthetic biology is attempting to overturn these traditional conventions by focusing on the construction of artificial circuits through the joining together of independent biological modules. Composed of individual biological devices that allow for the sensing and processing of inputs, these modules are expected to

[*]E-mail address: lsun@ecs.umass.edu, Phone: 413-5456143, Fax: 413-5451647. (Corresponding author)

function in defined ways to produce outputs that can directly trigger cellular responses or interact with other modules. To be effective, modules should function independently of other modules and of the host cell except through predetermined inputs and outputs. The goal of this method is to allow for the bottom-up construction of complex cellular behavior, and to bring traditional engineering principles such as standardization, abstraction, and de-coupling into the field of cellular engineering[1].

Cell-to-cell signaling modules are of particular interest to the field of synthetic biology as they allow for the construction of complex intercellular circuits and the programming of responses at the population-level. In bacterial systems, cell-to-cell signaling occurs through quorum-sensing mechanisms with the most prominent signal in Gram-negative bacteria being acylated homoserine lactones (AHLs)[2]. Quorum-sensing systems that use AHLs as the signaling molecule have relatively simple structures with the most basic systems composed of three main components: a signal synthase that synthesizes the AHL signal, an AHL responsive transcription factor, and a promoter regulated by the transcription factor. Owing to the simple structure of the quorum-sensing mechanism, many groups have examined the properties of different quorum-sensing modules and how these modules can be utilized in artificial genetic networks to program complex intercellular responses.

Quorum Sensing

Intercellular communication between bacteria was originally discovered through studies of the marine bacterium *Vibrio fischeri,* which is involved in symbiotic relationships with a variety of fishes and squids. In these relationships, *V. fischeri* are taken in by their hosts and grown in specialized light organs, where at high cellular densities they produce luminescence ($>10^{10}$ cells/mL)[2]. The signaling mechanism responsible for the luminescence response was termed quorum sensing because of the high cellular densities of *V. fischeri* that were required to trigger luminescence. Since its discovery in *V. fischeri*, quorum sensing has been shown to be conserved in a large number of bacteria and involved in a variety of important biological process including virulence and biofilm formation[3].

The quorum-sensing response in *V. fischeri* is controlled by the LuxR transcriptional activator and the LuxI synthase (Figure 1). At low cell densities, basal expression of LuxI results in a small amount of N-3-oxohexanoyl-L-homoserine lactone (OHHL) being synthesized and freely diffusing into the extracellular environment. As the cell population grows, extracellular accumulation of OHHL results in slower diffusion of OHHL out of the cell and allows for a critical intracellular concentration to be reached. At this critical concentration, OHHL binds LuxR forming a complex that causes expression from the *luxI* promoter (P_{luxI}) by binding to a *lux* box site centered at 42.5 base pairs upstream of the transcriptional start site[4]. Activation of P_{luxI} results in expression of the luminescence genes (*luxCDABEG*), and enhancement of the global quorum-sensing response through positive feedback on *luxI*. This general mechanism is conserved in all quorum-sensing systems found in Gram-negative bacteria, with specificity between each of the systems achieved through the synthesis and detection of unique AHLs by LuxI and LuxR homologs. The AHL signals are unique in the length and degree of saturation of their acyl side chains[2]. Individual quorum-sensing systems also have additional sources of regulation that influence their responses.

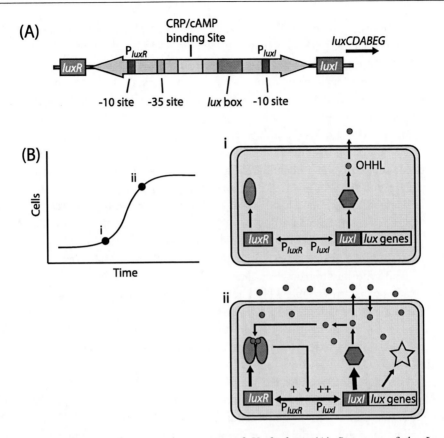

Figure 1. The LuxI/LuxR quorum-sensing system of *V. fischeri*. (A) Structure of the LuxI/LuxR regulatory region. (B) Regulation of the quorum-sensing response. Basal expression from P_{luxI} is weak, preventing luminescence until a critical concentration of OHHL is reached. At this critical concentration, activation of P_{luxI} results in luminescence and positive feedback on LuxI, increasing system activation. Additional feedback on LuxR increases the sensitivity of the response.

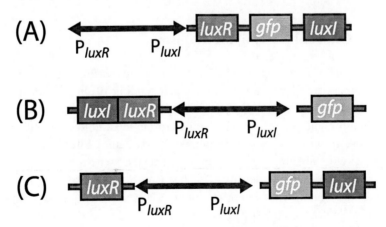

Figure 2. Rearrangements of the LuxI/LuxR system used to determine effect of architecture on system response. (A) Both LuxI and LuxR under P_{luxI}-regulated positive feedback. (B) Both LuxI and LuxR under constitutive P_{luxR} expression. (C) Natural architecture of the LuxI/LuxR quorum-sensing system. System response was measured using expression of a green fluorescent protein (GFP) from P_{luxI}.

While OHHL is freely diffusible, efflux pumps have been implicated in the transport of some larger, more hydrophobic AHLs across the cellular membrane, thereby increasing the complexity of the basic quorum-sensing mechanism in these systems[5]. Regulation of the LuxR homologs also differ between quorum-sensing systems, with the native *luxR* promoter (P_{luxR}) being regulated by the cAMP-CRP activator complex[6], and capable of both positively and negatively regulating its own expression level once activated[7, 8].

Studies into LuxR and its homologs have shown that all LuxR-type transcriptional activators share a common structure with a helix-turn-helix (HTH) DNA binding motif in the carboxy-terminal domain, and a ligand binding site in the amino-terminal domain[9]. Binding of the cognate signal molecule to the amino-terminal domain of a LuxR-type protein is thought to cause conformational changes that lead to multimerization and relieve repression of the carboxyl-terminal domain allowing for DNA binding. Studies of LuxR and its homolog, TraR, have shown that the mechanisms for binding of the AHL signal molecules differ between LuxR homologs with binding of OHHL by LuxR being reversible by dilution[10], while the binding between TraR and its signal molecule, N-3-oxooctanoyl-L-homoserine lactone, is irreversible[11]. The specificities of the LuxR homologs for their cognate signal molecules is high with even small changes to the length or saturation of the acyl side chain resulting in at least 10-fold decreases in activity[12]. After signal binding, however, the activated LuxR-type protein complexes can bind certain *lux*-type boxes nonspecifically[13].

LuxI and its homologs synthesize AHL signal molecules using acylated acyl carrier proteins (acyl-ACPs) and S-adenosylmethionine (SAM) as substrates[14, 15]. The specificity of LuxI and its homologs is high, but secondary, low-level synthesis of AHLs distinct from the primary signaling molecule does occur for any given LuxI-type protein[16]. Specificity of LuxI and its homologs for the synthesis of specific AHLs is thought to be caused by the size and structure of their acyl-ACP binding pockets[17, 18]. While LuxI homologs show only limited homology, conserved regions and specific amino acid residues that are critical for AHL synthesis have been identified[17, 19].

Analysis of the Quorum-Sensing Mechanism

For most biological circuits, the complex and nonlinear nature of the interactions that occur between components limits an intuitive understanding of circuit function. Therefore, coupling experimental measurements with models detailing the interactions of the components is helpful, and often necessary, to determine the architecture and properties of a genetic circuit that result in a desired response. Of particular interest in the response of quorum-sensing circuits are the properties that lead to the switch-like response that occurs once the cells reach a critical cell density. This has lead researchers to use a combination of experiments and mathematical modeling to examine how interactions between the quorum-sensing components determine the system's response.

Using the LuxI/LuxR module as a basis for study, the effects of circuit architecture on the quorum-sensing response has been examined by shuffling the regulation of LuxI and LuxR between P_{luxR} and P_{luxI} (Figure 2)[20]. In creating the shuffled systems, it was assumed that expression from P_{luxR} was effectively constitutive because of the comparatively small amount of activation that occurs for P_{luxR} compared to P_{luxI} upon induction of the quorum-sensing response[8, 21]. Therefore, regulation of LuxI and LuxR differed between being constitutive or under positive feedback depending on circuit architecture. By combining steady-state analysis of deterministic differential equations and experimental measurements, it was determined that while all of the shuffled architectures resulted in functional population sensors, only the dual feedback system (P_{luxI}: *luxR, luxI*) was capable of hysteresis and bistability. In comparison, the natural architecture of the quorum-sensing system (P_{luxR}: *luxR*, P_{luxI}: *luxI*) resulted in a threshold response, and the response of the constitutive system (P_{luxR}: *luxR, luxI*) was graded.

A combination of modeling and experimental analysis has also been used to test the assumption of constitutive expression from P_{luxR}, and to determine the actual impact of LuxR positive feedback on circuit dynamics. Using analytical solutions to steady-state deterministic differential equations, theoretical results showed that positive feedback on the LuxR protein was required to achieve bistability in the quorum-sensing response in agreement with what was observed for the shuffled quorum-sensing modules. However, the results predicted that feedback present in the regulation of P_{luxR} should be sufficient to cause bistability. This was tested experimentally using a chromosomally maintained copy of the *lux* regulatory region in *E. coli* cells grown in minimal media. The use of minimal media allowed for full activity of P_{luxR} to both cAMP-CRP activation and LuxR feedback by preventing catabolite repression. Under these conditions, bistability and hysteresis was most prominent at high levels of P_{luxR} activity upon induction with OHHL, confirming the importance of P_{luxR} mediated feedback for the establishment of bistability in the natural LuxI/LuxR system.

Along with showing the importance of circuit architecture on the response of quorum-sensing modules, the studies of the LuxI/LuxR system also show the importance of the expression levels and activities of the regulatory proteins. While both studies examined the natural LuxI/LuxR system, the role of LuxR feedback was not observed for the shuffled systems because the expression levels of LuxR were repressed by the rich media used to grow the cultures. The result of this repression was that instead of demonstrating a switch-like response capable of bistability, the system instead showed a threshold response. Interestingly, bistability and hysteresis were also absent in a minimal positive feedback motif in which LuxR was expressed from P_{luxI}[22, 23]. Thus, when constructing quorum-sensing modules to be used in artificial genetic circuits the expression levels and regulatory mechanisms of the quorum components must be carefully considered and tuned to achieve the desired responses.

Engineering of the Quorum-Sensing Response

In the construction of artificial genetic circuits, it is common that a proposed circuit design does not behave as expected when implemented into a biological host. This occurs because desired behaviors are typically only observed for specific properties of the circuit components, and the properties required for the proper function of an artificial circuit are often different from the naturally evolved properties of the components. Theoretical predictions are also based on incomplete knowledge of the *in vivo* parameters and interactions that govern the behavior of a circuit in a recombinant host, preventing optimization of a design prior to implementation. These limits require that we have reliable *in vivo* methods to tune the properties of genetic circuits so as to obtain desired behaviors. Common methods for tuning the responses of a circuit include altering of the *cis*-regulatory and ribosome binding sites that control protein expression; and using protein engineering techniques to change component activities. Of these options, changing the translational rate of a circuit component by altering its ribosome binding site (RBS) is probably the most widely-used, as alterations to the RBS allow for the expression level of a component to be changed without changing its regulation or the circuit architecture. The relative expression levels of a protein can also be changed by several orders of magnitude by mutating a small number of bases in its RBS[24]. Further modification of a protein's expression level can by obtained by mutating the *cis*-regulatory elements controlling transcription. This methods is particularly attractive for well-studied promoters like P_{luxI}, as extensive analysis of P_{luxI} has resulted in the identification of a series of mutated promoters that show a significant range of activities[25].

Along with altering a component's expression level, directed evolution has become a popular approach for tuning the properties of artificial genetic circuits because it does not require a complete understanding of the protein components, or their interactions, to achieve functional systems. Directed evolution also allows for the rapid generation of diversity in the response of a circuit component, which is helpful for determining the behavior of a genetic circuit and improving theoretical predictions[20]. The use of directed evolution for altering circuit properties is especially relevant for the tuning of quorum-sensing modules as few complete structures are available for quorum-sensing components[17, 18, 26], preventing the extensive use of rational protein engineering methods for altering system behavior.

Methods for the directed evolution of quorum-sensing components are well-established, with previous studies demonstrating the isolation of mutants with altered signal specificities and activities. The ability to alter the specificity of quorum-sensing components allows for the minimization of cross-talk between different quorum-sensing modules, and can be used for the creation of additional signaling pathways. To achieve high levels of specificity, a dual selection method is required to isolate mutants that only show activity in the presence of the desired signaling molecule. A dual selection method for LuxR has been demonstrated, and was successfully used to increase the specificity of a broad-specificity LuxR mutant to N-octanoyl-L-homoserine lactone(OHL)[27, 28]. To create the broad-specificity LuxR mutant, a directed evolution library was screened for activity in the presence of OHL[27]. An analogous approach has been used generate a broad-specificity RhlI mutant. RhlI typically synthesizes N-butryl-L-homoserine lactone, but a mutant capable of synthesizing AHLs with longer chain lengths was isolated by screening an RhlI mutant library for the ability to activate LuxR[29].

While altering the specificities of quorum-sensing components allows for the construction of discrete signaling modules, altering the activities of these components allows for the responses of quorum-sensing modules to be tuned[30]. The ability to use directed evolution to increase the sensitivity of LuxR-type proteins to their cognate signal molecules was initially shown during screening of libraries for mutants with altered signal specificities[27]. Because of the value of these mutants for tuning the responses of quorum-sensing modules, the original screening method was modified to allow for the identification of additional hypersensitive LuxR mutants[22]. In addition, a genetic selection for altering the enzymatic activity of LuxI has also been demonstrated and was used to isolate a LuxI mutant with an 80-fold increase in the yield of OHHL after two rounds of selection[31].

The output from a quorum-sensing module determines how it will interact with other genetic modules or regulate protein expression. While the form and strength of this output can be modified by changing the regulatory mechanisms and properties of the quorum-sensing components, completely novel responses can also be created by incorporating the *lux* box into hybrid promoter regions that contain operator sites for additional regulators. The ability to construct complex responses through the combination of *cis*-regulatory elements has been demonstrated by the combinatorial synthesis of hybrid promoters incorporating operators for the AraC, LacI, TetR, and LuxR transcriptional regulators[32]. One clear property of all the hybrid promoters was the presence of logic. This property has been examined in more detail for a hybrid *luxI-lacO* promoter ($P_{luxI-lacO}$) that was capable of establishing AND logic for induction with OHHL and Isopropyl β-D-1-thiogalactopyranoside (IPTG) by integrating the activities of LuxR and LacI (Figure 3)[33]. Tuning of the AND response was also shown through the use of LuxR mutants with altered sensitivities to OHHL. In addition to using additional *cis*-regulatory elements to change the response of a hybrid quorum-sensing promoter, it has also been demonstrated that LuxR can be used as a transcriptional repressor by positioning the *lux* binding site upstream of the -35 site in an artificial promoter[34]. By inverting the quorum-sensing regulatory response, such novel promoters could expand the possible designs and uses of quorum-sensing modules in artificial genetic circuits.

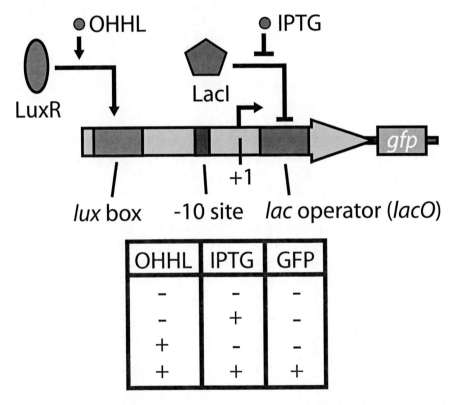

Figure 3. Generation of logic in a hybrid $P_{luxI-lacO}$ promoter. Activation of LuxR binding by OHHL, and deactivation of LacI binding by IPTG activates expression from $P_{luxI-lacO}$. The relative binding strengths of the LuxR and LacI proteins are balanced to prevent significant expression in the absence of either inducer. Homologous systems can be constructed using alternative transcriptional activators and repressors.

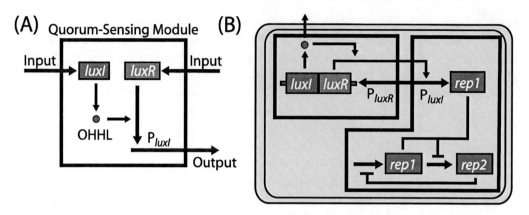

Figure 4. Interfacing quorum-sensing modules to additional cellular modules. (A) Inputs and outputs of a basic LuxI/LuxR quorum-sensing module. The response of a LuxI/LuxR quorum-sensing module can be controlled by regulating the expression levels of either the LuxI or LuxR proteins. Output from the quorum-sensing module is in the form of transcription from the P_{luxI} promoter. (B) Example of module integration. A genetic toggle switch was integrated with a LuxI/LuxR quorum-sensing module by using the module's output to increase the expression level of one of the toggle switch's repressors.

Achieving Spatiotemporal Regulation in Artificial Circuits Using Quorum-Sensing Modules

At its most basic, quorum sensing is meant to trigger the coordinated expression of genes in a cellular population once a critical cell density is reached. One clear application of this coordinated response is the use of quorum-sensing modules for the autonomous regulation of recombinant protein expression. By delaying induction to higher cell densities, quorum-sensing modules allow for the effects of stress caused by the over-expression of recombinant proteins, such as depressed growth rates[35], to be minimized. Low basal expression rates also allow for the expression of proteins that are toxic to the host cell. When expressing toxic proteins, circuit architecture is a particularly important consideration as a coordinated, switch-like response will maximize the yield of the recombinant protein before cellular death[36].

Moving beyond simple recombinant protein production, quorum-sensing modules can be used to regulate genes that cause specific cellular responses or can be integrated with additional cellular modules to program complex behaviors. One method to achieve module integration is to regulate the expression or activity of the quorum-sensing components using the output from another module. In turn, the output of the quorum-sensing module, in the form of expression from the regulated promoter, can be used to regulate another module's components. This is demonstrated for the LuxI/LuxR system in Figure 4. Theoretically, any circuit that results in transcription as an output, or can use transcription as an input, can be combined with a quorum-sensing module. This "plug-and-play" ability has been demonstrated by combining a quorum-sensing module with a genetic toggle switch (Figure 4B)[36].

The ability of quorum-sensing modules to regulate genes that cause specific cellular responses was shown by the construction of a circuit capable of regulating cellular growth through the expression of a toxic protein[37]. In this circuit, bicistronic expression of LuxI and LuxR from a hybrid *lac/ara-1* promoter ($P_{lac/ara-1}$) was used to establish the quorum-sensing response and regulate the expression of a lacZα–ccdB killer gene. With this design, the circuit could be turned off and on by the addition of IPTG, and the regulated cellular density was tunable by altering the degradation rate of the OHHL signal molecule using the pH of the media. At higher media pHs, OHHL degradation was increased resulting in the regulated cultures reaching higher cell densities. Observation of the regulated cells in both macro-scale batch cultures and microchemostats showed that the system was fairly stable with the microchemostat cultures maintaining regulated population levels for over 200 hours[37, 38].

Heterogeneity across the cellular population was essential for the correct functioning of the population control circuit, as cellular heterogeneity allowed for a portion of the cells to remain viable after the critical cellular density had been reached. In general, positive feedback on the LuxI-type synthase limits heterogeneity in the response of natural quorum-sensing systems by causing the synthesis of large amounts of the signal molecule. The influx of the signaling molecule ensures all cells become active despite any heterogeneity in their responses. As this feedback was removed in the population control circuit by expressing LuxR and LuxI from $P_{lac/ara-1}$[37], the circuit was able to exploit population heterogeneity to maintain function. This approach is counter to the traditional goal of using quorum-sensing modules to synchronize cellular responses at the population level, and emphasizes the importance of circuit architecture in obtaining desired responses.

A particularly active area of research in synthetic biology is on the creation of modules that are capable of synchronizing cellular oscillations, with the goal of determining the mechanisms that lead to the stable oscillations in cellular populations. To achieve this synchronization a number of theoretical designs have been proposed based on the integration of quorum-sensing modules with different positive and negative feedback loop modules capable of driving oscillations[39-41]. Key to these designs is the incorporation of the LuxI-type synthase into one of the feedback loops to couple each cell's state to the entire population. In addition to these proposed designs, a number of studies have also used models incorporating stochasticity to more accurately determine how cellular variability and noise affects synchronization of coupled cellular populations[42, 43].

Quorum-sensing modules have also been proposed as mechanisms for achieving specificity in the use of bacterial cells as targeted delivery systems for the treatment of tumors. To demonstrate the usefulness of quorum sensing for this targeted delivery, the output of a LuxI/LuxR quorum-sensing module was used to express the *inv* gene from *Yersinia pseudotuberculosis*, which causes adhesion and invasion of mammalian cells when expressed in *E. coli*[44]. Though the system was implemented in *E. coli*, the cell density of circuit activation (3×10^8 CFU/mL) was noted to be in the range between the densities observed for *Salmonella* in tumors (10^9) and healthy tissues (10^3-10^6) in mice. As *E. coli* have also been shown to localize to tumors[45], it could be possible to make the circuit discriminate between healthy and diseased cells by tuning the cell density at which it activates. Additional work has shown how the specificity of the invasion response can be further improved by using the quorum-sensing module as one leg of a genetic AND gate capable of integrating two distinct environmental signals[46].

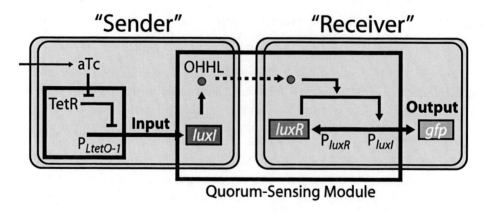

Figure 5. Establishment of intercellular signaling between distinct cellular populations. Signal generation in sender cells is dependent on the output of a hybrid phage lambda-*tetO* promoter ($P_{LtetO-1}$) regulated by the Tet repressor. Upon generation, OHHL diffuses through media to receiver cells, activating LuxR and causing expression from P_{luxI}.

The systems discussed above relied on the synthesis of the signal molecule to time the induction of a genetic circuit maintained in all cells of the cellular population. Alternatively, it is also possible to use quorum-sensing modules to establish communication between distinct cellular populations. This was first demonstrated by Weiss et al., who created distinct "receiver" and "sender" cells by transforming different cell strains with either receiver plasmids containing LuxI/LuxR regulatory region with the *lux* operon replaced by a detectable marker (GFP(LVA)), or sender plasmids containing LuxI under the control of an inducible promoter (Figure 5)[47]. By splitting the quorum-sensing module between the two cellular populations, the responses of the receiver cells was dependent on the signals generated in the sender cells. Therefore, the module is no longer acting as a method to coordinate the responses of a cellular population, but instead is acting as communication module.

Building on this relatively simple communication module, pulse-generating and band-detect circuits have been constructed by tying the output of the communication module to additional regulatory modules. For the pulse-generating network the downstream module contained an incoherent feed-forward motif based on a hybrid *luxI/cI-O_R1* promoter ($P_{luxI/cI-OR1}$)[48]. In the circuit, slow expression of the CI repressor from P_{luxI} resulted in the eventual repression of GFP expression from $P_{luxI/cI-OR1}$, creating a pulse of fluorescence. In order to achieve functional circuits, it was necessary to express CI from a weak RBS and decrease its binding strength by mutating its binding site in $P_{luxI/cI-OR1}$. The band-detect circuit was constructed by using the output of the communication module to regulate a feed-forward motif where the activation level of LuxR determined if GFP production was repressed by one of two LacI proteins, one directly activated by LuxR and the other repressed by a CI repressor controlled by LuxR[49]. Due to the different repression strengths of the LacI and CI repressors, the circuit could be tuned to respond between specific concentrations of the OHHL signal molecule. Tuning of the circuit was done by altering the copy number of the plasmid used to express the LuxR protein consequently changing its expression level, or by using a high-sensitivity LuxR mutant. To obtain programmed pattern formation, different variants of the band-detect circuits were plated onto solid media with multiple populations of sender cells. Diffusion of OHHL from the signal cells resulted in gradients of the signal molecule across the media, creating regions where each of the band-detect variants was active.

Coupling the designs of the intercellular communication module and the population control circuit, a synthetic predator-prey ecosystem was constructed in co-cultured cells[50]. To create this intercellular circuit, the signaling and response components of LuxI/LuxR and LasI/LasR quorum-sensing modules were split between distinct 'predator' and 'prey' cells, thereby establishing bi-directional communication. In the prey cells, intercellular signaling caused expression of CcdB resulting in cell death. For predator cells, intercellular signaling acted to rescue the cells by expressing an antidote (CcdA) to $P_{lac/ara-1}$-expressed CcdB. The regulators for the quorum-sensing modules were expressed from $P_{lac/ara-1}$ in the prey cells (LuxI, LasR) and from a constitutive promoter in the predator cells (LasI, LuxR). With this design, the two cell populations showed typical predator-prey oscillations when grown in a microchemostat. The behavior of the circuit could be tuned by changing the dilution rate in the microchemostat, or by altering the expression levels of the $P_{lac/ara-1}$-regulated quorum-sensing components in the prey cells and $P_{lac/ara-1}$-regulated CcdB in the predator cells using IPTG. No nonspecific interactions were observed between the signaling molecules and LuxR-type proteins of the LuxI/LuxR and LasI/LasR modules.

Bidirectional communication was also established between cells as a mechanism to generate a logical AND response[51]. The design of this 'consensus' circuit was similar to the predator-prey system with plasmids being used to split two unique quorum-sensing modules between two different cellular populations. As the modules were split between the two cellular populations, neither system could respond in the absence of the other cellular system. The quorum-sensing components used to establish this dependency were taken from the LasI/LasR and RhlI/RhlR systems of the opportunistic human pathogen *Pseudomonas aeruginosa*[52]. To minimize cross-talk between the two modules, expression of either signal synthase was controlled by the other systems transcriptional activator, thus minimizing synthesis of the signal molecules in the absence of the other cellular population.

Construction of Artificial Quorum-Sensing Modules

Quorum-sensing modules are of great interest because of their ability to program complex intercellular responses using a minimal number of components. This property has prompted some researchers to try and emulate the quorum-sensing mechanism using novel cellular components in both prokaryotic and eukaryotic organisms. By using such novel components, researchers not only hope to isolate the communication modules from other cellular processes and from each other, but also create universal signals that can be used for interkingdom signaling.

Artificial quorum-sensing networks have been constructed in bacteria[53], yeast[54], and mammalian cells[55]. Methods for constructing these artificial networks have included the repurposing of an existing metabolite as an intercellular signal[53], and the construction of hybrid networks that incorporated non-native elements into existing cellular pathways[54]. As these systems rely on the use of native cellular components, it has generally been necessary to modify the cellular hosts to prevent undesired interactions between the artificial signaling networks and the host organisms. For instance, in the construction of an artificial quorum-sensing module using acetate as a signal molecule in *E. coli*, acetate production had to be disconnected from cellular metabolism by deletion of the *pta ack* pathway[53]. This deletion allowed for acetate accumulation to be directly proportional to cell growth and not influenced by the metabolic state of the cells.

The ability to create artificial quorum-sensing modules that can function between different organisms was demonstrated by connecting a novel airborne signaling device with a hybrid eukaryotic promoter[55]. The signaling device used recombinant expression of mouse alcohol dehydrogenase (ADH) to convert ethanol into acetaldehyde, which then functioned as a volatile signaling molecule. ADH was shown to be expressed and active in yeast, bacteria, plant, and mammalian cells. The acetaldehyde signal was processed in Chinese hamster ovary (CHO) cells transfected with a plasmid containing a hybrid acetaldehyde-inducible promoter[56]. Using this novel module, interkingdom signaling could be achieved by growing the different sender cells in neighboring wells to the CHO receivers on multi-well plates.

Another method that has been examined for the construction of interkingdom signaling modules is the construction of hybrid bacterial quorum-sensing components that are active in mammalian cells[57-59]. To construct these chimeric transactivators, full-length LuxR-type proteins were fused to different eukaryotic transactivator domains. When expressed in mammalian cells, these chimeric proteins activate transcription by binding to hybrid eukaryotic promoters containing their cognate *lux*-type boxes. The binding ability of each of the transactivators was dependent on the presence of their cognate signaling molecules. While no attempt was made to connect these eukaryotic receiver cells to bacterial sender cells to construct an interkingdom signaling module, the construction of such modules would be straight-forward.

Conclusion

The diversity of the genetic circuits that have been constructed using quorum-sensing modules demonstrates the utility of these modules for the programming of complex cellular responses. Through the construction of these circuits, researchers have gained a better understanding of how the properties of quorum-sensing modules determine their outputs, and have used this understanding to control these outputs in time and space. While the current quorum-sensing derived circuits represent the first generation of complex intercellular circuits, a number of potential applications have already become apparent. In addition to the targeted treatment of cancer cells discussed above, other biomedical applications include the use of the intercellular communication modules to direct the fabrication of biomaterials or in tissue engineering[49]. For biotechnology, the ability to program interdependency between two cell populations could allow for the coculturing of organisms that normally could not be cultured together. An immediate application for such cocultures would be the processing of cellulose for the production of biofuels.

Moving ahead from our current ability to program cellular behavior with quorum-sensing modules will require both the creation of new signaling modules and a more complete understanding of the properties of the current systems. Currently, only a handful of quorum-sensing components have been characterized and used to construct circuit modules. As circuit complexity increases it will be necessary to use multiple intercellular signaling modules that exhibit minimum cross-talk. To meet this demand, it will be necessary for circuit designers to characterize additional quorum-sensing components and create novel signaling systems. While nature provides an immense range of possibilities for the construction of additional quorum-sensing modules, the challenge is in characterizing the properties of these modules and their components so as to allow for easy integration into larger genetic circuits. Currently, the construction and integration of a quorum-sensing module into a larger genetic circuit is a time intensive process that requires many rounds of iterative design and testing. Overcoming this challenge will require a deeper understanding of how modules interact with each other and the host cell, and necessitate the creation of standard methods to measure the activities of biological modules and components[60].

References

[1]   Endy, D. Foundations for engineering biology. *Nature,* 2005, 438(7067), 449-453.
[2]   Fuqua, C; Greenberg, EP. Listening in on bacteria: Acyl-homoserine lactone signalling. *Nat. Rev. Mol. Cell Biol.,* 2002, 3(9), 685-695.
[3]   Whitehead, NA; Barnard, AML; Slater, H; Simpson, NJL; Salmond, GPC. Quorum-sensing in Gram-negative bacteria. *FEMS Microbiol. Rev.,* 2001, 25(4), 365-404.
[4]   Egland, KA; Greenberg, EP. Quorum sensing in *Vibrio fischeri*: Elements of the *luxl* promoter. *Mol. Microbiol.,* 1999, 31(4), 1197-1204.
[5]   Pearson, JP; Van Delden, C; Iglewski, BH. Active efflux and diffusion are involved in transport of *Pseudomonas aeruginosa* cell-to-cell signals. *J. Bacteriol.,* 1999, 181(4), 1203-1210.
[6]   Dunlap, PV; Greenberg, EP. Control of *Vibrio fischeri* luminescence gene expression in *Escherichia coli* by cyclic AMP and cyclic AMP receptor protein. *J. Bacteriol.,* 1985, 164(1), 45-50.
[7]   Shadel, GS; Baldwin, TO. The *Vibrio fischeri* LuxR protein is capable of bidirectional stimulation of transcription and both positive and negative regulation of the *luxR* gene. *J. Bacteriol.,* 1991, 173(2), 568-574.
[8]   Shadel, GS; Baldwin, TO. Positive autoregulation of the *Vibrio fischeri luxR* gene: LuxR and autoinducer activate cAMP-catabolite gene activator protein complex-independent and -dependent *luxR* transcription. *J. Biol. Chem.,* 1992, 267(11), 7696-7702.
[9]   Stevens, AM; Greenberg, EP. Transcriptional activation by LuxR. In: Dunny GM, Winans SC, editors. *Cell-Cell Signaling in Bacteria.* Washington, DC: ASM Press; 1999, 231-242.
[10] Urbanowski, AL; Lostroh, CP; Greenberg, EP. Reversible acyl-homoserine lactone binding to purified *Vibrio fischeri* LuxR protein. *J. Bacteriol.,* 2004, 186(3), 631-637.
[11] Zhu, J; Winans, SC. The quorum-sensing transcriptional regulator TraR requires its cognate signaling ligand for protein folding, protease resistance, and dimerization. *Proc. Natl. Acad. Sci. U.S.A.,* 2001, 98(4), 1507-1512.
[12] Schaefer, AL; Hanzelka, BL; Eberhard, A; Greenberg, EP. Quorum sensing in Vibrio fischeri: Probing autoinducer-LuxR interactions with autoinducer analogs. *J. Bacteriol.,* 1996, 178(10), 2897-2901.

74   Daniel J. Sayut, Pavan K.R. Kambam, William G. Herrick et al.

[13] Gray, KM; Passador, L; Iglewski, BH; Greenberg, EP. Interchangeability and specificity of components from the quorum-sensing regulatory systems of *Vibrio fischeri* and *Pseudomonas aeruginosa*. *J. Bacteriol.*, 1994, 176(10), 3076-3080.

[14] Schaefer, AL; Val, DL; Hanzelka, BL; Cronan, JE; Greenberg, EP. Generation of cell-to-cell signals in quorum sensing: Acyl homoserine lactone synthase activity of a purified *Vibrio fischeri* LuxI protein. *Proc. Natl. Acad. Sci. U.S.A.*, 1996, 93(18), 9505-9509.

[15] Parsek, MR; Val, DL; Hanzelka, BL; Cronan, JE; Greenberg, EP. Acyl homoserine-lactone quorum-sensing signal generation. *Proc. Natl. Acad. Sci. U.S.A.*, 1999, 96(8), 4360-4365.

[16] Fuqua, C; Winans, SC; Greenberg, EP. Census and consensus in bacterial ecosystems: The LuxR-LuxI family of quorum-sensing transcriptional regulators. *Annu. Rev. Microbiol.*, 1996, 50, 727-751.

[17] Watson, WT; Minogue, TD; Val, DL; von Bodman, SB; Churchill, MEA. Structural basis and specificity of acyl-homoserine lactone signal production in bacterial quorum sensing. *Mol. Cell,* 2002, 9(3), 685-694.

[18] Gould, TA; Schweizer, HP; Churchill, ME. Structure of the *Pseudomonas aeruginosa* acyl-homoserinelactone synthase LasI. *Mol. Microbiol.*, 2004, 53(4), 1135-1146.

[19] Fuqua, C; Eberhard, A. Signal generation in autoinduction systems: Synthesis of acylated homoserine lactones by LuxI-type proteins. In: Dunny GM, Winans SC, editors. *Cell-Cell Signaling in Bacteria*. Washington, DC. ASM Press; 1999, 211-230.

[20] Haseltine, EL; Arnold, FH. Synthetic gene circuits: Design with directed evolution. *Annu. Rev. Biophys. Biomol. Struct.*, 2007, 36, 1-19.

[21] Sitnikov, DM; Shadel, GS; Baldwin, TO. Autoinducer-independent mutants of the LuxR transcriptional activator exhibit differential effects on the two *lux* promoters of *Vibrio fischeri*. *Mol. Gen. Genet.*, 1996, 252(5), 622-625.

[22] Sayut, DJ; Niu, Y; Sun, L. Construction and engineering of positive feedback loops. *ACS Chem. Biol.*, 2006, 1(11), 692-696.

[23] Sayut, DJ; Kambam, PKR; Sun, L. Noise and kinetics of LuxR positive feedback loops. *Biochem. Biophys. Res. Commun.*, 2007, 363(3), 667-673.

[24] Barrick, D; Villanueba, K; Childs, J; Kalil, R; Schneider, TD; Lawrence, CE, et al. Quantitative analysis of ribosome binding sites in *E. coli*. *Nucl. Acids Res.*, 1994, 22(7), 1287-1295.

[25] Antunes, LC; Ferreira, RB; Lostroh, CP; Greenberg, EP. A mutational analysis defines *Vibrio fischeri* LuxR binding sites. *J. Bacteriol.*, 2008, 190(13), 4392-4397.

[26] Vannini, A; Volpari, C; Gargioli, C; Muraglia, E; Cortese, R; De Francesco, R, et al. The crystal structure of the quorum sensing protein TraR bound to its autoinducer and target DNA. *EMBO J.*, 2002, 21(17), 4393-4401.

[27] Collins, CH; Arnold, FH; Leadbetter, JR. Directed evolution of *Vibrio fischeri* LuxR for increased sensitivity to a broad spectrum of acyl-homoserine lactones. *Mol. Microbiol.*, 2005, 55(3), 712-723.

[28] Collins, CH; Leadbetter, JR; Arnold, FH. Dual selection enhances the signaling specificity of a variant of the quorum-sensing transcriptional activator LuxR. *Nat. Biotechnol.*, 2006, 24(6), 708-712.

[29] Kambam, PKR; Eriksen, DT; Lajoie, J; Sayut, DJ; Sun, L. Altering the substrate specificity of RhlI by directed evolution. *Chembiochem,* 2009, 10(3), 553-558.

[30] Yokobayashi, Y; Collins, CH; Leadbetter, JR; Arnold, FH; Weiss, R. Evolutionary design of genetic circuits and cell-cell communications. *Adv. Complex Syst.,* 2003, 6(1), 37-45.

[31] Kambam, PKR; Sayut, DJ; Niu, Y; Eriksen, DT; Sun, L. Directed evolution of LuxI for enhanced OHHL production. *Biotechnol. Bioeng.,* 2008, 101(2), 263-272.

[32] Cox, RS; Surette, MG; Elowitz, MB. Programming gene expression with combinatorial promoters. *Mol. Syst. Biol.,* 2007, 3: 145.

[33] Sayut, DJ; Niu, Y; Sun, L. Construction and enhancement of a minimal genetic AND logic gate. *Appl. Environ. Microbiol.,* 2009, 75(3), 637-642.

[34] Egland, KA; Greenberg, EP. Conversion of the *Vibrio fischeri* transcriptional activator, LuxR, to a repressor. *J. Bacteriol.,* 2000, 182(3), 805-811.

[35] Dong, H; Nilsson, L; Kurland, CG. Gratuitous overexpression of genes in *Escherichia coli* leads to growth inhibition and ribosome destruction. *J. Bacteriol.,* 1995, 177(6), 1497-1504.

[36] Kobayashi, H; Kaern, M; Araki, M; Chung, K; Gardner, TS; Cantor, CR, et al. Programmable cells: Interfacing natural and engineered gene networks. *Proc. Natl. Acad. Sci. U.S.A.,* 2004, 101(22), 8414-8419.

[37] You, L; Cox, RS, III; Weiss, R; Arnold, FH. Programmed population control by cell-cell communication and regulated killing. *Nature,* 2004, 428(6985), 868-871.

[38] Balagadde, FK; You, L; Hansen, CL; Arnold, FH; Quake, SR. Long-term monitoring of bacteria undergoing programmed population control in a microchemostat. *Science,* 2005, 309(5731), 137-140.

[39] McMillen, D; Kopell, N; Hasty, J; Collins, JJ. Synchronizing genetic relaxation oscillators by intercell signaling. *Proc. Natl. Acad. Sci. U.S.A.,* 2002, 99(2), 679-684.

[40] Alexey, K; Mads, K; Nancy, K. Synchrony in a population of hysteresis-based genetic oscillators. *SIAM J. App. Mat.,* 2004, 65(2), 392-425.

[41] Garcia-Ojalvo, J; Elowitz, MB; Strogatz, SH. Modeling a synthetic multicellular clock: Repressilators coupled by quorum sensing. *Proc. Natl. Acad. Sci. U.S.A.,* 2004, 101(30), 10955-10960.

[42] Koseska, A; Zaikin, A; Garcia-Ojalvo, J; Kurths, J. Stochastic suppression of gene expression oscillators under intercell coupling. *Phys. Rev. E Stat. Nonlin. Soft Matter Phys.,* 2007, 75(3), 031917.1-031917.9.

[43] Li, C; Chen, L; Aihara, K. Stochastic synchronization of genetic oscillator networks. *BMC Syst. Biol.,* 2007, 1: 6.

[44] Anderson, JC; Clarke, EJ; Arkin, AP; Voigt, CA. Environmentally controlled invasion of cancer cells by engineered bacteria. *J. Mol. Biol.,* 2006, 355(4), 619-627.

[45] Yu, YA; Shabahang, S; Timiryasova, TM; Zhang, Q; Beltz, R; Gentschev, I, et al. Visualization of tumors and metastases in live animals with bacteria and vaccinia virus encoding light-emitting proteins. *Nat. Biotechnol.,* 2004, 22(3), 313-320.

[46] Anderson, JC; Voigt, CA; Arkin, AP. Environmental signal integration by a modular AND gate. *Mol. Syst. Biol.,* 2007, 3: 133.

[47] Weiss, R; Knight, T. In *DNA Computing*. Heidelberg: Springer Berlin; 2001, 1-16.

[48] Basu, S; Mehreja, R; Thiberge, S; Chen, M-T; Weiss, R. Spatiotemporal control of gene expression with pulse-generating networks. *Proc. Natl. Acad. Sci. U. S. A.,* 2004, 101(17), 6355-6360.

[49] Basu, S; Gerchman, Y; Collins, CH; Arnold, FH; Weiss, R. A synthetic multicellular system for programmed pattern formation. *Nature,* 2005, 434(7037), 1130-1134.

[50] Balagadde, FK; Song, H; Ozaki, J; Collins, CH; Barnet, M; Arnold, FH, et al. A synthetic *Escherichia coli* predator-prey ecosystem. *Mol. Syst. Biol.,* 2008, 4: 187.

[51] Brenner, K; Karig, DK; Weiss, R; Arnold, FH. Engineered bidirectional communication mediates a consensus in a microbial biofilm consortium. *Proc. Natl. Acad. Sci.* U.S.A., 2007, 104(44), 17300-17304.

[52] Pesci, EC; Pearson, JP; Seed, PC; Iglewski, BH. Regulation of *las* and *rhl* quorum sensing in *Pseudomonas aeruginosa. J. Bacteriol.,* 1997, 179(10), 3127-3132.

[53] Bulter, T; Lee, SG; Woirl, WWC; Fung, E; Connor, MR; Liao, JC. Design of artificial cell-cell communication using gene and metabolic networks. *Proc. Natl. Acad. Sci. U.S.A.,* 2004, 101(8), 2299-2304.

[54] Chen, M-T; Weiss, R. Artificial cell-cell communication in yeast *Saccharomyces cerevisiae* using signaling elements from *Arabidopsis thaliana. Nat. Biotechnol.,* 2005, 23(12), 1551-1555.

[55] Weber, W; Daoud-El Baba, M; Fussenegger, M. Synthetic ecosystems based on airborne inter- and intrakingdom communication. *Proc. Natl. Acad. Sci.* U. S. A., 2007, 104(25), 10435-40.

[56] Weber, W; Rimann, M; Spielmann, M; Keller, B; Baba, MD-E; Aubel, D, et al. Gas-inducible transgene expression in mammalian cells and mice. *Nat. Biotechnol.,* 2004, 22(11), 1440-1444.

[57] Weber, W; Schoenmakers, R; Spielmann, M; El-Baba, MD; Folcher, M; Keller, B, et al. Streptomyces-derived quorum-sensing systems engineered for adjustable transgene expression in mammalian cells and mice. *Nucl. Acids Res.,* 2003, 31(14): e71.

[58] Neddermann, P; Gargioli, C; Muraglia, E; Sambucini, S; Bonelli, F; De Francesco, R, et al. A novel, inducible, eukaryotic gene expression system based on the quorum-sensing transcription factor TraR. *Embo Rep.,* 2003, 4(4), 439-439.

[59] Williams, SC; Patterson, EK; Carty, NL; Griswold, JA; Hamood, AN; Rumbaugh, KP. *Pseudomonas aeruginosa* autoinducer enters and functions in mammalian cells. *J. Bacteriol.,* 2004, 186(8), 2281-2287.

[60] Canton, B; Labno, A; Endy, D. Refinement and standardization of synthetic biological parts and devices. *Nat. Biotechnol.,* 2008, 26(7), 787-793.

In: Synthetic and Integrative Biology
Editor: James T. Gevona, pp. 77-91

Chapter 4

SYNTHETIC MORPHOLOGY: MODULES FOR ENGINEERING BIOLOGICAL FORM

Jamie A. Davies[*]

Centre for Integrative Physiology, University of Edinburgh,
EH8 9XB, Scotland, UK

Abstract

Synthetic morphology is a coupling of synthetic gene networks to output modules that change the shape or the morphogenetic behaviour of cells. In other words, it is the engineering of biological form. It differs from traditional surgical and tissue engineering approaches in that it is not restricted to forms that exist in nature and it works by making cells organize themselves into the desired form, rather than by manual manipulation of tissues. Synthetic biology has uses in basic science (eg testing hypotheses in developmental biology), industry (eg altering microbial associations and behaviours to improve the efficiency of fermentation, drug production and remediation of polluted soils) and medicine (engineering cell collectives for ex-corporo organ substitutes, engineering novel cell arrangements for repair of tissues or interfacing with artificial devices). This chapter introduces morphogenetic 'primitives' that can be used, in different combinations and sequences, to produce engineered forms and that can be invoked by the expression of single molecules. Both bacterial and mammalian systems are described.

Introduction

So far, efforts in synthetic biology have centred on three main aims. One has been the creation of novel biosynthetic pathways, for example to produce drugs or biofuels[1-4]. Another has been to make novel biosensor-reporter networks so that cells can report the presence of trace chemicals, such as toxins, or physical conditions such as light and electric currents[5-9]. A third has been the construction of cellular information-processing 'logic circuits', oscillators etc[10-15]. All of these are important and offer considerable promise both to biotechnological industries and to medicine. All, though, tend to view cells as genetic

---

[*] E-mail address: jamie.davies@ed.ac.uk

or chemical reactors, the form of which is irrelevant to the function of their introduced synthetic biological systems. This chapter introduces a fourth and relatively new aim of synthetic biology; the production of 'designer' shapes and arrangements of cells and tissues, a field that is becoming known as 'synthetic morphology'[16].

Why Bother?

Why, given the immense diversity of evolved biological forms, might it be valuable to engineer ones under the control of synthetic biological systems? There are a number of reasons, some to do with basic scientific knowledge and some to do with medical and industrial applications.

At the level of basic science, synthetic morphology will be an immensely powerful addition to the existing toolkits of conventional developmental biology. For many centuries, natural philosophers, anatomists, embryologists and developmental biologists (the names change with the times) have been struggling to understand how biological form arises. Although much remains to be discovered, decades of molecular analysis have brought us to thinking that we have at least an outline understanding of morphogenesis during animal, plant and fungal development, generally in the form of 'stories' of cause and effect[17-19] and occasionally in the form of formal mathematical models[20]. Developmental biologists can be sure that they understand the principles of morphogenesis, though, only if they can take them and use them to create forms of our own design. If everything works as designed, then we can be fairly certain that we have understood the principles well; if it does not, then we know we have more to learn about one of the processes we have tried to use.

Beyond this basic interest, synthetic morphology is likely to have both medical and industrial applications. Medically, a synthetic morphology approach offers a number of potential advantages over tissue engineering based on the endogenous developmental programme that already exists within cells. To begin with, there are aspects of regenerative medicine that require the construction of structures that fall outside the normal developmental programme of the body. Some may be wildly unnatural, for example interfaces between body tissues and artificial limbs of organs of sensation. Some may be less drastic modifications of normal structures; for example, clusters of cells, engineered to secrete insulin, that can embed themselves in other tissues to substitute for damaged pancreatic islets in type I diabetes. Some may be effectively natural structures but produced out of embryonic sequence; for example a tissue needed in a new-born child in whom that tissue is congenitally missing or in an adult from which a tissue has had to be removed because of injury or cancer. The problem here is that, though the normal developmental programme of cells (be they stem cells or other cells) includes the making of that structure in the context of, and in the spatial scale of, a developing embryo, it does not necessarily include the ability to make the structure in the quite different environment of an already-born child or an adult. In such an environment, the surrounding tissues will be mature, the space to be filled will be larger, and most of the signals characteristic of the embryo will be absent. Indeed, there may be some signals present in the adult body that are positively antagonistic to development of the new tissue. Cells engineered to organize themselves using their own signals, not normally present in a mammalian body, would be immune from interference by these.

Synthetic morphology also offers potential advantages in extracorporeal medical devices such as artificial livers, kidneys etc. It is already well-understood that purely physical mechanisms, such as dialysis filters, cannot replicate all of the biological activities of the organs that they are intended to replace. For this reason, experiments have been done in which simple devices such as dialysis machines are enriched with extra chambers that contain living cells to provide a more realistic organ substitute[21;22]. The problem is that such cells do not live long in such an alien environment and many cell types have yet to be cultured at all. Providing synthetic gene circuits to drive the appropriate survival, multiplication and arrangement of these cells in the engineered environment of an extracorporeal culture chamber might be a much more promising route than trying to find ways of keeping natural cells alive and happy in such a place. Being extracorporeal, this type of application has the advantage that no engineered cells will be introduced into the body, which will be less worrying from a bio-safety point of view.

The possible industrial applications of synthetic morphology are varied, although early ones will probably be connected more with prokaryotes and fungi than with animals and plants. Engineering novel and controllable morphologies into prokaryotes could make substantial alterations in the way in which they flow past or adhere to surfaces. This could be used both to improve bioreactor dynamics in industries such as fermentation and drug production and to change the dynamics of microbes in applications such as remediation of polluted soils or in biofuel manufacture. Altering and controlling fungal morphology, for example the degree of branching and entanglement of hyphae, can be used for similar purposes and also in the food industry, either in improvement in bioreactor dynamics[23] or even directly in controlling the texture of foods made from fungi, for example.

A General Approach to Synthetic Morphology

Whether being tailored to prokaryotes, fungi, plant or animal cells, the general approach to synthetic morphology advocated here has two main features[16];

(a) it should be done, as far as possible, by the use of interchangeable genetic modules that can be connected in a simple manner to existing sensory, logic and control modules.

(b) Morphogenesis should be achieved, as much as possible, by the sequential activation of a number of basic, primitive morphogenetic mechanisms each of which can be driven by one genetic module.

These two related features encourage the flexible use of a standard range of parts and should help to reduce the need for genetic engineers to be continuously 're-inventing the wheel'. Fortunately, evolution itself seems to have proceeded along broadly similar lines, a few basic morphogenetic events being used over and over again in different orders and in the contexts of different tissues. This means that, in each kingdom of life, there is a set of basic morphogenetic primitives[24] that can be adapted to be the basis of synthetic morphology, the necessary adaptation being mainly concerned with isolating them from their normal control connections and connecting them instead to synthetic control systems (this is important so that their operation is not affected by, and does not trigger, events in a cell's endogenous genetic programme).

The primitives differ in each of the Kingdoms, as do the synthetic genetic logic and control circuits that have already been developed for them. The rest of this chapter will therefore consider two kingdoms, eubacteria and animals, in isolation, before all of the ideas are brought together for in a brief summary.

Synthetic Morphology in Prokaryotes

Prokaryotes are not renowned for producing structures of great morphological complexity but they still offer several basic morphogenetic processes that can be useful to synthetic biologists; indeed, it might be argued that their simplicity might make them very much more predictable and therefore easier to use. Taking the enterobacterium *Eschericia coli* as a model organism, the obvious possibilities are;

- Living in free suspension
- Forming an aggregate
- Forming chains
- Actively swimming
- Chemotaxis (an addition to the swimming process)
- Lysis ('morphogenetic' in the sense that it can create cavities and holes)
- Alteration of cell shape.

In standard media, eg Luria broth or DMEM, living in free suspension is the default behaviour for *Fim⁻* lab strains of this organism, eg *E. coli* JM109 [25]. Expressing *Fim* causes auto-aggregation in DMEM. Agregation of even *Fim⁻* strains can be driven, however, by their expressing the *YapC* gene from *Yersinia pestis* (another enterobacterium). This autoaggregation effect is so marked that the bacteria fall out of solution as large aggregates over the course of 15-30 minutes[26]. When out of solution, on a surface, the *YapC* expressing bacteria form adherent biofilms. There is a family of similar molecules, such as AIDA, TibA and Ag43, collectively known as the self-associating autotransporters[27], and expression of any of them causes bacteria to adhere to one another.

Like other bacteria, *E. coli* is equipped with an internal targeting system that can cause some proteins to be localized only to the two ends, or 'poles', of the rod-shaped cell. This system can be used by researchers to target other proteins, that are tagged with the correct targetting domain, to the poles of the cell too. The construct $IcsA_{507-620}$-GFP, for example, contains green fluorescent protein (GFP) joined to a targetting domain from the Shigella ICSA outer membrane-located, actin-organizing protein. When expressed in *E. coli*, the protein is located only at the two ends of a cell [28]. Making chimaeric constructs between this ICSA-derived targetting domain and an adhesion protein, such as the YapC mentioned above, would render only the ends of the *E. coli* cells adhesive and would therefore promote the formation of chains rather than bulk aggregates.

Active movement of bacteria such as *E. coli* is achieved by the rotation of flagella, powered by an electrostatic motor complex in the membranes of the cell[29]. Construction of motile flagella depends on the presence of the FliA protein and FliA⁻ strains are immotile[30].

They can be made motile, though, by expression of FliA or *Bacillus subtilis* σ^D. Placing one of these factors under the control of a promoter controlled by synthetic genetic networks will therefore allow these networks to switch motility on and off.

Bacteria normally couple swimming to chemotactic guidance. In swimming *E.coli,* this guidance is normally achieved by natural signal transduction systems in the cell controlling how much time the cell spends in each of two modes of flagellar beat. In one mode, the bacterium is propelled in a more-or-less straight line with high efficiency, while in the other mode it tumbles randomly. If a cell finds itself in a rising concentration of a chemoattractive molecule, which would happen only if it is swimming up a gradient to the source, it remains in the straight line mode of swimming (each flagellum beating anti-clockwise). If the concentration ceases to increase, then clockwise flagellar rotation, and consequent tumbling, resumes again, interspersed with short periods of straight swimming which will be maintained if they happen to result in rising concentrations of attractant. By using changes of concentration of time, bacteria therefore succeed in moving appropriately in space[31].

There are at least three ways in which *E. coli* might be engineered to undergo chemotaxis in response to a synthetic genetic system. One would be to activate chemotaxis by expressing natural chemoreceptors (of which there are five) and to engineer the metabolisms of other cells in the system to produce the chemoattractant. Another would be to mutate one of the chemoreceptors to render it sensitive to a novel chemoattractant, such as an industrial pollutant or a compound released by tumour cells. Some success has already been achieved in altering chemoreceptor specificity[32].   Another, very different approach, is to control directly the expression of the protein CheZ, which converts tumbling swimming to the straight form (bacteria with no CheZ tumble all the time). This has been demonstrated elegantly by Topp and Gallivan, who made an RNA aptamer-based combined-CheZ-mRNA-and-theophylline-receptor. In the absence of theophylline, the aptamer portion of the RNA makes a hairpin and it is not translated. If theophylline is present, it can bind to the RNA aptamer and cause it to open up, allowing ribosomes to access the ribosome binding site and translate the CheZ open reading frame. Between zero and saturation, the amount of CheZ protein, and therefore the proportion of time bacteria spend swimming straight, is a positive function of the local concentration of theophylline. The cells therefore tend to move up-gradient. Theophilline also allows them to respond to their normal chemottractants[33].

Self-triggered lysis of a bacterial cell can be achieved by the expression of bacteriophage holin genes, for example the S protein from bacteriophage lambda. Driven from a variety of promoters, their expression results in the destruction of cells by the time as few as 1000 molecules of holin have been translated[34]. Placing holin expression under the control of sensors for chemicals, surfaces or light, could be morphogenetically useful by clearing cells away from particular places such as the centres of cell aggregates or any place on a biofilm on which light is projected. It can also be used to dispose of engineered bacteria when their task is done.

Cell shape in *E. coli* is controlled, at least in part, by the expression levels of the filament-forming protein, RodZ. Deletion of RodZ results in loss of the coliform morphology and the production of spherical cells while over-expression of RodZ causes cells to become over-long[35]. Changes in cell shape can be combined with at least some of the manipulations mentioned above, such as adhesion and filament formation, to create further variety of bacterial morphology and dynamics.

Synthetic Morphology Using Animal Cells

The cells of animals differ from those of bacterial and fungal species in that they have plasma membranes but no cell walls. This makes them very much more flexible in terms of shape so that they are able to alter their outline millisecond-by-millisecond and thus engage in behaviours such as crawling. It also allows the membranes of adjacent cells to interact directly with each other to form a variety of adhesive and signalling complexes, junctions and synapses. For this reason, the development of multicellular animals has been able to evolve to include a bewildering variety of morphogenetic events and consequent tissue types. Even these events, though, seem to rest mainly on about ten basic mechanisms which, while they cannot be used to construct every type of animal morphogenesis seen, do underlie most of them and are flexible enough to be used as a basis of a rich variety of engineered structures. These ten basic mechanisms are cell death, cell proliferation, cell fusion, cell locomotion, directed locomotion, cell adhesion/ condensation, cell sorting, epithelial-mesenchymal transition, mesenchymal-epithelial transition and epithelial folding[16;24].

Each of these events can be induced, in specific types of cells, by normal developmental signals such as those provided by growth factors, hormones etc. The central idea of synthetic morphology, though, is to be able to invoke morphogenetic mechanisms independently of any endogenous developmental programme so that we can build patterns, structures and tissues that may not exist in a normal body. This means finding ways of driving these morphogenetic mechanisms by – ideally - a single protein, whose expression can be switched on by the action of a synthetic genetic network and which is sufficient to activate the desired morphogenetic process. A search of the cell biology and virology literature has identified a number of morphogenetic 'master regulator' proteins that seem to be promising candidates for driving each of the ten basic processes listed above[16] (Figure 2). Expression of *C. elegans* Nedd2 in a variety of mammalian cells, for example, causes them to undergo elective cell death[36]. Proliferation is the natural behaviour of cell lines that grow in culture, so control of proliferation in response to synthetic genetic networks will generally be a question of turning proliferation off when it is not needed rather that turning it on when it is. Expression of p17^{kip} is sufficient to block cell proliferation in fibroblasts and probably in other mammalian cells too[37]. Fusion between cells, to make a syncytium, can be driven by expression of the gH/gL glycoproteins from cytomegalovirus[38]. Sedentary fibroblasts, and probably other cells too, can be made motile by expression of Crk[39]. Fibroblasts can be made to adhere to one another by expression of E-cadherin[40] while making different cells express different amounts of this protein, or making come express a different cadherin such as P-cadherin, will make the two cell types sort out from one another, the more highly adhesive population being engulfed by the less adhesive[41-43]. Heterophilic adhesion can be induced by the expression of CD2 on one cell and CD28 on another, while expression of Alfacept will destroy CD2/CD28 adhesion[44;45]. Folding of epithelial sheets can be driven by expression of Shroom in the cells along the site at which folding is required[46-48] and epithelial cells can be induced to break up into mesenchyme by expression of LMP1[49], while adenovirus E1a makes mesenchymal cells epithelial[50].

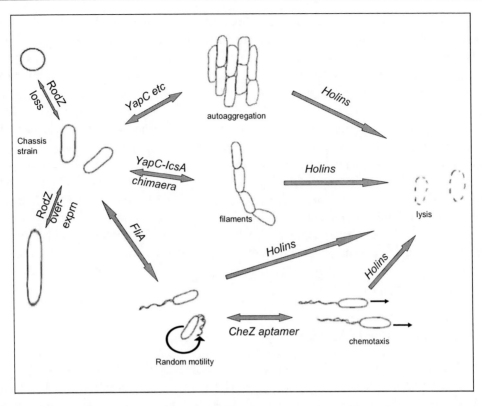

Figure 1. some possibilities for synthetic morphology in the prokaryote *E. coli*. For this diagram, the 'chassis strain' is assumed to be FliA⁻ Fim⁻ CheZ⁻

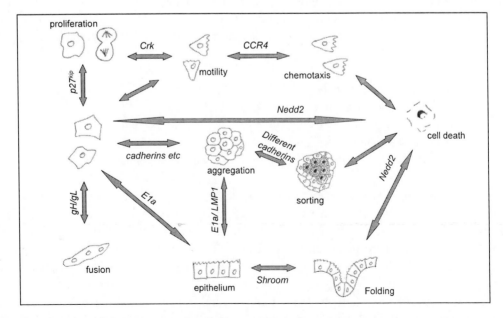

Figure 2. Some possibilities for synthetic morphology in mammalian cells. The driver genes, in italics above the arrows, are explained in more detail in the main text.

Making cells migratory, by expression of Crk as described above, will not of itself impart any sense of direction. Migration can be directed by either chemotaxis or haptotaxis. Where cells will be used outside the body, and cross-talk between engineered and the natural systems of specialist body cells will not therefore be a problem, chemotactic behaviour can be induced by expression of the cytokine receptor CCR4, which makes cells chemotactic for the cytokine CKLF1 (which could itself be expressed by other cells under control of synthetic genetic networks)[51]. Similarly, once a cell is made motile by expression of Crk, it will naturally undergo haptotaxis on a gradient of any extracellular matrix compound (eg fibronectin, collagen) for which it already expresses integrin receptors, and most cells express these[52;53]. If the intention is to use engineered cells in the context of living tissues, though, expression of mammalian cytokines and receptors can't be used (because they would recruit normal body cells, for example of the immune system) and nor can guidance by normal matrix unless it is intended that engineered cells follow normal paths in the body. Instead, receptors would need to be mutated so that they recognize only molecules that are not native to, and are inert in, the normal body, or signal-receptor pairs could be sourced from phylogenetically very distant organisms.

First Steps in Synthetic Morphology

At the beginning of this article, in the section headed 'Why bother?', I set out some of the reasons that adding synthetic morphology modules to existing synthetic biology parts registries and tool boxes might ultimately be a very valuable thing to do for intellectual, medical and industrial reasons. There is, however, clearly a very large gap between the current state of the field, which is still mainly speculation with only some actual experimentation, and the useful applications mentioned. How should that gap be bridged? There are probably at least as many strategies as scientists involved, but here is one possible way forward, the numbered steps being discussed in more detail in the paragraphs that follow them;

1. Construct the basic modules.
2. Test whether modules work in most cells in most states
3. Perform proof-of-principle experiments in which the modules are used to control morphology through synthetic genetic networks.
4. When the proofs of principle are done, work towards real applications.

Construction of modules: The modules should be constructed in a way that maximizes their compatibility with existing synthetic biology modules already constructed for that type of organism. In the case of bacteria, in particular, there is already a substantial registry of synthetic biology standard parts run by the BioBricks foundation (http://partsregistry.org/). These include basic 'chassis' organisms (eg strains of *E. coli*), plasmid backbones, and a large and growing variety of sensor, information-processing and output modules. Given the engineering spirit of the whole synthetic biology enterprise, it would make most sense to construct synthetic morphology effector modules for prokaryotes in a way that allows them to work with existing BioBrick parts, and to become BioBrick parts themselves, available 'off-the-shelf'. Yeast cells are also somewhat supported by the BioBricks registry. Mycelial fungi, animals and plants are not yet well supported by any registry but it is again sensible to use promoters, etc, that are as compatible as possible with existing synthetic biology sensory and logic modules, for example the mammalian set developed by the Fussenegger group[13-15].

Initial testing of the modules: In general, synthetic morphology effector modules will be most useful if they work in all cells (of their intended organism type), in all cell states. Ones that only work in some cell types or in cells in only some states are likely to be less useful, although this property might be used as a means of regulation. For initial testing, the modules should be connected to a very simple and reliable type of contingency. They might be placed, for example, under the control of a promoter that can be induced by a simple drug such as tetracycline. They should then be introduced into a large variety of cell types, which for *E coli* might mean bacteria in different growth phases and in different solid or liquid media, and for mammals might mean in a variety of different types of cell line (fibroblasts, epithelials, neurons, ES cells etc). The operation of the module should then be tested to determine how restricted it is by cell type or state.

Proofs of principle: The object of this step is to demonstrate that morphogenetic behaviour can be controlled by synthetic genetic networks, such as existing BioBricks modules. For proofs of principle, synthetic morphology modules tested under simple contingency systems should be placed under the control of more complex contingencies, mediated by (mainly existing) sensory and information-processing modules.

Bacteria have already been engineered with sensory systems for light[9] (ref) and for trace chemicals, that activate the expression of enzymes such as beta-galactosidase as a reporter. One simple set of proofs of principle for prokaryotes would be to couple one of two of these systems to morphogenetic effectors. Coupling the light sensor of Levskaya et al.[9] to an adhesion effector would, for example, cause illuminated bacteria to form an autoaggregating biofilm whereas ones raised in the dark would not: one could even use this to 'print' an image on to a surface the lit areas retaining a film of adherent bacteria resistant to being washed off. It could also be used to cause a suspension of bacteria to aggregate and settle out on illumination of their broth. If the effector module were one that causes lysis of the bacteria, rather than adhesion, then illumination would clear a bacteria-laden broth of living cells.

Another possibility would to be connect a chemical sensor module to an effector module for chain formation, so that the bacteria would form long chains when the trigger chemical is present but not when it is absent. Given that individual bacteria would be expected to be more mobile than those in chains, even without induction of flagellar motility in the absence of the trigger chemical (this feature could be added to the system if desired), the effect would be for bacteria to move freely as individuals in areas of the trigger chemical's absence but to form chains, which would tangle with each other and reduce motility, in its presence. If the chemical were a nutrient, this could even give the bacteria a new strategy for better exploiting their environments, because it would keep them where the nutrient is and then allow them to disperse when it runs out, perhaps to find another source. Such a system might also be used in microbial remediation of polluted soils etc, to encourage bacteria to remain where there is pollutant to be metabolized until it has run out, and then to move on. This type of synthetic system is, arguably, very close to creating a synthetic multicellular organism with a definite life cycle that alternates, much like that of organisms such as *Dictyostelium discoideum,* between individual and multicellular phases.

There are, of course, many more possible proofs of principle for prokaryotic synthetic biology, which might couple sensors for all kinds of physical and chemical triggers to cell death, adhesion and motility so that bacteria move towards or away from stimuli or make biofilms or networks at different concentrations of stimulus. One important caveat should, however, be borne in mind; the ability to produce biofilms, and particularly to adhere to mammalian cells, is frequently what makes the difference between a harmless bacterium and a pathogen[54;55]. Even when using the 'harmless' strains of *E. coli*, such as JM109, that are the normal laboratory types, it should always be borne in mind that a change in morphology may make them more able to try to live on or in a human. It should be borne in mind that, if microbiological practice is sloppy, there may always be a risk of wild-type *E. coli*, already capable of living in the human gut, moving from experimenter into experiment, becoming engineered, then moving back. It would therefore be sensible to regard synthetic morphology of bacteria as potentially more hazardous than engineering oscillators, switches, light sensors etc, and for adequate microbiological practice to be followed with great care.

Proofs of principle for synthetic morphology in mammalian cell lines are very unlikely to raise safety concerns, such cells being incapable of colonizing a human with a normal immune system. Again, the fastest routes to proof of principle would be to couple existing synthetic biology sensor and information-processing modules to the novel morphogenetic effector modules. Existing latch modules, that can be set by a transient pulse of erythromycin and reset by a transient pulse of pristinamycin, might for example be used to switch cells between motile (Crk-on, cadherin-off) and adherent (Crk-off, cadherin-on) states: and I have described one design for this in detail elsewhere[16].

Another proof of principle, which would be immediately useful to test some hypotheses about cell sorting and boundary population, would be to engineer one population of weakly-adherent cells (eg L929) to express CD2 and green fluorescent protein and the other CD58 and the red fluorescent protein, dsRed. As mentioned above, CD2 and CD58 form a heterophilic adhesion system so that green cells will bind to red strongly, but green to green weakly and red to red weakly. If cell arrangements can be explained purely on the grounds of minimization of free energy, then mixing the cells in different ratios should result in predictable and ratio-dependent patterns (Figure 3). Making expression of CD2 and CD58 inducible by, say, erythromycin would allow an experimenter to test whether an established monolayer of cultured cells could re-sort itself when it acquires new adhesive differences. Putting alfacept expression under the control of, say, pristinamycin would allow the heterophilic adhesion system to be later destroyed.

A more complex example, again akin to building an artificial multicellular system with a defined life cycle, might be made by engineering cells that grow in suspension culture and have components of the Wnt pathway (eg B16 cells) to express Wnt1 and CD2 constitutively, to express the transcription factor PIP-KRAB and alfacept under the control of the Wnt-sensitive TOP-FLASH promoter and to express CD58 under a promoter inhibited by PIP-KRAB (the PIP-KRAB system is already much-used in mammalian synthetic biology) (Figure 4). The Wnt made by isolated cells and very small aggregates will diffuse away easily so PIP-KRAB and alfacept will be expressed only weakly, CD58 will be expressed strongly and the cells will be adherent. The aggregate will therefore grow by accretion and proliferation. As it enlarges, though, more Wnt gets trapped, CD58 falls and alfacept production rises to block adhesion and cause the aggregate to fall apart in the stirred culture. Each of its cells, now in free solution, will then be able to begin an aggregate again.

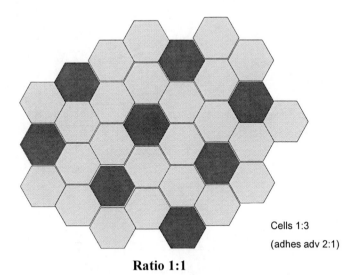

Blue expresses cd2

Yellow expresses cd58

Cells 1:3

(adhes adv 2:1)

Ratio 1:1

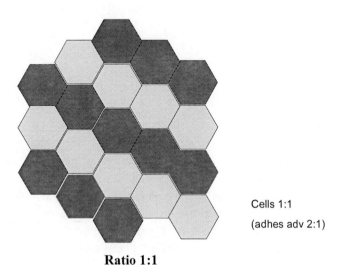

Blue expresses cd2

Yellow expresses cd58

Cells 1:1

(adhes adv 2:1)

Ratio 1:1

Figure 3. Expected self-organizing patterns for cells expressing CD2 (blue) and its adhesion receptor CD58 (yellow), when mixed in different ratios.

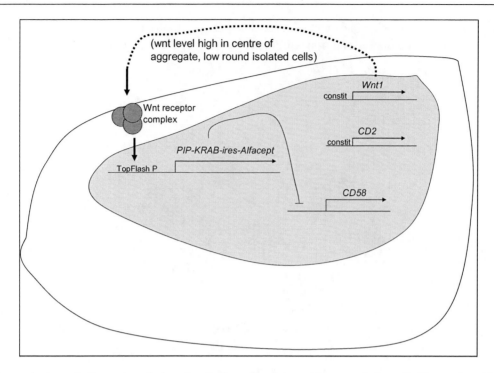

Figure 4. A synthetic system designed to make cells alternate between being adhesive and making aggregates and being unadhesive and living alone. In this system, which has not yet been completed in wet-ware, adhesion is mediated by CD58/ CD2 heterophilic interactions. CD2 is always expressed, as is the secreted signalling protein Wnt1. CD58 is expressed until blocked by PIP-KRAB. Wnt1 will diffuse easily away from isolated cells but will build up in the middle of growing aggregates. When it does, it causes production of PIP-KRAB to inhibit CD58 production and it also drives production of alfacept, which diffuses from the cells and blocks CD2/CD58 adhesion, affecting even cells on the outside of the aggregate.

Conclusion

This chapter is, necessarily, a rather short introduction to a very new field of research. Nevertheless, I hope that it has demonstrated that the coupling of synthetic biological approaches to the field of morphogenesis offers a powerful way of making designer anatomies, very crude at first but potentially more subtle as we learn more. In the far distance there are a number of medical and industrial applications, while even from the first experiments it may be possible to use the techniques to test ideas in basic science, as in the cell sorting example described above. Getting synthetic morphology off the ground will require some commitment by funding bodies as well as by scientists and the state of synthetic biology as a whole should make this very timely. The current spirit of hyperbole about them notwithstanding, stem cells cannot do everything we want to do in tissue engineering, and in industry it may be easier to engineer the morphology of micro-organisms that already have useful metabolic properties, than to engineer the metabolisms of morphologically suitable organisms. Development of synthetic morphology is therefore a rational component of the development of biotechnology as a whole.

References

[1] Lee, S. K., Chou, H., Ham, T. S., Lee, T. S. & Keasling, J. D. (2008). Metabolic engineering of microorganisms for biofuels production: from bugs to synthetic biology to fuels *Curr. Opin. Biotechnol.,* **19**, 556-563.

[2] Keasling, J. D. (2008). Synthetic biology for synthetic chemistry *ACS Chem Biol,* **3**, 64-76.

[3] Ro, D. K. et al. (2006). Production of the antimalarial drug precursor artemisinic acid in engineered yeast *Nature,* **440**, 940-943.

[4] Savage, D. F., Way, J. & Silver, P. A. (2008). Defossiling fuel: how synthetic biology can transform biofuel production *ACS Chem Biol,* **3**, 13-16.

[5] Weber, W. et al. (2009) A synthetic mammalian electro-genetic transcription circuit *Nucleic Acids Res,* **37**, e33.

[6] King, K., Dohlman, H. G., Thorner, J., Caron, M. G. & Lefkowitz, R. J. (1990). Control of yeast mating signal transduction by a mammalian beta 2-adrenergic receptor and Gs alpha subunit *Science,* **250**, 121-123.

[7] Chen, M. T. & Weiss, R. (2005). Artificial cell-cell communication in yeast Saccharomyces cerevisiae using signaling elements from Arabidopsis thaliana *Nat Biotechnol.,* **23**, 1551-1555.

[8] Looger, L. L., Dwyer, M. A., Smith, J. J. & Hellinga, H. W. (2003). Computational design of receptor and sensor proteins with novel functions *Nature,* **423**, 185-190.

[9] Levskaya, A. et al. (2005) Synthetic biology: engineering Escherichia coli to see light *Nature,* **438**, 441-442.

[10] Stricker, J., Cookson, S., Bennett, M. R., Mather, W. H., Tsimring, L. S. & Hasty, J. (2008) A fast, robust and tunable synthetic gene oscillator *Nature,* **456**, 516-519.

[11] Elowitz, M. B. & Leibler, S. (2000) A synthetic oscillatory network of transcriptional regulators *Nature,* **403**, 335-338.

[12] Tan, C., Song, H., Niemi, J. & You, L. (2007). A synthetic biology challenge: making cells compute *Mol. Biosyst.,* **3**, 343-353.

[13] Kramer, B. P., Viretta, A. U., Daoud-El-Baba, M., Aubel, D., Weber, W. & Fussenegger, M. (2004). An engineered epigenetic transgene switch in mammalian cells *Nat Biotechnol.,* **22**, 867-870.

[14] Kramer, B. P., Fischer, C. & Fussenegger, M. (2004). BioLogic gates enable logical transcription control in mammalian cells *Biotechnol. Bioeng.,* **87**, 478-484.

[15] Kramer, B. P. & Fussenegger, M. (2005). Hysteresis in a synthetic mammalian gene network *Proc Natl. Acad Sci* U. S. A, **102**, 9517-9522.

[16] Davies, J. A. (2008). Synthetic morphology: prospects for engineered, self-constructing anatomies *J Anat.,* **212**, 707-719.

[17] Gilbert, S. (2003). *Developmental Biology*. Sinauer, Sunderland, Massachusetts.

[18] Wolpert, L. (1998). *Principles of development*. Current Biology: Oxford University Press.

[19] Gilbert, S. & Raunio, A. (1997). Embryology: constructing the organism ppIX-X pp. IX-X. Sinauer.

[20] Forgacs, G. & Newman, S. A. (2005) *Biological Physics of the Developing Embryo*. Cambridge University Press.

[21] Humes, H. D. et al. (2002). Metabolic replacement of kidney function in uremic animals with a bioartificial kidney containing human cells *Am J Kidney Dis.*, **39**, 1078-1087.

[22] Sauer, I. M. et al. (2002). Primary human liver cells as source for modular extracorporeal liver support--a preliminary report *Int. J Artif. Organs*, **25**, 1001-1005.

[23] Wiebe, M. G., Blakebrough, M. L., Craig, S. H., Robson, G. D. & Trinci, A. P. (1996). How do highly branched (colonial) mutants of Fusarium graminearum A3/5 arise during Quorn myco-protein fermentations? *Microbiology*, **142**, (Pt 3), 525-532.

[24] Davies, J. (2005). *Mechanisms of Morphogenesis*. Academic Press.

[25] Huang, Y. J., Liao, H. W., Wu, C. C. & Peng, H. L. (2009). MrkF is a component of type 3 fimbriae in Klebsiella pneumoniae *Res Microbiol.*, **160**, 71-79.

[26] Felek, S., Lawrenz, M. B. & Krukonis, E. S. (2008). The Yersinia pestis autotransporter YapC mediates host cell binding, autoaggregation and biofilm formation *Microbiology*, **154**, 1802-1812.

[27] Klemm, P., Vejborg, R. M. & Sherlock, O. (2006). Self-associating autotransporters, SAATs: functional and structural similarities *Int. J Med. Microbiol.*, **296**, 187-195.

[28] Nilsen, T., Yan, A. W., Gale, G. & Goldberg, M. B. (2005). Presence of multiple sites containing polar material in spherical Escherichia coli cells that lack MreB *J Bacteriol.*, **187**, 6187-6196.

[29] Terashima, H., Kojima, S. & Homma, M. (2008). Flagellar motility in bacteria structure and function of flagellar motor *Int. Rev Cell Mol. Biol*, **270**, 39-85.

[30] Chen, Y. F. & Helmann, J. D. (1992). Restoration of motility to an Escherichia coli fliA flagellar mutant by a Bacillus subtilis sigma factor *Proc Natl. Acad Sci* U. S. A, **89**, 5123-5127.

[31] Wadhams, G. H. & Armitage, J. P. (2004). Making sense of it all: bacterial chemotaxis *Nat Rev Mol. Cell Biol*, **5**, 1024-1037.

[32] Derr, P., Boder, E. & Goulian, M. (2006). Changing the specificity of a bacterial chemoreceptor *J Mol. Biol*, **355**, 923-932.

[33] Topp, S. & Gallivan, J. P. (2007). Guiding bacteria with small molecules and RNA *J Am Chem Soc*, **129**, 6807-6811.

[34] Smith, D. L., Chang, C. Y. & Young, R. (1998). The lambda holin accumulates beyond the lethal triggering concentration under hyperexpression conditions *Gene Expr.*, **7**, 39-52.

[35] Shiomi, D., Sakai, M. & Niki, H. (2008). Determination of bacterial rod shape by a novel cytoskeletal membrane protein *Embo J*, **27**, 3081-3091.

[36] Kumar, S., Kinoshita, M., Noda, M., Copeland, N. G. & Jenkins, N. A. (1994). Induction of apoptosis by the mouse Nedd2 gene, which encodes a protein similar to the product of the Caenorhabditis elegans cell death gene ced-3 and the mammalian IL-1 beta-converting enzyme *Genes Dev*, **8**, 1613-1626.

[37] Vlach, J., Hennecke, S., Alevizopoulos, K., Conti, D. & Amati, B. (1996). Growth arrest by the cyclin-dependent kinase inhibitor p27Kip1 is abrogated by c-Myc *Embo J* **15**, 6595-6604.

[38] Kinzler, E. R. & Compton, T. (2005). Characterization of human cytomegalovirus glycoprotein-induced cell-cell fusion *J Virol.*, **79**, 7827-7837.

[39] Klemke, R. L., Leng, J., Molander, R., Brooks, P. C., Vuori, K. & Cheresh, D. A. (1998). CAS/Crk coupling serves as a "molecular switch" for induction of cell migration *J Cell Biol*, **140**, 961-972.

[40] Nagafuchi, A., Shirayoshi, Y., Okazaki, K., Yasuda, K. & Takeichi, M. (1987). Transformation of cell adhesion properties by exogenously introduced E-cadherin cDNA *Nature,* **329**, 341-343.

[41] Nose, A., Nagafuchi, A. & Takeichi, M. (1988). Expressed recombinant cadherins mediate cell sorting in model systems *Cell* **54**, 993-1001.

[42] Friedlander, D. R., Mege, R. M., Cunningham, B. A. & Edelman, G. M. (1989). Cell sorting-out is modulated by both the specificity and amount of different cell adhesion molecules (CAMs) expressed on cell surfaces *Proc Natl. Acad Sci U. S. A,* **86**, 7043-7047.

[43] Collares-Buzato, C. B., Jepson, M. A., McEwan, G. T., Hirst, B. H. & Simmons, N. L. (1998). Co-culture of two MDCK strains with distinct junctional protein expression: a model for intercellular junction rearrangement and cell sorting *Cell Tissue Res,* **291**, 267-276.

[44] Wang, J. H. et al. (1999). Structure of a heterophilic adhesion complex between the human CD2 and CD58 (LFA-3) counterreceptors *Cell,* **97**, 791-803.

[45] Dustin, M. L. et al. (2007). Quantification and modeling of tripartite CD2-, CD58FC chimera (alefacept)-, and CD16-mediated cell adhesion *J Biol Chem,* **282**, 34748-34757.

[46] Haigo, S. L., Hildebrand, J. D., Harland, R. M. & Wallingford, J. B. (2003). Shroom induces apical constriction and is required for hingepoint formation during neural tube closure *Curr. Biol.,* **13**, 2125-2137.

[47] Hildebrand, J. D. & Soriano, P. (1999). Shroom, a PDZ domain-containing actin-binding protein, is required for neural tube morphogenesis in mice *Cell,* **99**, 485-497.

[48] Hildebrand, J. D. (2005). Shroom regulates epithelial cell shape via the apical positioning of an actomyosin network *J Cell Sci,* **118**, 5191-5203.

[49] Horikawa, T. et al. (2007). Twist and epithelial-mesenchymal transition are induced by the EBV oncoprotein latent membrane protein 1 and are associated with metastatic nasopharyngeal carcinoma *Cancer Res,* **67**, 1970-1978.

[50] Frisch, S. M. (1994). E1a induces the expression of epithelial characteristics *J Cell Biol,* **127**, 1085-1096.

[51] Wang, Y. et al. (2006). Chemokine-like factor 1 is a functional ligand for CC chemokine receptor 4 (CCR4) *Life Sci,* **78**, 614-621.

[52] Rhoads, D. S. & Guan, J. L. (2007). Analysis of directional cell migration on defined FN gradients: Role of intracellular signaling molecules *Exp Cell Res.*

[53] Sells, M. A., Boyd, J. T. & Chernoff, J. (1999). p21-activated kinase 1 (Pak1). regulates cell motility in mammalian fibroblasts *J Cell Biol,* **145**, 837-849.

[54] Wright, K. J. & Hultgren, S. J. (2006). Sticky fibers and uropathogenesis: bacterial adhesins in the urinary tract *Future. Microbiol.,* **1**, 75-87.

[55] Sherlock, O., Vejborg, R. M. & Klemm, P. (2005). The TibA adhesin/invasin from enterotoxigenic Escherichia coli is self recognizing and induces bacterial aggregation and biofilm formation *Infect. Immun.,* **73**, 1954-1963.

In: Synthetic and Integrative Biology
Editor: James T. Gevona, pp. 93-103

ISBN: 978-1-60876-678-9
© 2010 Nova Science Publishers, Inc.

Chapter 5

RESULTS OF THE ELECTRON MICROSCOPIC STUDY OF THE ANTARCTIC SPECIES CONOTROCHAMMINA ANTARCTICA SAIDOVA, 1975 (FORAMINIFERA)

A.-V. Mikhalevich[*]
Zoological Institute RAS, Universitetskaya naberezhnaya,
1, S. Petersburg, Russia

Summary

The study of the shell wall of Antarctic species *C. antarctica* Saidova, 1975 in SEM was carried on for the first time. The character and disposition of sand particles, pseudopore openings and inner and outer organic linings and thin structure of the apertural collar was revealed. The character and position of the aperture of this species and of the genus *Conotrochammina* on which there were some contradictory data in the previous literature was clarified. The taxonomic position of the genus was changed: it was moved from the subclass Textulariana to the subclass Hormosinana according to the terminal position of its aperture beginning from the initial stage of its shell.

Introduction

The species *Conotrochammina antarctica* Saidova, 1975 was described by Saidova (1975) from the shelf Antarctic waters in the Pacific sector of Antarctica near the Oates Coast, Northern part of the Victoria Land from the depth 695 meters ("Ob", station 336). The species is widely distributed in the Antarctic area in sublittoral and upper bathyal subzone (Fillon, 1974, Saidova, 1975, Milam & Anderson, 1981, Igarashi et al., 2001, Mikhalevich, 2004a and many others) though in some works it was attributed to different genera (see below). The inner structure of the shell and the ultrastructure of the shell wall of this species were not investigated previously, even the data on the position and structure

---

[*]E-mail address: mikha07@mail.ru. (Corresponding author)

of its aperture were contradictive. The study of all of these specific features in the Electron Microscope was the purpose of the present study.

Material and Method

The material at our disposal was that one gathered by "Ob" in 1956- 1972 years from the collections of the Zoological Institute of the Russian Academy of Sciences in S. Petersburg and from the collections of the Shirshov Institute of Oceanology of the Russian Academy of Sciences in Moscow kindly presented for this study by Chadyzhat Magomedovna Saidova. The value of her material is of a special significance concerning the fact that it included the topotypes of her new species. The studied specimens were picked up from the samples of the stations 336, 69^0 36'S, $161^0$50'E, "Ob", 1958, 650 – 700 m depth.

The shell and wall structure were studied under magnifications from 50 to 8000 times. The inner structure of the wall and apertures was studied on the breakings of the shell. Observations were carried out on the SEM Hitachi, model S – 570 with the assistance of the engineer T.K. Tsoegoev (Zoological Institute, RAN) and partly on Philips XL-20 (Institute of Paleobiology, PAN).

Results

1. Details of the Shell and Apertural Structures

The thorough study of the external character of 15 exemTablars of the species designated by Kh. M. Saidova as *Conotrochammina antarctica* in the light and electronic microscopes had unexpectedly showed that nearly half of them lack the outer aperture (Table 1, Figures 1 a, b, c; 2) while in the others the clear areal aperture could be discovered (Table 1, Figures 3a,b; Table 2; Table 2, Figure 1 a, b). In the shells without external aperture the internal apertures were clearly seen in all the inner chambers of the broken shells (Table 2, Figures 2 - 7; Table 3, Figure 4, 5). The series of successive breakings of the same shell (Table 2, Figures 2 - 7) permit to reveal the inner apertures of the shell up to the initial chamber (Table 2, Figure 7). All of them have areal position and are represented by the oval opening surrounded externally with rather high very thin and delicate white collar (or neck) (Table 2, Figures 2 – 7; Table 3, Figures 1, 2; Table 4, Figure 1, 6) constituted by very thin (pelite) fine sand material with no special characters when viewed from the inside of the chamber (Table 2, Figure 6; Table 3, Figure 5). This collar could be clearly seen only in SEM, in the light microscope the aperture looks as being flash with the surface. And the photographs in SEM show that the collar of the inner aperture is higher and best developed than in the outer aperture of the last chamber when present. The distance of the apertural position from the base of the chamber varies strongly from being placed in the center of the chamber (Table 2, Figures 2,4,6) to being situated more closely to its base (Table 1, Figure 3a, b; Table 2, Figure 1a, b). In the case when the aperture is very close to the sutural line it looks from some angles of view like interiomarginal aperture and could be erroneously taken for such base opening (Table 1, Figure 3a).

The trochoid spire of the whole shell varies from rather low (Tabl 2, Figure 1) to rather high, with the shell height and breadth nearly equal (Table 1, Figures 1 a, b; Table 2, Figure 7) and sometimes the spire is more prominently elongated with the height slightly exciding the breadth of the shell (Table 2, Figure 2). From three to four or rarely five globular chambers are visible from the apertural side (Table 1, Figure 1a, b, 2, 3; Table 2, Figure 1; Table 4, Figure 7), the fifth chamber may have less regular form (Table 1, Figures 2, 3a).

Table 1.

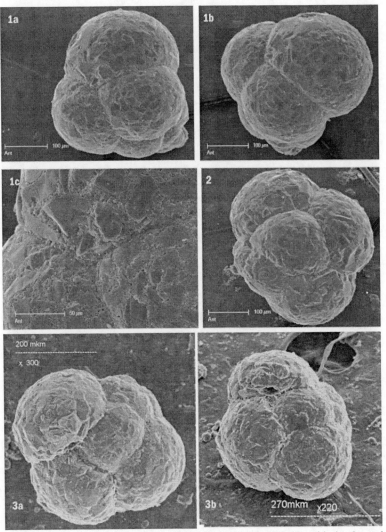

1a, b, c – view of the shell from the different positions of the "apertural" side with the three chambers in the final whorl but aperture absent ("Ob" 1958, station 336), 1a,b – x 250, 1c – x 500; 2 – view of another specimen from the "apertural" side with the five final chambers visible, aperture absent ("Ob" 1958, st. 336); 3a, b – view form the different positions of another specimen with five final chambers visible from the apertural side with the aperture present, 3a – from this position aperture looks as a narrow slit and seems to be placed at the base of apertural face – x 300, 3 b – from the position of the shell little changed aperture looks as oval opening only slightly elevated above the suture ("Ob" 1958, station 336).

Table 2.

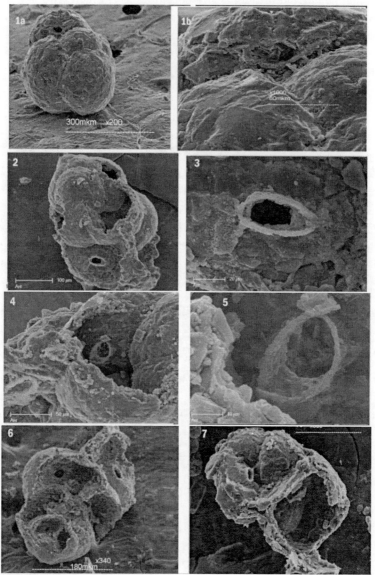

1a, b – the apertural side of the same specimen as Tabl. 1, Figure 3a, b from little changed positions: 1 a – x 200, 1 b – x 1000, mark the size of the sutural openings at the different sutures ("Ob" 1958, st. 336); 2 – the broken specimen, mark two inner apertures with the collars from the outer side of the chambers, character of the inner shell wall, transverse breaking of the shell and character of the circular openings of the broken wall at the left side of the shell near the junction with the nearest chamber (openings resembling that ones of canaliculated wall when the cutting goes perpendicular to canaliculi) – x 250, ("Ob" 1958, st. 336); 3 – part of the Figure 2 enlarged showing the inner aperture viewed from the outer side of the chamber – x 1250; 4 – the same shell as on the Figure 2 after the next breaking showing two inner apertures with the collars at the outer side of the chambers – x 500 (mark the character of the wall at transverse breaking showing the regular openings above the aperture); 5 – inner aperture from the outer chamber side from the Figure 4 enlarged, x 2500; 6 – another shell broken up to the initial chamber with inner apertures seen from the outer chamber surface and from the inside of the chamber – x 340 (mark the character of the transverse breakings of the wall and its openings) ("Ob" 1958, st. 336); 7 – part of the successive breaking of the exemplar of the Figure 6 revealing the aperture of the initial chamber (mark the character of the transverse breaking of the wall in the meadle part of the picture) – x 800.

Table 3.

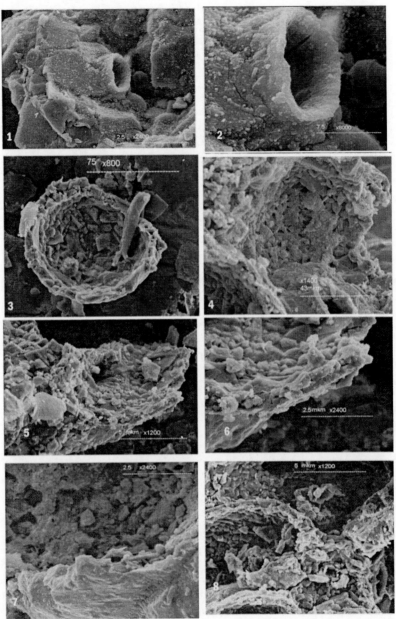

1 - the outer collar of the inner aperture of the initial chamber of the Figure 7 (Tabl. 2) – x 2400; 2 – the same, enlarged – x 8000; 3 – a piece of the broken initial chamber showing the structure of the inner wall and transverse breaking of the wall (mark the character of the openings at the upper part of the piece going in radial direction and white line of inner organic lining at the right side) – x 800; 4 - part of the Figure 6 (Tabl. 2) showing the inner aperture from the outer chamber side and the structure of the inner shell wall - x 1400; 5 – another piece of the broken shell of Figure6 (Tabl. 2) showing the inner aperture from the inside, the transverse section of the wall (lower part) with radial openings and outer organic lining (white) and rough inner wall of the chamber – x 1200; 6 – the same, enlarged – x 2400; 7 – the breaking of the same shell showing the structure of the inner and outer wall and the suture – x 2400; 8 – another place of breaking showing the structure of the transverse wall (central part of the picture) with the thick outer layer of the flat surface particles – x 1200.

Table 4.

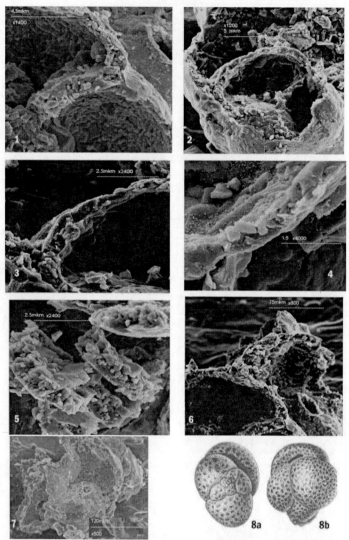

1 – details of the rough inner wall and of the transverse section of the wall (mark the radial openings below the pierced outer wall of fine material at the very upper part of the picture and at the left part of the middle septa and thick roof of the flat sand particles at the lower right side of transverse section) – x 1400; 2 – details of the wall structure at the transverse breakings of the initial chambers (mark the thin inner organic lining, the radial fissures at the left and right parts of the transverse section and longitudinally going spaces in the septa dividing two lower chambers) – x 1200; 3 – details of the transverse breaking of the septa (mark thin white lines of the outer and inner organic lining and dark spaces where the bigger sand particles are broken off) – x 2400; 4 – details of the transverse breaking of the septa with occasional radial openings – x 4000; 5 – details of the transverse breakings of the wall in the three small fragments (mark the outer organic lining in the lower and middle pieces, inner organic lining and roof layer in the middle piece, and openings in the upper piece resembling the transverse cutting of canaliculi in canaliculated wall) – x 2400; 6 – details of the transverse breakings of the wall (mark occasional radial openings) – x 800; 7 – initial part of the broken shell with a clear row of sutural openings (right side) and clear subcircular openings seen between the particles of the inner wall (mark also radial openings in the upper right part of the transverse breaking of the wall) – x 500; 8 a,b – holotype of *Conotrochammina antarctica* Saidova (after Saidova, 1975), "Ob", 1958, station 336 – x 40.

Sutures are deep and narrow, and in some places show the rows of the openings somewhat bigger than pseudopore openings of the wall. Such sutural openings could be seen from outside (Table 2, Figure 1b) and inside the shell (Table 4, Figure 7) only under the bigger SEM magnifications. Most of the sutures show only a series of minute openings or lack even such minute spaces (Table 3, Figure 7).

2. Details of the Shell Wall Ultrastructure

The shell wall of *Conotrochammina antarctica* was considered previously as noncanaliculate (Loeblich & Tappan, 1987), much earlier such wall was called imperforate.

In the light microscope the outer shell wall of this species looks as very smooth, nearly polished and solid, without any openings, formed by the sand particles of the middle size (Table 4, Figure 8a, b). In SEM it also looks smooth and polished, encrusted by the sand particles of ordered orientation, having angular or irregular outline and turned to the outer surface by their flat sides, with very thin pelite material between them (Table 1, Figure 1c). These pelite areas as well as the sutures are pierced by the small pseudopore openings of subcircular (in the middle part of pelite areas) or irregular (around the bigger sand particles) form. In some places such openings in the sutures form a row of bigger subcircular openings resembling the sutural additional apertures but in this species they are not regular for all the sutures (Table 2, Figure 1 b; Table 4, Figure 7). In the places where the outer flat sand particles were detached the more coarse and regular pseudopore openings could be observed.

The inner shell surface opposite to the outer one is rough with the sand particles turned to the inner surface by their acute angles (Table 2, Figure 6; Table 3, Figures 3 – 7; Table 4, Figure 7). This surface is pierced by the regular dense subcircular or irregular in form openings (Table 3, Figure 4; Table 4, Figure 7).

On the transverse breakings of the wall in some places the band of the upper flat sand grains could be seen (Table 4, Figures 1, 5) somewhat resembling the dense roof layer of miliolid wall. Below it a layer of angular sand grains is situated though these rather big grains are broken off the wall in the process of fracturing or of making slides of the shell leaving the yawning cavities (Table 4, Figure 3). Nevertheless the clear spaces piercing the transverse wall section could be seen in many places (Table 2, Figures 2, 4, 6, 7; Table 3 , Figures 3, 8; Table 4, Figures 1, 2, 4 - 7) which occasionally look as going the radial direction (Table 2, Figure 4; Table 3, Figures 3, 5; Table 4, Figures 1, 2, 4, 7). In the case the breaking of the wall goes another direction (not strictly perpendicular) the dense subcircular openings could be seen resembling those of the sections of canaliculate wall when the cutting goes perpendicularly to canaliculi (Table 2, Figure 2; Table 4, Figure 5 – the upper piece). Nevertheless these occasional features of the wall ultrastructure resembling occasionally some places of canaliculate wall could not be attributed to true canaliculated type. These more regularly organized spaces are usually met in the areas of the finer material. The SEM photographs of the shell wall of the species studied resembles in many features (rough sand grains in the middle part of the transverse wall section easily broken off, the rough character of the inner chamber wall) wall structure of *Saccaminella salsa* in the work of Bronniman et al., 1992 (Table XIX, Figures 1, 3, 7) differing from it in its smooth outer wall. Even some radially going spaces between sand particles were also met by the above authors (Bronnimann et. al., 1992, Table XIX, Figure 8, right lower part of the picture).

The very thin organic lining on the outer and inner wall surface could also be seen in the transverse breakings as a thin white line (Table 3, Figure 3; Table 4, Figures 2, 3, 5).

Thus in reality the wall of this species is not solid and is fully permeable.

Under the bigger magnifications up to x 2400 and 8000 the ultrathin structure of the collar of the inner aperture could also be seen. It consists of the minute white particles arranged in radial direction (Table 3, Figures 1, 2).

Discussion

The type species of the genus *Conotrochammina* - *C. whangaia* Finlay, 1940 was described as having areal aperture. But Bronnimann et al., 1983 didn't find an apparent aperture in the topotypes and paratypes of the type species. This was the cause for these authors to suppose the aperture as being interiomarginal and obscured by the rough sand particles of the wall. Loeblich & Tappan (1987) confirmed the presence of areal aperture in this species. As it turned out in our material nearly half of the exemplars of the species definitely lack any aperture at their last chamber (Table 1, fig 1a – c). But in the broken specimens of such forms inner arial aperture with a distinct collar was discovered through the series of breakings in all the previous chambers up to the initial one. The only possible suggestion in this case might be that the aperture is formed later in the fully performed last chamber though this could be hardly imagined in the agglutinated forms. The indirect confirmation of such supposition could be the fact that the apertural collar of the series of the inner apertures is higher and more strongly developed (Table 2, Figures 2 – 7; Table 3, Figures 1, 2) than the slight low rim of the outer aperture of the last chamber when present (Table 2, Figures 1 a, b). The terminal rather than interiomarginal position of the aperture and may be its later formation after the last chamber of the shell is fully formed distinguishes this genus and species from the true trochamminids where the next chamber is formed simultaneously with its aperture (Angel, 1990). The latter is interiomarginal and positioned at the base of the last chamber. Loeblich & Tappan had moved the genus *Conotrochammina* from trochamminids to verneuilinids (to the former superfamily Verneuilinacea Cushman, 1911, later the order Verneuilinida Mikhalevich et Kaminski, 2004). But the typical verneuilinids have interiomarginal aperture at least initially. Their aperture becomes terminal at the later stages of shell development. In the species studied the aperture is areal from the very beginning of the shell. The same situation is in the genera of the family Reophacellidae Mikhalevich et Kaminski, 2004. The conical shell and the character of the chambers also resemble more *Reophacella* or *Uvigerinammina* than true trochamminids though in these two genera their terminal aperture is elongated into more distinct neck. As these genera were moved from verneuilinids of the subclass Textulariana to the nouriids belonging to the subclass Hormosinana (Mikhalevich, 2004b) the taxonomic position of conotrochamminids was changed correspondingly.

Conotrochammina antarctica is widely distributed in the Antarctic waters though not rarely mentioned under the other names (e.g. – *Conotrochammina* sp. in Fillon, 1974, Tabl 2, Figure 4; *Trochammina conica* in Milam & Anderson, 1981, Table 3, Figure 5; and presumably *Paratrochammina scotiaensis* in Igarashi et al., 2001, Table 4, Figure 3 (photograph not quite clear).

Systematic Part

Phylum **Foraminifera** d'Orbigny, 1826
Class **Nodosariata** Mikhalevich, 1992
Subclass **Hormosinana** Mikhalevich, 1992
Order **Nouriida** Mikhalevich, 1980
Superfamily Nouriidoidea Chapman et Parr, 1936
Family Conotrochamminidae Saidova, 1981
Genus *Conotrochammina* Finlay, 1940
Type species: *Conotrochammina whangaia* Finlay, 1940, p. 448.
Syn: *Pseudotrochammina* Frerichs, 1969, type species *P. triloba* Frerichs, 1969, p. 1.
Trochammina conica Milam et Anderson, 1981, Table 3, Figure 5.

Diagnosis. Shell with low conical spire of about two to seven coils, from a few (three to six) chambers per whorl, with chambers inflated to subsphaerical; aperture arial, wide slit to oval or circular opening, often with a distinct collar. Paleocene to Holocene.

Remarks. Such features as the degree of the wall roughness and correlated with it clearly visible or obscure sutures usually mentioned in the diagnosis of this genus ought to be considered as having specific rank. The main taxonomically important features of the genus *Conotrochammina* are the conical form of its shell and areal aperture. The genus *Pseudotrochammina* described later does not principally differ in these features from the *Conotrochammina* and is regarded here as its synonym.

Conotrochammina antarctica Saidova, 1975
C. antarctica Saidova, 1975, p. 105, Table XCIX, Figure 6.
Conotrochammina sp. Fillon, 1974, Tabl 2, Figure 4.

Diagnosis. Shell very small (0.45 – 0. 5 mm), conical and slightly asymmetric, with five to seven coils of spiral and mostly three but rarely up to five chambers per whorl, chambers strongly inflated, subsphaerical, quickly enlarging in size as added, last chambers may be somewhat irregular in growth and position, sutures narrow, distinct, occasionally with pseudopore openings; wall externally smooth, mosaic, with flat middle sized sand grains of angular or irregular form and thin pelite material between them, areas of thin material rather densely pierced by pseudopores, inner wall surface rough, pierced by subcircular pseudopores, transverse sections of the wall shows flat "roof" sand particles with middle sized sand grains below alternating with areas of fine material and pierced through by the empty spaces everywhere (pseudopore passages going under the bigger flat particles as well); aperture areal, somewhat irregularly widely oval, may be slightly curved or subcircular, encircled by very thin white collar constituted by extremely thin grains, apertural opening situated variably – close to the suture or nearly at the center of the chamber outer surface. Holocene.
Distribution. All around Antarctic at the shelf and upper subzone of the bathyal zone.

Remarks. Among our material nearly half of the specimens have no apparent aperture. The same was observed in another Conotrochamminid species - *C. whangaia* by Bronnimann et al., 1983. The successive series of breakings of such shells up to the very initial chambers shows the presence of distinct areal apertures encircled by the thin fragile collar in all of them. This fact permits to suppose that their aperture may be formed later after the ultimate chamber is composed. At least the collar of the inner apertures is higher and more developed than the low rim around the external aperture when it is present. Rather rough sand grains in the middle part of the broken wall are often broken off. The wall could be considered as noncanaliculate as some occasional radial passages in the wall are not regular.

Conclusion

The study of the wall of Antarctic species *C. antarctica* in SEM revealed its ultrastructural character. Its agglutinated wall is smooth and mosaic externally consisting of oriented flat sand particles of middle size with thin pelite material between them pierced by the pseudopore openings. From the inner side of the chamber the wall looks rough and also having the pseudopores. The thin layers of the inner and outer organic lining usually covering each type of the wall were discovered as well. In nearly half of the specimens studied the apparent external aperture was absent presenting in all their previous chambers up to the initial one. The character and position of the aperture of this species and this genus on which there were some contradictory evidence in the previous literature was clarified. The aperture of *Conotrochammina* is definitely areal and has a fragile collar surrounding it. The ultrastructure of this collar was also studied. The taxonomic position of the genus concerning the structure of its aperture was changed: the genus was transferred from the order Verneuilinida (subclass Textulariana) to the order Nouriida (subclass Hormosinana).

Acknowledgments

The author is deeply grateful to Dr. Khadyzhat Magomedovna Saidova kindly presenting her topotype material of her new species and permitting to copy the pictures of holotype, to Dr. Danuta Peryt for her assistance in the part of SEM work and to Dr. Olga Kamenskaya helping in the legalization of the necessary papers permitting the copy of the pictures according to the copyright rules.

References

Angell, RW. Observations on reproduction and juvenile test building in the foraminifer *Trochammina inflata. Journal of Foraminiferal Research*, 1990, 20, (3), 246 - 247.
Bronnimann, P; Zaninetti, L; Whittaker, JE. On the classification of the Trochamminacea (Foraminiferida). *Journal of Foraminiferal Research*, 1983, 13, 202-218.
Bronnimann, P; Whittaker, JE; Zaninetti, L. Brackish water foraminifera from mangrove sediments of Southwestern Viti Levu, Fiji Islands, Southwest Pacific. *Revue de Paleobiologie*, 1992, 11(1), 13-65.
Fillon, RH. Late Cenozoic foraminiferal paleoecology of the Ross Sea, Antarctica. *Micropaleontology,* 1974, 20(2), 129-151.

Igarashi, A; Numanami, H; Tsuchiya, Y; Fukuchi, M. Bathymetric distribution of fossil foraminifera within marine sediment cores from the eastern part of Lutzow-Holm Bay, East Antarctica, and its paleoceanographic implications. *Marine Micropaleontology*, 2001, 42, 125-162.

Loeblich, AR; Jr., Tappan, H. *Foraminiferal genera and their claassification*. Department of Earth and space sciences and center for the study of evolution and origin of the life. Univ. California. Los Angeles. Van Nostraand Company. N.Y., 1, 2, 1988.

Mikhalevich, VI. The general aspects of the distribution of Antarctic foraminifera. *Micropaleontology*, 2004a, 50(2), 179-194, 5 Tablates.

Mikhalevich, VI. On the heterogeneity of the former Textulariina (Foraminifera). In: M; Bubik, MA; Kaminski, (Eds),. *Proceedings of the Sixth International Workshop on Agglutinated Foraminifera*. Grzybowski Foundation Special Publication, 2004b, 8, 317-349.

Milam, RW; Anderson, JB. Distribution and ecology of recent benthonic foraminifera of the Adelie-Georg V continental shelf and slope. *Marine Micropaleontology*, 1981, 6, 297-325.

Saidova Kh. M. *Bentosnye foraminifery Tikhogo Okeana* [Benthonic foraminifera of the Pacific Ocean]. 3 vol. Moscow, Institut Okeanologii PP. Shirshova, Akademiya Nauk SSSR, 1975, (in Russian).

In: Synthetic and Integrative Biology
Editor: James T. Gevona, pp. 105-121

Chapter 6

State-Dependency of Process Rates: A Clear Concept of Feedback in Biology

Jon Olav Vik[1] and Stig W. Omholt[2]

[1] Centre for Integrative Genetics (CIGENE),
Department of Mathematical Sciences and Technology,
Norwegian University of Life Sciences, Norway
[2] Centre for Integrative Genetics (CIGENE),
Department of Animal and Agricultural Sciences,
Norwegian University of Life Sciences, Norway

Abstract

Characteristics of feedback loops, i.e. closed interaction chains, can often be used as indicators of the kinds of dynamics a biological system can exhibit. However, published definitions of feedback vary widely, especially in their verbal descriptions of feedback. In particular, opinions differ as to whether the sign of links in a causal chain are given by the direction of the *processes themselves*, or *how process rates respond* to changes in system state. In the latter case, a self-effect (the direct effect of a state variable on itself) may appear qualitatively different depending on whether one considers the state-dependency of the *relative* or the *absolute* rate-of-change of the variable. A fourth definition uses "feedback" as a summary measure of all disjunct loops of action in the system.

For a system of ordinary differential equations, our evaluation favors a definition of "the action of state variable x on y" as being positive if an increase in x causes an increase in the rate-of-change of y. Thus, the sign of an action is given by the corresponding element in the Jacobian matrix, evaluated at the current state of the system. No predictive power seems to be lost by abandoning the competing definitions of feedback, because all authors base their mathematical treatment on the Jacobian matrix.

Although many useful quantities can be derived from a dynamical model, not all of them should be called feedback. In our opinion, a positive or negative term in the rate-of-change should be called just that. Similarly, per capita growth rates may often be adequately

---

[1] E-mail address: jonovik@gmail.com. Fax: +47 6496 5101. P.O. Box 5003 N-1432 AAS Norway (Corresponding author.)

characterized as positively or negatively density-dependent. Lumping disjunct causal loops in a single feedback term seems misleading, because disjunct loops are not causally interconnected.

The state-dependence of process rates is a fundamental feature of natural dynamical systems, which makes this notion of feedback widely applicable. This suggests that verbal and conceptual explanations focussing on how process depends on state will be heuristically useful.

Introduction

The complexity of dynamical biological systems motivates a search for invariant patterns (signatures) that indicate which categories of dynamics a system can exhibit, without requiring a complete analysis of the system. The concept of mutual causality, or "feedback", has proved essential in uncovering such generic principles. Negative feedback is recognized as the essence of homeostatic, "deviation-counteracting" mechanisms (e.g. Milsum, 1968a). By contrast, the nature and function of positive feedback is less well understood. One important feature is that it may enable alternative stable states (multiple attractors), a phenomenon of great importance in biological conservation, environmental protection, ecology and biochemistry (insect pest outbreaks, Holling, 1973;   minimum viable populations, Gilpin & Soulé, 1986; gene regulatory networks, Thomas & D'Ari, 1990; lake turbidity, Scheffer *et al.*, 1993). In the same vein, positive feedback facilitates differentiation, at scales ranging from individual cells (Thomas & Kaufman, 2001a; 2001b) to vegetation communities (Sutherland, 1974; Wilson & Agnew, 1992). Most natural systems have a complex interplay of positive and negative feedback mechanisms. For instance, such feedback regulation may explain the genetic phenomena of dominance, additivity and epistasis (Omholt *et al.*, 2000).

There is an obvious need for a widely applicable, clear-cut definition of feedback, on which one can build theories, both mathematically and conceptually. Presently, however, several disparate definitions of feedback abound in the literature (reviews from various viewpoints include Milsum, 1968b; Puccia & Levins, 1985; DeAngelis *et al.*, 1986; Thomas & Kaufman, 2001a; 2001b). Most authors agree that feedback refers to a closed chain of causal connections, involving specific state variables of the system. These causal connections involve state-dependent process rates, so that a change in state affects the further development of the system. However, opinions differ as to whether the links in the causal chain are the *processes themselves*, or *how process rates respond* to changes in system state. In the latter case, a self-effect (the direct effect of a state variable on itself) may appear qualitatively different depending on whether the state-dependency considered is of the *relative* (e.g. Abrams, 2001) or *absolute* (e.g. Thomas & Kaufman, 2001a) rate-of-change of the variable.

These differences affect how one frames verbal and conceptual explanations of complex dynamic phenomena such as alternative stable states. For example, Petraitis and Latham (1999) and Wilson and Agnew (1992) hold that positive feedback, in addition to driving a shift from one stable species assemblage to another, serves to stabilize the new state. Similarly, positive feedback has been viewed as a "life-support mechanism" for consumer populations whose resource supply may increase as consumer density increases (Bianchi *et al.*, 1989; Stone & Weisburd, 1992). Other authors equate positive feedback with closed loops of state-dependent flow such as nutrient cycles (Stone & Weisburd, 1992) or life cycles

(DeAngelis *et al.*, 1986:129; Ulanowicz, 1995). We challenge these views, and intend to show that much confusion can be resolved by a few simple conceptual clarifications.

This paper documents the subtle differences between many of the published usages of "feedback", often even between the verbal and mathematical description of feedback mechanisms adopted in the same publication. We demonstrate some of the resulting inclarities and inconsistencies, and argue for a definition that focuses on how process rates respond to changes in state, whilst retaining the analytical power of competing definitions. Finally, we discuss how this feedback concept can be generalized to dynamical systems on different levels of aggregation and in other mathematical frameworks.

Alternative Definitions of Feedback

A serviceable concept of feedback should satisfy several requirements besides the obvious ones of predictive and heuristic usefulness. It should be mathematically unambiguous and clearly expressible verbally, once a mathematical model for the system has been specified. Thus, once the state variables for the system have been chosen, its feedback signature ought to be invariant under a change of reference frame (scaling, translation, transformation). The definition of feedback should have a real-world interpretation that relates clearly to empirically observable quantities or processes. Preferably, it should generalize to interactions between an arbitrary number of state variables whilst retaining intuitive properties such as the deviation-counteracting effects of negative feedback on small deviations from equilibrium. In this section, we summarize and evaluate four different views of interactions and feedback loops, assuming an autonomous system of two ordinary differential equations (ODEs) with state variables x and y. Definitions of feedback for other mathematical frameworks are considered in the next section.

Common Vocabulary and Examples

The basic ingredient in feedback is the effect, widely speaking, of one state variable on another. This has variously been termed an "action" (e.g. Omholt & Plahte, 1994), a "link" (Puccia & Levins, 1985), or an "interaction" (e.g. Abrams, 2001). We use "action" rather than "interaction" to emphasize that it is a directed relationship, which may or may not be reciprocated.

The term "feedback loop" (or "circuit", or just "feedback") usually denotes a closed action chain among specific state variables (e.g. Milsum, 1968a). However, "feedback" is also sometimes used for influences or functional relationships in general, as in "the feedback of population size on individual growth". As used in this paper, an action chain does not constitute feedback unless the chain is a closed loop. A third use of "feedback" is as a summary measure of all the action chains in a system (Puccia & Levins, 1985).

The Jacobian matrix is a mathematical tool common to most published treatments of feedback. Its elements (i,j) are the partial derivatives of the rate-of-change of variable x_i with respect to variable x_j. Classically, it is used to evaluate the local stability of single-point equilibria, for instance in terms of eigenvalues, the Routh-Hurwitz criteria, and "qualitative stability" (e.g. Murray, 1993).

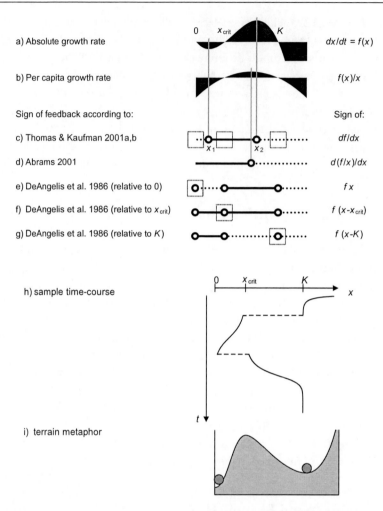

Figure 1. Alternative stable states result when there is a minimum population size below which net reproduction is negative. The x axis shows population size. Figures a and b show growth rates for the whole population and per individual, respectively. Figures c-g show how the sign of feedback varies with population size under various definitions. Solid and dotted lines indicate positive and negative action of x on itself, respectively. Figures e-g are "relative to" three different reference states (DeAngelis et al., 1986); near each reference state this almost agrees with figure c (indicated by dotted boxes). Figures h and i illustrate the dynamics and attractor structure of the system. a) The population net growth rate, $dx/dt = f(x)$, as a function of x. There are stable equilibria at $x = 0$ and $x = K$; their domains of attraction are separated by an unstable equilibrium at $x = x_{crit}$. b) The per capita net growth rate, $f(x)/x$, is an increasing function of population size at low values of x, in contrast to population growth rate, which is a decreasing function of x at low x. c) Feedback as determined by df/dx (Thomas & Kaufman, 2001a) is positive for $x_1 < x < x_2$, and negative elsewhere. Thus, feedback is negative in the neighbourhood of the stable equilibria and vice versa. d) The action of x on itself according to Abrams (2001), determined by $d(f/x)/dx$. Note that it is positive near the stable zero equilibrium. Figures e-g show whether dx/dt points towards or away from a reference state (negative and positive feedback, respectively, according to DeAngelis et al., 1986). Three reference states are used for illustration, namely zero, x_{crit}, and carrying capacity K. Note that a change of reference frame inverts feedback in the region traversed by the moving reference point. h) Time-course showing attraction to different stable states depending on initial population size. i) Metaphorical terrain where a "hill" of positive feedback (sensu Thomas & Kaufman, 2001a) separates two "valleys" (attractors) stabilized by negative feedback.

To exemplify the differences between competing usages of "feedback", we use a simple model with alternative stable states. Figure 1 describes the dynamics of a population whose density must be above some threshold for the birth rate to exceed the death rate, and density-dependent regulation limits population growth at high densities (Allee, 1931; Dennis, 1989). Assume that the net birth rate, dx/dt, is a function $f(x)$ of population size x, as shown in Figure 1a. In this simple example, investigating the sign of the rate-of-change dx/dt suffices for a global qualitative analysis. Population density decreases for $0 < x < x_{crit}$, increases for $x_{crit} < x < K$, and decreases for $x > K$ (Figure 1e). Hence, there are stable equilibria at 0 and K, whereas the one at x_{crit} is unstable. The population growth rate is an increasing function of population size in a region containing the unstable equilibrium; elsewhere dx/dt is a decreasing function of x (Figure 1a,c). The per capita growth rate, on the other hand, has a qualitatively different dependence on population size (Figure 1b,d). It is an increasing function of x at low to moderate population densities, and decreasing at higher densities. Figure 1h shows attractor shifts resulting from perturbations, which will be described to in the next chapter.

Definition 1. How Process Rates Respond to Changes in State

A definition of "action" widely used in regulatory cell biology (reviewed by Thomas, 1998; Thomas & Kaufman, 2001a) is that the action of x on y is positive if the partial derivative $(\partial/\partial x)(dy/dt)$ is positive, and vice versa. That is, x acts positively on y if an increase in x would modify the rate-of-change of y in the positive direction. (Conversely, a decrease in x would decrease the rate-of-change of y.) Under this definition, the signs of elements in the interaction matrix are given by the Jacobian of the system, evaluated at its current state. (Hence, we will sometimes refer to this as the Jacobian-based definition.)

Thomas' definition is the basis for many results on the correspondence between the feedback structure of a system and its dynamical properties. For instance, positive feedback is required for the existence of multiple stable points (Plahte *et al.*, 1995; Snoussi, 1998; Gouze, 1998). A negative feedback loop of length two or more is required for a stable periodic orbit (Snoussi, 1998; Gouze, 1998). Some examples of chaotic dynamics are robust to details of the system once a basic feedback structure is in place (Thomas, 1999). However, these results are mostly qualitative, as the definition specifies only the sign and not any absolute magnitude of feedback.

Important advantages of the Jacobian-based definition are its reference-frame independence and scale invariance. A shift of the coordinate system does not affect the entries of the Jacobian (because they describe the change in the rate-of-change of y per unit *change* in x), and a scaling preserves the sign of the Jacobian elements. Reversing the coordinate axis of a state variable will not affect the sign of feedback loops, either. This is because such an inversion inverts all actions *of* and *on* the inverted state variable, so the sign inversions cancel in all loops of which the variable is part. (Self-effects remain unchanged, because this is an action *of* a variable *on* itself.) Although independent of reference frame, this definition makes obvious that actions among state variables depend on the state of the system (except in purely linear systems), a point that is easy to overlook when restricting attention to single-point equilibria or linear systems (see criticism by Abrams, 2001). State-independent terms do not contribute to feedback. While this is intuitively reasonable, it does imply that feedback alone will not, for instance, determine the existence of equilibria. Constant input to a system may enable or eliminate some equilibria, although the feedback at a given state is unchanged (Thomas & Kaufman, 2001a).

Some characteristics of a system can be stated in terms of sets of disjunct loops that, together, include all the variables in a system (Thomas & Kaufman, 2001a). Such a set is called a "full-circuit" by Thomas & Kaufman (2001a). However, the word "circuit" seems inappropriate, because disjunct loops are obviously not causally connected with each other. (These sets correspond to the terms in the determinant of the Jacobian matrix, each of which has exactly one element from each row and column. Thus, each variable is represented by exactly one outgoing and one incoming action, so that any loops that can be formed from these elements must be disjunct.)

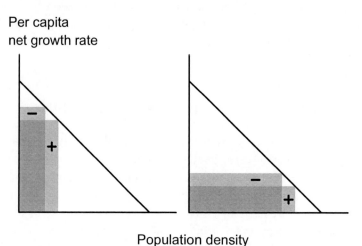

Figure 2. The feedback of population size on itself may have opposite sign than the density-dependence of per capita growth rate. In the logistic model, the per capita growth rate decreases linearly with population size. However, population size is the integral of the *population* growth rate, not the per capita rate. However, population size is the integral of the *population* growth rate, not the per capita rate. Hence, the former is required to link population size to itself, and the feedback of population size depends on a combination of change in population size and change in per capita rates. The figures show gains (+) and losses (–) in population growth rate due to an increase in population size from low vs. high densities (left vs. right figure). The population growth rate equals the product of population size and per capita net growth rate, shown by the shaded rectangles. Even though per capita growth shows purely negative density-dependence, population size exerts positive feedback on itself at low densities (left figure). ,This is because the gain in growth due to the added number of individuals more than outweighs the loss due to reduced individual reproduction. However, the situation is opposite at high densities (right figure).

Definition 2. How Per Capita Process Rates Respond to Changes in State

In community ecology, "interactions" between species are often defined in terms of how a change in the density of one species affects the *per capita* (i.e. relative) growth rate of another (Abrams, 1987; 2001). It can be shown that this agrees with the Jacobian-based definition on the sign of actions between distinct state variables. However, this may not be the case for self-loops. For instance, in a population that grows logistically from a density near zero, the population growth rate increases whereas the per capita growth rate decreases (Figure 2). A per-capita-based definition of feedback has some counterintuitive implications. For instance, the logistic equation shows only negative "per capita feedback" around the unstable zero equilibrium, whereas the Allee-effect system shows only positive "per capita feedback" near the stable zero equilibrium (Figure 1*d*; Figure 2). Both of these results disagree with common usage of feedback. Furthermore, relative rates have a real-world interpretation only for physical quantities whose scale has an absolute zero, such as molar concentrations and population sizes.

An emphasis on per capita rates is often highly useful for biological interpretation and model construction (Abrams, 2001). However, a self-loop must describe the action on *a state variable* by itself. State variables such as population size take their values from the integral of *absolute*, not relative, rates of change. Thus, there is no direct causal chain between a change in state, a change in relative rates, and the further change in state. The overall effect on population rates-of-change depends both on how the number of individuals change, and how each individual's per capita reproduction changes (Figure 2).

Definition 3. Whether Processes Work Towards or Away from a Reference State

The book on positive feedback by DeAngelis et al. (1986) seems not to provide any single, general definition of the term. As applied to single-variable systems in their initial description (pages 2-5), state-dependent terms in dx/dt are characterized as positive or negative feedback depending on whether they amplify or counteract the current deviation from some reference state (DeAngelis *et al.*, 1986, D.L. DeAngelis, personal communication). Thus, the sign of feedback is determined by the current direction of a process, rather than by how its rate is affected by changes in state. Furthermore, the choice of reference state affects how feedback appears (Figure 1*e-g*), as emphasized by DeAngelis et al.

Comparison [of the logistic equation in terms of population size vs. deviations from carrying capacity] underscores an important 'relativistic' effect in modeling feedback. In the reference frame of the original variable [population size], the equilibrium point is at K and represents a balance between positive and negative feedbacks. However, in the reference frame of the substitute variable [deviation from K], the equilibrium point is at 0 and the feedback is purely negative. [...]

Often the choice of a particular frame of reference may obscure what is actually happening biologically. In this case the representation [the logistic equation in terms of deviation from carrying capacity] of the population as acted on simply by negative feedback is misleading. A stable, steady-state population represents a balance between positive feedback (births) and negative feedback (deaths). This is not an exercise in hairsplitting, the choice of a frame of reference that accentuates negative feedback mechanisms may cause one to ignore the positive feedbacks that may become important under changed circumstances.

(DeAngelis *et al.*, 1986:5)

The arbitrariness of a reference-frame dependent feedback concept seems to give little hope of obtaining generic relationships between feedback structure and dynamical patterns, because changing the reference state will invert the sign of feedback in the part of state space traversed by the moving zero-point (Figure 1e-g). Furthermore, the above description of birth and death processes as positive and negative feedback *per se* seems incompatible with DeAngelis et al.'s later exemplification of regulation in a metabolic pathway:

a A negative feedback loop, where [...] the end product [...] inhibits further production [of the precursor]

b A positive feedback loop, where [...] one of the end products [...] stimulates further production [of the precursor]

(DeAngelis *et al.*, 1986:53)

In this quotation, what determines the sign of feedback is clearly *how* a process rate changes when a state variable changes, *not* the process rate itself (which is always nonnegative). This notion of feedback is used of biochemical regulation e.g. by Murray (Murray, 1993:144), and matches the Jacobian-based definition exactly. In fact, DeAngelis et al. (1986:22) identify feedback in a two-variable system from the sign of entries in the Jacobian – which summarize precisely how process rates are affected by changes in state. It seems that DeAngelis et al. sometimes confuse the regulation of a state-dependent flow with the flow itself, and that their usage is inconsistent. What predictive power they do achieve is apparently based on analyses of the Jacobian matrix, despite their claim that using a nonzero equilibrium as a reference state is biologically misleading (DeAngelis *et al.*, 1986:5, quoted above).

There is almost agreement between the Jacobian-based and process-direction-based definitions in the particular case of a single-variable system initially at equilibrium, where state is measured as a deviation from that equilibrium. Because in this case state variable and rate-of-change both start at zero, a small, positive perturbation of x will cause x to start moving away from zero if and only if the Jacobian (i.e. the slope of dx/dt as a function of x) is positive (e.g. x_{crit} in Figure 1c and *f*). The remaining disagreement is that DeAngelis et al. describe equilibrium as "zero net feedback", whereas the Jacobian is usually nonzero at equilibrium. Of course, the definitions may disagree fundamentally outside the neighborhood of the equilibrium, and will certainly do so for any choice of reference state except the equilibrium (compare feedback at x_{crit} in Figure 1c vs. *e-g*).

Definition 4. Feedback as the Sum of Products of Disjunct Loops

The "loop analysis" of Puccia & Levins (1985) deals mainly with systems near an equilibrium point (Puccia & Levins, 1985:194). They, too, rely heavily on the Jacobian, and indeed state that "the loop diagram has a one-to-one correspondence with [...] the Jacobian" (Puccia & Levins, 1985:159). However, Puccia & Levins's definition of "feedback" does not refer to specific state variables. Instead, "Feedback is defined in terms of *disjunct loops*" (Puccia & Levins, 1985:17). Technically,

Feedback at level k is found by determining all the loops of length k or products of disjunct loops that have a combined length of k, and then adding them together. In formula this is

$$F_k = \sum_{m=1}^{k} (-1)^{m+1} L(m,k)$$

where $L(m, k)$ is the notation meaning m disjunct loops with k elements.

(Puccia & Levins, 1985:19)

This means that the feedback at level k is the coefficient for the term λ^{n-k} in the characteristic polynomial for the Jacobian of a system at equilibrium having n variables (Puccia & Levins, 1985:164, corrected for two typographical errors). Note that the terms in the sum for F_n are what Thomas & Kaufman (2001a) call "full-circuits".

Regrettably, Puccia & Levins' verbal description of actions (Puccia & Levins, 1985:12ff) seems to contravene their claim of correspondence between actions and entries in the Jacobian. Like DeAngelis et al., they seem to focus on the actual direction of processes rather than their regulation. Their first example is a negative link from a predator to its prey, "readily interpreted to mean that the predator consumes its prey" (Puccia & Levins, 1985:12). However, the reason why the corresponding Jacobian element will often be negative is not that "the predator consumes it prey", but rather that an increase in the number of predators (a change in state) will usually result in a higher total rate of predation (a change in process). In principle, predator interference could be so strong that a higher number of predators would have a lower total rate of consumption. If so, the corresponding entry in the Jacobian would show a positive action of predator density on prey density, but the predator would still be consuming its prey.

The description of self-effects is particularly cryptic:

> Self-effects come about either because the growth rate of a variable depends on its own density [...] or because there is a source for a continuous supply of the variable from outside the system being modeled; hence, a self-effect can be independent of its own density [...] Self-effects are absent when the growth of a species is proportional to its own abundance, so that the *rate* per individual is independent of its own abundance; there is no outside supply and the growth rate can depend only on other variables.

(Puccia & Levins, 1985:13)

The assertion that state-dependence is not required for feedback contrasts with both the Jacobian-based definition and DeAngelis et al. (1986:2). As previously noted, the suggestion that self-effects are defined based on per capita rather than absolute growth rates also disagrees with the definition of the Jacobian. It seems their claim that "a self-effect can be independent of its own density" refers to a particular kind of model (Puccia & Levins, 1985:160), which can be exemplified as

$$dx/dt = I + x\,(a-by) \qquad\qquad \text{(Equation 1)}$$

where x and y are species densities, I is a constant input to x, and the per capita growth rate of x (disregarding I) depends on y but not on x. Puccia and Levins remark that "An input in the functional growth rate equation of x_1 will cause self-damping on x_1 even though there is no direct density-dependent regulation!" (Puccia & Levins, 1985:161; we use the symbol x instead of x1). However, this is a marginal phenomenon and the explanation is simple. In this system, the Jacobian element for the action of x on itself is nonzero in all state space except the line $y = a/b$; any external forcing will simply move the equilibrium away from that line and to a part of state space where x does act on itself. In our opinion, it is wrong to portray this as the external input "causing" a self-effect on x, because the self-effect is present almost everywhere in state space regardless of whether there is any external input. Restricting attention only to equilibria makes it easy to forget that feedback usually varies across state space.

The statement that "self-effects are absent when the growth of a species is proportional to its own abundance" does hold for systems like Equation 1. However, this rule seems disproved by simple exponential growth, $dx/dt = rx$. The "Jacobian" of this system is r, and so it seems that self-effects are *not* absent even though x has no effect on its relative growth rate.

Despite these problems with their verbal definition, the mathematical analysis which follows from the Jacobian is of course sound. As with the term "full-circuit", however, we find it misleading to use the term "feedback" for a sum of all possible products of disjunct loops, because these are not causally connected with each other, and thus it seems there is no feeding "back" among them.

Summary of Definitions

In summary, many useful quantities can be derived from a dynamical model, but not all of them should be called feedback. In our opinion, a positive or negative term in the rate-of-change (DeAngelis *et al.*, 1986) should be called just that. Similarly, per capita growth rates may often be adequately characterized as positively or negatively density-dependent. The coefficients of the characteristic polynomial of a linearized system (Puccia & Levins, 1985) do not represent closed causal chains, and so we believe this should not be called feedback either. What goes to the core of dynamical systems is how process rates change when the system state changes. This is what is represented by the Jacobian-based definition (Thomas, 1998; Thomas & Kaufman, 2001a; 2001b), which has an impressive track record of generic results concerning the feedback structures required for particular kinds of dynamics. It allows the conceptualization of a complex system as the set of its interacting feedback loops, rather than as the set of its individuals elements (Thomas, 1998). Typically, the number of loops is fairly small compared to the number of possible interactions in the system. Understanding the relationships between feedback structure and qualitative dynamics may also allow "reverse logic" (Thomas & Kaufman, 2001b), i.e. designing a model to fit an observed pattern (cf. Grimm *et al.*, 1996).

Our preferred feedback definition relates easily to the classic stability analyses based on the Jacobian matrix, which form the basis for all the useful results of DeAngelis et al. (1986) and Puccia & Levins (1985). However, the verbal descriptions these authors give of feedback seem at variance with the definition of the Jacobian, with each other, and with themselves. We propose that further use of the feedback concept should focus on how change-in-state causes change-in-process. For nonlinear systems it is essential to realize that the feedback structure of the system changes as the system evolves, so that even the sign of a feedback loop can vary across state space (Omholt & Plahte, 1994; Thomas & Kaufman, 2001a). Finally, we note the inherent asymmetry in the definition of action. The causal chain is not directly between state variables, but from state variable to process, in each link in the chain (Milsum, 1968a:28; Thomas & Richelle, 1988).

The Nature and Function of Positive Feedback

The real-world implications of this feedback concept shed some light on the nature and function of positive feedback. Positive feedback seems to be the least well understood aspect of feedback, and cultivating understanding of it appears essential in identifying signatures for different kinds of complex dynamics, such as alternative stable states (a.k.a. multiple attractors).

Figure 1h shows attractor shifts resulting from perturbations. In this example, a population initially regulated near its carrying capacity is reduced to below its critical size. This perturbation is amplified by positive feedback, because a reduction in the size of the population reduces its growth rate (an 'extinction vortex' in the sense of Gilpin & Soulé, 1986), and the population dwindles towards extinction. However, a pulse of immigration can bring population density above the threshold. In this case, the population growth rate increases as population density increases, and the positive-feedback loop now mediates a shift from the attractor at $x = 0$ to $x = K$. Thus, positive feedback constitutes the "hill" separating two valleys in the oft-used metaphor of state space as an undulating landscape (Figure 1i). The negative feedback stabilizing a population at carrying capacity (e.g. competition) is different from this positive-feedback mechanism (e.g. less efficient resource utilization at low population density).

This demonstrates the general principle that the mechanisms maintaining a new state differ from those that drove the shift. Petraitis and Latham (1999) emphasized the need to distinguish between the origin of a new stable state (a perturbation) and its maintenance (allegedly by positive feedback), but seem to overlook the general fact that the feedback structure of a nonlinear system is a function of its state. The strength of interactions, and possibly even their sign, will change as the system evolves. A perturbation may be reinforced by positive feedback, but the ensuing change cannot go on forever. Consequently, we must distinguish not only between origin and maintenance, but between the *origin, shift, and maintenance* of a stable state.

Failing to make this distinction may lead one to attribute each positive feedback loop to only one of the stable states. However, a positive feedback loop may cut both ways. The so-called "life-support system" of positive feedback between resource supply and consumer density (Bianchi *et al.*, 1989; Stone & Weisburd, 1992) can equally well cause a collapse, if a population falls below a threshold density required for efficient resource exploitation. Thus, positive feedback does not of necessity help a population "over the hill". Rather, it is *part of* the hill (Figure 1c,h,i). Such a mechanism pertains to both of the attractor basins that it separates.

Finally, it is essential to distinguish between loops of physical flow (e.g. of individuals or nutrients) and loops of action. In our opinion, the usage of "positive feedback" to denote closed loops of state-dependent flow such as life cycles (DeAngelis *et al.*, 1986:129) or nutrient cycles (Stone & Weisburd, 1992; Ulanowicz, 1995) is conceptually misleading (Ringelberg, 1993; Omholt & Plahte, 1994). A simple example is the regulation of biochemical processes: production rates are nonnegative, yet may be subject to negative feedback.

Generalizing the Feedback Concept

One may ask if an unambiguous concept of feedback is at all possible, given that different viewpoints may give contrasting pictures of feedback. For example, predation is often part of a negative feedback mechanism at the level of predator and prey populations, but may involve positive feedback on the level of individual predators. The population-level negative feedback results from prey mortality being higher when predators are abundant, and predators reproducing better when prey are abundant. On the individual level, a positive feedback of body size on itself (Cushing, 1992) may result if prey availability increases with predator size (near a "feeding size threshold", Griffiths, 1994) and the predator grows faster when energy intake is high.

However, it is important to realize that the choice of state variables is a question separate from the definition of feedback. It is usually valuable to have several models that focus on different aspects of a phenomenon. A feedback definition should merely be required to be unambiguous once the form of the model is decided. If feedback appears differently in complementary models, then that should stimulate investigation of why this is so.

Our preferred definition of "action" implies that verbal explanations of feedback will focus on how process rates are affected by a change in system state. This kind of statement are among the most general that can be made about natural dynamical systems, because speaking about dynamics at all *requires* a concept of process rates. Hence, this feedback concept should generalize well to biological and mathematical settings beyond ordinary differential equations. For instance, the observation of a persistent shift in a system's state leads one to look for potentially self-reinforcing mechanisms that can cause such a shift. Thus, a clear feedback concept holds promise for heuristic understanding of complex dynamics even where rigorous mathematical proofs are not yet available.

Feedback at Different Levels of Aggregation

Research on spatial pattern formation has provided many insights into how large-scale patterns are generated from small-scale feedback interactions (e.g. Meinhardt, 1997; Perrimon & McMahon, 1999). This exemplifies a very general question: What characterizes low-level mechanisms that manifest themselves as a particular kind of feedback on higher levels? The feedback concept may not by itself suffice to understand this connection. Nevertheless, a necessary first step is to describe feedback at different levels of aggregation or organization.

Such an endeavour could be based on an individual-based model, in which each entity (e.g. molecule, cell, or individual) is represented separately in a computer simulation (an i-state configuration model, in the sense of Caswell & John, 1992). The very detailed state information of such a model could be sampled and aggregated at different resolutions with respect to time, physical space or individual-state space. Given some way to describe the state-dependence of process rates, one could estimate feedback at the various levels of the system. Opting for a system with alternative stable states would ensure a feedback structure that is strongly state-dependent, and therefore easy to study.

Individual-based models exemplify many challenges in defining feedback, e.g. by their inherent stochasticity (Metz & de Roos, 1992) and volatile number of state variables. They have been advocated as more realistic than "classical" models in some ways (Huston *et al.*, 1988), and have proved useful in many fields (ecology, DeAngelis & Gross, 1992; animal behaviour, Watts, 1998; molecular genetics, Fuchslin & McCaskill, 2001). The hope for identifying feedback in individual-based models is strengthened by recent advances in estimating population process rates from individual-based models (Fahse *et al.*, 1998), and in relating individual-based to "classical" population models (Wilson, 1998; Flierl *et al.*, 1999).

Other Mathematical Frameworks

"Logical networks" of gene regulation is the other main framework where feedback has established formal as well as heuristic utility (Thomas & Richelle, 1988; Thomas & D'Ari, 1990; Thomas & Kaufman, 2001b). Switch-regulated production, countervailed by exponential decay, is a generic feature of gene regulatory systems, and serves to coordinate physiological processes (Thomas, 1998). Thus, in logical regulatory networks, the state variables are concentrations of gene products, simplified to a boolean description of "present" (i.e. above the threshold for activating synthesis of some gene product) or "absent". The processes (synthesis of gene products) are similarly simplified as being "on" (saturating near a maximum production rate) or "off", depending on the system state. When there is a mismatch between the current state and the production pattern it causes (e.g. x is being produced but is still "absent", i.e. below threshold), there is a time-delay before the state is updated. However, the time-delays usually differ among interactions, and this asynchronism precludes two variables from changing at the exact same time. Hence, which production pattern comes next may depend crucially on which variable is the first to change (Thomas & Kaufman, 2001b).

This framework generalizes easily to state variables with discrete, but more than two, possible values. It allows powerful use of graph theory to investigate the relationship between feedback structure and dynamics, yet the qualitative results often transfer to corresponding ODE systems (Thomas & Kaufman, 2001b). The main mathematical differences between the logical framework and ODEs are that the system state is discrete and time is discrete/asynchronous. Thus, process rates are no longer differentiable functions of state variables. The verbal description transfers directly from ODEs, however, as in "x acts positively on y if an increase in x would cause an increase in the production rate of y".

In other mathematical frameworks, the feedback concept is as yet poorly expressed. Some fundamental challenges arise from stochasticity, time-delays, and systems whose state variables are continuous distributions or volatile configurations. Positive feedback in a stochastic sense might relate to how a given change in state enhances the probability of similar further change (e.g. Puccia & Levins, 1985:17). Time-delays in linear systems (Nisbet & Gurney, 1982) correspond in some sense to a long chain of connected compartments. Perhaps this or similar results can form a common basis for comparing time-delayed and direct actions in a set of delay-differential equations.

Discrete-time matrix models with continuous state variables (Caswell, 2001) invite a definition of feedback similar to that for ODEs (substituting Δy for dy/dt, so that the feedback structure is given by $J-I$, i.e. the Jacobian [a.k.a. the transition matrix] minus the identity matrix). Unfortunately, analytical results from ODEs do not carry over to difference equations in a straightforward fashion. However, the transition matrix of a system of difference equations already provides much insight into its dynamics (Caswell, 2001). Lessons from ODE models suggest that it could be worthwhile to extend the focus from how population growth depends on model parameters (e.g. elasticity analysis) to how the feedback structure depends on state variables (i.e. feedback). The problem of multiple attractors is even more challenging in discrete-time than in ODE models (Caswell, 2001). On the positive side, understanding feedback in difference equations should prove immensely useful in analyzing aggregated (i.e. categorized) data from more complex models such as individual-based models or partial differential equation (PDE) models.

In PDE models, individuals are not categorized but continually distributed along some axis, e.g. size (Metz & Diekmann, 1986). Hence, within-population feedback will have to be described in some continuous fashion. A few definitions are offered by De Roos (1997), but do little to meet this need. "Feedback loops" are loosely defined as interactions with the environment, whereas "feedback functions" denote statistics of a population that enter directly into its governing equations. No advice is given on how to assign strength and sign to the actions among subgroups of the population. However, one might imagine an "action density function" $a(x_1, x_2)$ describing the action of individuals of size x_1 on individuals of size x_2. Hills or valleys in a plot of this function could be interpreted as positive or negative action of a group of individuals on another. However, *chains* of action are hard to define in this setting, as there would be an infinite number of possible action chains from one size-value to itself. This problem applies to individual-based models as well.

Physiologically structured population (PSP) models represent a population by a set of cohorts, each represented e.g. by the (common) size of its individuals, the number of individuals in the cohort, and equations governing the change in numbers and the change in individual-state (de Roos, 1997). It should in principle be possible to describe the action of one cohort on another. However, which cohorts are in the model changes over time, as cohorts are discarded when their abundance is negligible.

At present, the most feasible approach may be one based on aggregation to a moderate number of state variables. Most of the above frameworks rely on a "law of large numbers", so that state variables can be reckoned on a continuous scale (Metz & de Roos, 1992). However, a stochastic concept of feedback, based on how probabilities of change depend on the system state, should be able to deal with discrete state variables and handle issues such as demographic stochasticity in small populations.

Conclusion

A clear concept of feedback enables generic insights in the dynamics of biological systems ranging from molecular reactions, via pattern formation and population dynamics, to ecosystem function. The most successful definition of feedback describes the links in a closed action chain by how change-in-state causes change-in-process (Thieffry, 2007). This differs subtly from the common notion that a change-in-state causes further change-in-state directly.

In particular, it is essential to distinguish between loops of flow (e.g. of individual or nutrients) and loops of action (Ringelberg, 1993). Many general results, on how feedback corresponds to dynamics, now exist for two quite different mathematical settings: logical networks, and systems of differential equations. This brings hope for providing rigorous definitions for other mathematical frameworks. Equally importantly, this notion of feedback is widely applicable because the state-dependence of process rates is a fundamental feature of natural dynamical systems. This suggests that verbal and conceptual explanations focussing on how process depends on state will be heuristically useful.

References

Abrams, P. A. (1987). On classifying interactions between populations. *Oecologia,* **73**, 272-281.

Abrams, P. A. (2001). Describing and quantifying interspecific interactions: a commentary on recent approaches. *Oikos,* **94**, 209-218.

Allee, W. C. (1931). *Animal aggregations. A study in general sociology.* Chicago: University of Chicago Press.

Bianchi, T. S., Jones, C. G. & Shachak, M. (1989). Positive feedback of consumer population density on resource supply. *Trends Ecol. Evol.* **4**, 234-238.

Caswell, H. (2001). *Matrix population models: construction, analysis, and interpretation.* Sunderland, MA, USA: Sinauer.

Caswell, H. & John, A. M. (1992). From the individual to the population in demographic models. In: *Individual-based Models and Approaches in Ecology: Populations, Communities and Ecosystems* (DeAngelis, D. L. & Gross, L. J., eds) pp. 36-61. London: Chapman & Hall.

Cushing, J. M. (1992). A size-structured model for cannibalism. *Theor. Pop. Biol.,* **42**, 347-361.

de Roos, A. M. (1997). A gentle introduction to physiologically structured population models. In: *Structured-population models in marine, terrestrial and freshwater systems* (Caswell, H. & Tuljapurkar, S., eds) pp. 119-204. New York: Chapman & Hall.

DeAngelis, D. L. & Gross, L. J. (Eds.) (1992). Individual-based models and approaches in *ecology: populations, communities, and ecosystems.* Chapman and Hall, London.

DeAngelis, D. L., Post, W. M. & Travis, C. C. (1986). *Positive Feedback in Natural Systems.* Berlin: Springer-Verlag.

Dennis, B. (1989). Allee effects: population growth, critical density, and the chance of extinction. *Nat. Res. Mod.,* **3**, 481-538.

Fahse, L., Wissel, C. & Grimm, V. (1998). Reconciling classical and individual-based approaches in theoretical population ecology: A protocol for extracting population parameters from individual-based models. *Amer. Natur.* **152**, 838-852.

Flierl, G., Grunbaum, D., Levin, S. & Olson, D. (1999). From individuals to aggregations: The interplay between behavior and physics. *J. Theor. Biol.,* **196**, 397-454.

Fuchslin, R. M. & McCaskill, J. S. (2001). Evolutionary self-organization of cell-free genetic coding. *Proc. Natl. Acad. Sci.* USA, **98**, 9185-9190.

Gilpin, M. E. & Soulé, M. E. (1986). Minimum viable populations: processes of species extinction. In: *Conservation biology: the science of scarcity and diversity* (Soulé, M. E., ed) 19-34. Sunderland, Massachusetts: Sinauer Associates.

Gouze, J. L. (1998). Positive and negative circuits in dynamical systems. *J. Biol. Syst.,* **6**, 11-15.

Griffiths, D. (1994). The size structure of lacustrine Arctic charr (Pisces: Salmonidae) populations. *Biol. J. Linnean Soc.,* **51**, 337-357.

Grimm, V., Frank, K., Jeltsch, F., Brandl, R., Uchmanski, J. & Wissel, C. (1996). Pattern-oriented modelling in population ecology. *Sci. Total Environ.,* **183**, 151-166.

Holling, C. S. (1973). Resilience and stability of ecological systems. *Ann. Rev. Ecol. Syst.,* **4**, 1-24.

Huston, M., DeAngelis, D. L. & Post, W. (1988). New Computer Models Unify Ecological Theory. *BioScience,* **38**, 682-691.

Meinhardt, H. (1997). Biological pattern formation as a complex dynamic phenomenon. *Int. J. Bifurc. Chaos,* **7**, 1-26.

Metz, J. A. J. & de Roos, A. M. (1992). The role of physiologically structured population models within a general individual-based modeling perspective. In: *Individual-based Models and Approaches in Ecology: Populations, Communities and Ecosystems* (DeAngelis, D. L. & Gross, L. J., eds) pp. 88-111. London: Chapman & Hall.

Metz, J. A. J. & Diekmann, O. (Eds.) (1986). *The dynamics of physiologically structured populations.* Springer, Berlin.

Milsum, J. H. (1968b). Mathematical introduction to general system dynamics. In: *Positive feedback: a general systems approach to positive/negative feedback and mutual causality* (Milsum, J. H., ed) 23-65. Oxford: Pergamon Press.

Milsum, J. H. (Eds.), (1968a). *Positive feedback: a general systems approach to positive/negative feedback and mutual causality.* Pergamon Press, New York.

Murray, J. D. (1993). *Mathematical Biology.* Berlin: Springer-Verlag.

Nisbet, R. M. & Gurney, W. S. C. (1982). *Modelling fluctuating populations.* Chichester: Wiley.

Omholt, S. W. & Plahte, E. (1994). Feedback confusions. *J. Theor. Biol.,* **168**, 231-231.

Omholt, S. W., Plahte, E., Øyehaug, L. & Xiang, K. F. (2000). Gene regulatory networks generating the phenomena of additivity, dominance and epistasis. *Genetics,* **155**, 969-980.

Perrimon, N. & McMahon, A. P. (1999). Negative feedback mechanisms and their roles during pattern formation. *Cell,* **97**, 13-16.

Petraitis, P. S. & Latham, R. E. (1999). The importance of scale in testing the origins of alternative community states. *Ecology,* **80**, 429-442.

Plahte, E., Mestl, T. & Omholt, S. W. (1995). Feedback loops, stability and multistationarity in dynamical systems. *J. Biol. Syst.,* **3**, 409-413.

Puccia, C. J. & Levins, R. (1985). *Qualitative modeling of complex systems: an introduction to loop analysis and time averaging.* Cambridge, Massachusetts: Harvard University Press.

Ringelberg, J. (1993). A fed-back flow does not make a feedback. *Trends Ecol. Evol.,* **8**, 35-36.

Scheffer, M., Hosper, S. H., Meijer, M. L., Moss, B. & Jeppesen, E. (1993). Alternative equilibria in shallow lakes. *Trends Ecol. Evol.,* **8**, 275-279.

Snoussi, E. H. (1998). Necessary conditions for multistationarity and stable periodicity. *J. Biol. Syst.,* **6**, 3-9.

Stone, L. & Weisburd, R. S. J. (1992). Positive feedback in aquatic ecosystems. *Trends Ecol. Evol.,* **7**, 263-267.

Sutherland, J. P. (1974). Multiple stable points in natural communities. *Amer. Natur.,* **108**, 859-873.

Thieffry, D. (2007). Dynamical roles of biological regulatory circuits. *Briefings in Bioinformatics,* **8**, 220-225.

Thomas, R. (1998). Laws for the dynamics of regulatory networks. *International Journal of Developmental Biology,* **42**, 479-485.

Thomas, R. (1999). Deterministic chaos seen in terms of feedback circuits: Analysis, synthesis, "labyrinth chaos". *Int. J. Bifurc. Chaos,* **9**, 1889-1905.

Thomas, R. & D'Ari, R. (1990). *Biological Feedback*. Boca Raton, Florida: CRC Press.

Thomas, R. & Kaufman, M. (2001a). Multistationarity, the basis of cell differentiation and memory. I. Structural conditions of multistationarity and other nontrivial behavior. *Chaos,* **11**, 170-179.

Thomas, R. & Kaufman, M. (2001b). Multistationarity, the basis of cell differentiation and memory. II. Logical analysis of regulatory networks in terms of feedback circuits. *Chaos,* **11**, 180-195.

Thomas, R. & Richelle, J. (1988). Positive feedback loops and multistationarity. *Discrete Applied Mathematics,* **19**, 381-396.

Ulanowicz, R. E. (1995). *Utricularia*'s secret: the advantage of positive feedback in oligotrophic environments. *Ecol. Modell.,* **79**, 49-57.

Watts, J. M. (1998). Animats: Computer-simulated animals in behavioral research. *J. Anim. Sci.,* **76**, 2596-2604.

Wilson, J. B. & Agnew, A. D. Q. (1992). Positive-feedback switches in plant communities. *Adv. Ecol. Res.,* **23**, 263-336.

Wilson, W. G. (1998). Resolving discrepancies between deterministic population models and individual-based simulations. *Amer. Natur.,* **151**, 116-134.

In: Synthetic and Integrative Biology
Editor: James T. Gevona, pp. 123-148

ISBN 978-1-60876-678-9
ⓒ 2010 Nova Science Publishers, Inc.

Chapter 7

TRANSLATIONAL RESEARCH: NOVEL TECHNOLOGIES, IMPACT ON SCIENCES AND POTENTIAL IN ALTERNATIVE MEDICINES

Christine Nardini
MPG-CAS PICB Shanghai, China

Abstract

Advances in biotechnology have and are providing -for the analysis of events occurring at the molecular genome-wide level- innovative tools which change deeply the scientific and medical landscape of this century. These tools in fact are not only offering more detailed and abundant data, but, also a different -systemic- vision on how molecular mechanisms operate, with direct impact on our way to perceive the chemophysical mechanisms that underlie drug discovery, therapy delivery, and ultimately medicine and health care. To effectively take advantage of the novel technologies, biology and medicine cannot be any longer two separate and distinct fields, they need to interact in order to bring the discoveries of the fundamental mechanisms of activity of the cells into applicative actions at the patients bedside. This is carried on by the so called *translational research*. This chapter will present an introduction on the technologies that are promoting these profound changes, an overview on some of the most striking changes occurring in biology, pharmacology and medicine, the areas most closely related to health care. All these concepts will be used as the rationale to deepen and promote the use of the scientific approach to complementary and alternative medicine, an area too poorly explored and yet bearing the promise to offer alternatives in our way to approach diseases. This chapter aims at providing the background necessary to understand the scientific bases and current evidence that allow to perceive this area as a promising area of development, along with the limitations and issues that need to be solved.

1. Introduction

Translational research is a novel approach to life sciences with the specific goal to enhance and accelerate their applications in healthcare. In particular, it focuses on multidisciplinary collaboration among life sciences, exact sciences and medicine, with the aim of advancing molecular-based medicine. In fact, it aims to enable physicians to leverage systems-biology approaches to allow early detection of complex diseases, increase efficiency in drug development and therapy testing, improve drug efficacy, and enable personalized medicine. Such an approach is necessary to narrow the gap existing between clinical practice and basic research, to accelerate the bidirectional flow of scientific discoveries into the clinic and of clinical findings into novel research directions, and to realize the return on investment made by private and public institutions on life science basic research. To fully realize this vision, translational research requires scientists and clinicians to have access to three types of information: (i) clinical information: including data contained in hospital systems and medical records, pathology reports and diagnostic labs, clinical trials systems and study participant questionnaires; (ii) biomolecular information: including genomics, proteomics, medical imaging and other high-throughput molecular and cellular research data; (iii) methods and tools: to synergistically process the data described above.

This chapter will expand the concepts introduced above: systems biology, drug development, and systems and personalized medicine, with special focus on their current evolution and changes and having a specific application target in view: the yet obscure and controversial area of Complementary and Alternative Medicine (CAM), focussing on acupuncture. The objective of this work is twofold: (1) offer a view of the breadth of the impact of the recent and revolutionary technological changes in life sciences, their connection to exact sciences and their impact on health care application, and (2) provide the reader with the knowledge and tools necessary to appreciate the importance of translational medicine and in particular its potential in the area of CAM, which could provide a large reservoir of untapped knowledge in the query of solutions for several challenges in health related problems.

The chapter is organized as follows: Section 2. introduces the new technologies responsible for the advancements of molecular biology, more emphasis will be given on this part as it represents the base on which the advances described in the following sections are based. Section 3. presents how these technologies change several scientific areas with emphasis in Section 3.1. on their impact on biology; in Section 3.2. on their impact on pharmacology with an introduction to the latest evolution in drug research from a systems perspective; in Section 3.3. on their impact on medicine with introduction to personalized and systems medicines. Section 4. will specifically deal with the application of these concepts to CAM and in particular acupuncture, with a case study for potential application: Rheumatoid Arthritis. Finally, Section 5. will summarize the introduced topics and discuss the problems and openings for future work.

2.   New Technologies

Current tools and technologies allow to screen the cell's molecular activity at the genome-wide level for all types of molecules involved in the cellular information processing. DNA, RNA and proteins are the fundamental actors of such system, and, through complex and highly non-linear mechanisms, they are used by the cell to exchange information and accomplish functions. Current tools allow the highly parallel monitoring of number of such functioning, involving sometimes different types of defects such as DNA mutation, RNA over/under-expression, disequilibria in protein patterns and more. To illustrate these tools and their relation to the activity of the cell, we base the following discussion on an extended version of the fundamental principle of molecular biology (see Figure 2), which in summary, indicates how the flow of information inside the cell moves from the the data encoded in the DNA to the information transcribed in mRNA and potentially translated into proteins, the more direct actuators of molecular functions, or silenced in some measure by miRNA, small RNAs whose potential and function are under active research, and that share the ability to modulate the final gene expression.

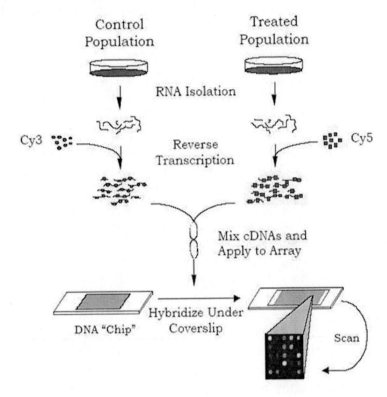

Figure 1. A schematic representation of a comparative genetic analysis performed with double channel microarrays. Two different cell populations are taken into consideration, one for analysis (for example after treatment) and one for control. Form both cell populations RNA is isolated, reversely transcribed, and labeled adding two different dyes (in this case Cy3, Cy5). The mixture of both labeled RNAs is then spread on the array, where competitive hybridization can take place. Scan of the slide is then performed to read out fluorescence corresponding to different expression activity. The same principle holds for DNA and miRNA arrays. Adapted from: www.uwec.edu, and further used with 2008 ACM, Inc. Included here by permission, [2].

Interactions among nucleic acids molecules (polynucleotides) include DNA, mRNA, miRNA interactions and exploit the same mechanism for recognition: *hybridization* that consists of the binding of complementary nucleotides from two different molecular sequences. This in fact takes advantage of the fundamental characteristic of polynucleotides, that makes these molecules so successful in the perpetuation of life, that is its ability to duplicate, using one strand of molecule, thanks to the fact that the 4 nucleotides (Adenine, Guanine, Cytosine, Thymine, A, G, C, T) pair spontaneously (A with T and C with G). In this process, the complementary segment (known, used as blueprint) can be shorter than the hybridizing molecules (often unknown). This phenomenon is exploited in arrayed analysis tools (also called chips) to test the level of complementarity between species immobilized on the array sites and species present in a solution, obtained from proper molecules extraction of cells of interest. DNA interactions are used to study mutations, mRNA and miRNA interactions for the observation of different modulations of genes expression. In this context, the more widespread screens are by far mRNA screens, appeared roughly 15 years ago [1], the basic functioning of this technology is given below for illustrative and also didactic purpose, as many of the polynucleotide microarray (and in particular recently miRNA arrays) based screens follow the same principles (for more technical details see [2]). The technical solutions used to perform parallel hybridization are numerous but can be grouped in 2 main categories, notably for the choice of the blueprint molecules on the chip. In the first type they are fragments of cellular extracts and their length goes from 20 to hundreds of base pairs (because they perform the comparative analysis of the molecules abundance in two cells populations they are called two channels); in the second type they are synthesized short probes ($15 - 25\ bp$) of known sequence which are able to capture specific fragments (these chips are called single-channel). The fragments diluted in the sample solution are pre-processed and coupled with a permanent marker molecule which, once the fragment has been captured by a complementary strand on the surface of the chip, is able to generate a localized detectable signal (hence the well known microarray heatmaps see Figure 1 for an example of the representation of the process). Although the reproducibility of the results is not perfect, the MicroArray Quality Control Project (MAQC), led by the U.S. Food and Drug Administration (FDA) [3] proved that findings can be shown to overlap, provided great care is used in the definition of the experimental protocols, and that results are compared in terms of genes functionalities. These problems may soon be overcome by broadly available and more precise sequencing technologies, able to offer quantitative information on the molecules' abundance. However, for differential analyses (i.e. identification of genome-wide differences in expression among samples taken from different patients, after different treatments, at different time points etc.) microarrays remain a yet cheaper and valuable approach [4, 5].

Proteomics (the study of proteins at genome-wide scale) represents a very complex area of research due to the large existing number of proteins (the estimate for the human proteome is $500,000$ proteins), to the complexity of the molecules' structure, and to the variety of interactions they can have. Nevertheless, there exist broadly used high-throughput techniques for proteomics, in particular: two-dimensional gel electrophoresis (2DE) and liquid chromatography-tandem mass spectrometry (LC-MS/MS).

2-DE couples two techniques for protein classification. The first is named *isoelectric focusing* (IEF), and uses an electric current applied to a gel matrix to separate protein based on electric charge. More precisely, a gradient of pH is applied to a gel and an electric potential is applied across the gel. At all pHs other than the one at which the protein carries no net electrical charge (isoelectric point) proteins will be charged and will be pulled towards the more positive or more negative end of the gel. The second technique, *SDS-PAGE* (sodium dodecyl sulfate polyacrylamide gel electrophoresis) is used to separate proteins based on their electrophoretic mobility, which is fundamentally a function of the length of the polypeptide chain (roughly proportional to its molecular weight when the protein is unfolded). SDS-PAGE unfolds the polypeptide chain, and each chain is processed in order to have the same mass-to-charge ratio (this is the result of attaching to each protein fragment a number of SDS negatively charged molecules proportional to the fragment length). When a second electric potential is applied to the gel (orthogonal to the one used for IEF), the proteins will derive in the gel, but will be slowed in their migration by frictional forces proportional to the length of the fragment (since the mass-to-charge ratio is approximately identical for all proteins). Ultimately then 2-DE allows the discrimination of protein bases on their electric charge and molecular weight, as it is shown in Figure 2.. Depending on the gel size and pH gradient used, 2-DE can resolve more than 5000 proteins simultaneously [6].

Mass spectrometry (MS, [7]) is a technique used for the identification of the composition of a molecule. Its principle consists of ionizing chemical compounds to generate charged molecules and measurement of their mass-to-charge ratios. MS instruments consist of three modules: an ion source, which can convert gas phase sample molecules into ions; a mass analyzer, which sorts the ions by their masses by applying electromagnetic fields; and a detector, which measures the value of an indicator quantity and thus provides data for calculating the abundances of each ion present. MS can be applied in several rounds (tandem mass spectrometry) usually separated by molecule fragmentation. When tandem mass spectrometry is used in combination with liquid chromatography (LC/MS or LC-MS) the molecules under study are chromatographically separated (thanks to the different speed at which the fragments of interest run through the chromatography column) before they are introduced to the ion source and mass spectrometer. This stream of separated compounds is fed into the ion source. Complex samples may be run in a modern LC-MS/MS system and result in over 1000 proteins being identified, provided that the sample was first separated for example on an SDS-PAGE gel, described above, a general illustration of the process is shown in Figure 2..

To screen protein-protein interaction yeast two hybrid assays (Y2H, [8]) are commonly used. This technique is based on the activation of a reporter gene due to the binding of a transcription factor onto a sequence upstream of the reporter gene (Upstream Activating Sequence, UAS). The transcription factor is split into two separate fragments, called the binding domain (BD) and activating domain (AD). The BD is the domain responsible for binding to the UAS and the AD is the domain responsible for the activation of transcription. The activation of the transcription is only possible if the two portions (AD and BD) are reunited. Y2H screens require in fact the preparation of two fusion proteins, one containing the AD domain with one of the two proteins of interest, and the other one containing the BD domain with the second protein on interest. Only if the 2 proteins of interest interact will the AD and BD domain be reunited and able to properly start the transcription. Thus, the activation of the gene downstream of the UAS will report the reunion of AD and BD proteins mediated by the binding of the two proteins of interest. This technique is also applied with high parallelism (HTP-Y2H) [9].

The interaction among DNA and proteins is relevant to understand how promoters interact with DNA allowing the expression of genes, to initiate, reinforce or interrupt specific molecular functions. The connection between DNA and proteins, in fact, represents a fundamental step in the regulation of cell activity, as follows: the structure of a gene includes not only the set of sequences that are actually transcribed (exons) and other non-coding regions (introns) but also the *promoter region*. This portion of the DNA is recognized by *transcription factors* (TF, a protein), that bind to the promoter sequences and recruit the RNA polymerase, the enzyme that allows the actual synthesis of mRNA. Promoter regions can also be assisted in the transcription process by other DNA sequences called enhancers or silencers (regions where proteins that enable or disable the actual transcription of the DNA can bind, facilitating or impeding the transcription process). The study of promoters and transcription factors is in close interaction with *histones*, the more abundant proteins that envelope the chromosomes and constitute the *chromatin*. Histones modifications are necessary for promoters, transcription factors and RNA polymerase to access the coiled DNA and start transcription. Some of these modifications can also be inherited, uncovering these mechanisms is the object of the study of *epigenomics* (see the Human Epigenome Project [10]).

Some techniques exist to analyze DNA-protein interactions, the most widespread is named ChIP-chip. Since the relation promoter-gene can be multiple (one promoter can bind in more than one location on the genome), this technique aims at the identification of one promoters and all its target genes (protein-DNA interaction) by associating a precipitation technique with microarray technology. First, the precipitation technique, namely Chromatin ImmunoPrecipitation (ChIP) is applied. In particular, DNA and promoter proteins are allowed to cross-link in vivo under suitable conditions to form a promoter-DNA complex. Then, antibodies (proteins that have the ability to target a specific 'coupled' protein, the antigen, an approach designed by the immune system for recognition and control of possibly harmful molecules) corresponding to the promoter proteins and associated to agarose beads are added to the mixture to capture the appropriate promoters-DNA complexes. Beads are precipitated by centrifugation along with the complexes bead-promoter-DNA, that are then separated from all other molecules. DNA is finally extracted and fragmented and fluorescently labeled. The technique is then coupled with a microarray approach: the device is exposed to a mixture of the input DNA labeled with a different fluorophores and of the DNA fragments obtained by immunoprecipitation. This technique reveals the binding position of specific promoters on the genome. Globally this screening is often referred to as ChIP-chip. Recently, another technique called Proteomics of Isolated Chromatin segments (PICh, [11]) has been proposed. PICh acts "in reverse", and it uses a specific DNA probe (instead of a specific antibody) to isolate proteins from fixed cells, which are then characterized using mass spectrometry described above. This overcomes the limitation of ChIP-chip that must rely on antibodies to known DNA-binding proteins. However, due to the use of MS it requires relatively large amounts of proteins.

Sequencing technologies have undergone a rapid evolution in the past few years, highly improving the precision and throughput of the previous methods, and can now be used to measure the abundance of several polynucleotides, improving on several of the techniques described above. The main technologies are briefly introduced below.

The first techniques adopted for sequencing were initiated by Maxam and Gilbert in the early '70s [12], and based on the cleavage of short polynucleotides, which were then identified thanks to their different migration characteristics in two dimensional paper chromatography. This technique was very time consuming, but achieved nevertheless the sequencing of the Lac Operon in *E. coli*. Later on in the mid '70s, Sanger et al. [13], gave the first fundamental impulsion to higher throughput for sequencing introducing the replication of the sample via the design of primers and the use of polymerase. Basically, the Sanger method requires a single-stranded DNA template, a DNA primer, a DNA polymerase, radioactively or fluorescently labeled nucleotides, and modified nucleotides that terminate DNA strand elongation. Each sample undergoes 4 sequencing reactions, each with all the regular nucleotides and only one of the four dideoxynucleotides (ddATP, ddGTP, ddCTP, or ddTTP) which are the chain-terminating nucleotides. Synthesis is performed and at the end of the process each of the 4 reactions will contain terminated DNA fragments of varying length. These fragments are separated in 2D gels, and as described above for proteins, longer polynucleotide molecules are also slowed down in their migration, then it is possible to read spatially the extended polynucleotides, and identify sequentially the nucleotides forming the chain, thanks to the fact they terminate the sequence at different points. In particular, the introduction of labeled (radio- or fluorescent-) nucleotide terminators improved the efficiency and permitted the automatization of the final readings. This approach and its automation have been the leading technology until the early 2000, when flow cell sequencing has changed the sequencing landscape. Broadly defined, a flow cell is a reaction chamber that contains templates attached to a solid support, to which nucleotides and necessary reagents are iteratively applied and washed away (with few exceptions, described below), with the goal of generating multiple copies of the template. Templates must be preprocessed (library construction) usually by attaching to the fragments of the polynucleotides to be read some flanking sequence able to bind to the primer that will initiate the amplification. Duplicate molecules are then sequenced by synthesis. There are currently 5 main technologies to achieve this [14, 15], summarized in Table 1.

The first (Roche GC-FLX, former GS20 by 454 Life Sciences, known as 454 sequencing) uses a flat fiber optic plate with 1.6 million 75-picoliter wells used as small test tubes. Ideally in each tube a different template is attached to a bead and amplified in a droplet of PCR reaction mixture within an oil emulsion. Sequencing is obtained by iterative pyrosequencing [16] which allows the sequencing of a single strand of DNA, thanks to the synthesis of the complementary strand along it. The method exploits the fact that at each iteration a buffer containing one of four nucleotides is passed horizontally over the wells, and is incorporated (when appropriate) into the growing complementary chain. The nucleotides used are in fact deoxyribonucleotide triphosphate (dNTPs), which, when incorporated by polymerase, release a pyrophosphate molecule. This molecule, when converted to ATP by sulfurylase, generates a luciferase-catalyzed luminometric signal detected by a charge coupled device (CCD) camera. After washout of residual nucleotides, the cycle is repeated with the next dNTP.

The second technology (1G Analyzer developed by Solexa and now distributed by Illumina) consists of a planar optically transparent surface on which oligonucleotides acting as primers for amplification of the templates are bound. Amplification is obtained with the so called solid-phase bridge PCR: each sample hybridizes to one of the primer on the planar surface, and once the hybridization cycle initiates, the sample will also tend to hybridize to the second primer, thus forming a bridge on the planar surface. Amplification is performed along this bridge, then, finally, denaturation leaves the planar surface populated with amplified samples, attached by either primer side and grouped in clusters. At the end of this amplification phase, sequencing is performed by synthesis using reversible four-color fluorescence (a mix of the four bases each labeled with a different cleavable fluorophore, such that they can be used simultaneously rather than sequentially). After base extension and recording of the fluorescent signal at each cluster, the sequencing reagents are washed away, labels are cleaved, and the 3' end of the incorporated base is unblocked in preparation for the next nucleotide addition.

The third technology is the SOLiD (Supported Oligonucleotide Ligation and Detection) from Applied Biosystems. Amplification is obtained by emulsion PCR (like in 454), and amplified templates are then immobilized with high density to a flow cell (like in Illumina). Each cycle of sequencing involves the ligation of fluorescently labeled octamers, where the fluorescent label correlates to the central (base 5) nucleotide. After ligation of the octamer to the template, images are acquired in four channels. These images collect data for the same base positions across all template-bearing beads. Then, the octamer is chemically cleaved between positions 5 and 6, removing the fluorescent label. Progressive rounds of octamer ligation enable sequencing of every 5th base. When this first cycle is completed, the sample amplified from the primer is denatured and the system is reset. At this point the process is repeated with an offset to read a different set of positions (from base 4 instead of base 5, with an offset of 5 as before). This technique can also allow the use of two-base encoding (i.e. the fluorescent label correlates with 4 out of 16 possible nucleotide couples, i.e. base 5 and 6), which provides an error-correction scheme. In this way, each base position is queried twice (once as the first base, and once as the second base, in a set of 2 bp interrogated on a given cycle) such that miscalls are easier to identify. This makes the SOLiD system one of the most accurate. The current technology is SOLiD 3. The Polonator (www.polonator.org) in Church laboratory at Harvard uses the same principle and off-the-shelf instrumentation and reagents [17]. The package is developed for commercial distribution by Danaher Motion, the technology is open source and economically very advantageous, however reads length is very short.

All these technologies require amplification in clusters in order to read the nucleotide synthesized and identify the sequence.

The fourth technology, Heliscope, does not need amplification, and performs sequencing on a single molecule. With this method, oligonucleotide fragments of $100 - 200$ bases are first attached along a substrate within a microfluidics flow cell. Nucleotides with a bright fluorophore (these are more readily detectable, and thus the system does not need amplification of the template) are introduced one species at a time and incorporated by DNA polymerase to the growing complementary strand. Again, images are then recorded and analysed to identify which nucleotide was incorporated into which growing strand, before the cycle is repeated with a different species of nucleotide.

Finally, the method developed by Pacific Biosciences also uses single molecules of DNA polymerase immobilized in 10^{-21} liter wells where labelled nucleotides are incorporated into a complementary strand. Because of the reduced volume of the wells, nucleotides concentration is very high, which results in fast synthesis and highly focused detection. Imaging is carried out continuously, thus, each newly incorporated base can be read in a short time. Finally, the approach uses of phospho-linked, (not base-labelled) nucleotides, in this way the preceding fluorophore is removed after incorporation of the next base and diffuses out of the detection volume, resulting in low background noise and high accuracy. This system can generate reads that are thousands of nucleotides long (at the expense of overall throughput).

Although sequencing was massively used for reading DNA molecules, the novel technologies all bear the strong limitation of generating short reads, which are not appropriate for genomes sequencings. Although this is improving at very fast pace, this limitation has in fact opened the doors to novel applications, in particular for RNA sequencing. It is then possible nowadays to sequence mRNAs and miRNAs, and, these approaches being more precise quantitatively ([4, 18]), they are likely to represent the future for transcriptomics (RNA-Seq). Based on the same rationale the chips used for DNA fragments detected in ChIP and now hybridized to a microarray may soon be sequenced (ChIP-seq).

Table 1. Principal sequencing technologies.

Platform	Sequencing by Synthesis	Template Preparation	Read Length
454 GS-FLX	Pyrosequencing	Emulsion PCR	250bp
Solexa	Polymerase with reversible terminators	Bridge PCR	36bp
SOLiD 3	Octamers ligation with 2 base-encoding	Emulsion PCR	35bp
Polonator	Nonamers ligation	Emulsion PCR	13bp
HeliScope	Polymerase with virtual terminators	-	30bp
Pacific Biosciences	Polymerase with phospho-linked nucleotides	-	1000bp

3. Applications to Sciences

3.1. Impact on Biology

Molecular biology describes and investigates the mechanisms regulating the chemical and functional interactions among the molecular actors playing in the cell. After the identification of the structure of DNA [20, 21], the first fundamental mechanisms of communication in the cell were uncovered (transcription, translation), and continuous improvements are made possible by concurrent technological advancements that enable the automated and high-throughput molecular analyses, described above. Thanks to these multiple advancements (which touched their highest diffusion in 2003 with the first complete draft of the decoding of the human genome, initiating the Genomic Era [22]) life sciences have undergone a major change, often defined as a paradigm shift from the *reductionist* to the *systemic* approach [23].

In fact, notwithstanding the fact that systems theory is a well established field, its application in life science had not been considered as a viable and systematic option to explain biological events beforehand. This novel perception of biological process as a *network* of

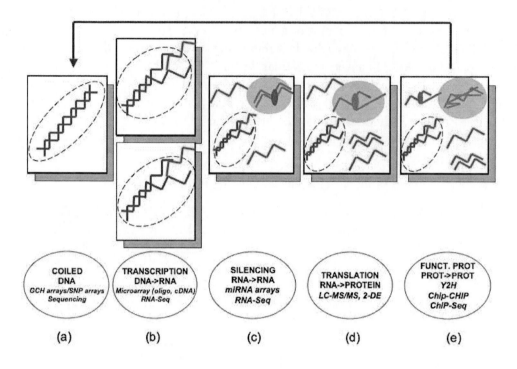

Figure 2. Flow of information in the cell, based on the fundamental principle of molecular biology. From left to right coiled DNA (blue, coiled, double-stranded molecule) is unfolded and transcribed into RNA (red, single-stranded molecule). Depending on the exact sequence of the encoding strands of DNA (exons) that are transcribed, the same gene can give rise to different proteins (variants of the gene), this fact is depicted with the two boxes in Panel (b). Once the mRNA molecule exits the nucleus (nucleus membrane represented by a dotted black line) it can be destroyed (degraded) by a complex mechanisms involving several molecules, highlighted in gray in Panel (c) (here oversimplified with a green molecule, representing the RISC complex responsible for the miRNA processing). If the RNA reaches the ribosome (purple dot, highlighted in gray) it can be translated into the corresponding sequence of aminoacids, Panel (d). Form there, with the help of other proteins (chaperone-proteins), if the aminoacids sequence is perfect, it is then folded in the appropriate 3-dimensional structure, highlighted in gray in Panel (e). The transcription process of a gene continues until the appropriate signal is not sent back to the DNA, through some specific inhibitory mechanism. Below each panel, in italic the platforms that allow high-throughput screen analyses. 2008 ACM, Inc. Included here by permission, [2].

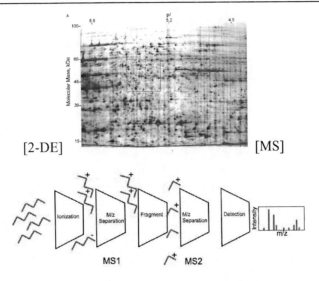

[2-DE]   [MS]

Figure 3. Figure 2. shows an example of output of 2-DE technology. In this assay a narrow pH range isoelectric focusing 2D gel (pH 4.95.5) is shown. Soluble yeast protein (500 μg) was loaded onto the gel. More than 1,500 features were visible by silver staining, the dotted square includes an arbitrary $4 - cm^2$ region of the gel that was selected for further analysis in [19] by the MS techniques. Copyright 2000 National Academy of Sciences, U.S.A. [19]. Schematic representation of a tandem mass spectrometer. Two stages of mass analysis (MS1, MS2) separation are accomplished with individual mass spectrometer elements separated in space.

events more than the sum of independent pathways, is leading to a more holistic view of diseases and is commonly referred to as the study of *omic* data [24]. This approach allows the definition of more comprehensive molecular portraits of diseases, and, importantly, permits to perceive both commonalities and differences among molecular profiles of individuals. This will lead, through the *translation* of the newly acquired knowledge into medicine, to personalized approaches in clinical diagnostics and therapy, through the individual monitoring at molecular level.

Systems Biology is the result of the effort of building an interdisciplinary approach to molecular biology to improve our understanding of the fundamental molecular mechanisms that regulate life. One distinctive characteristic of this area is its interdisciplinarity. In fact, in order to model the system, a continuous iteration between experimental and simulated data, empirical results and algorithms definition are used, with the aims of understanding more complex and dynamic relationships among genes activity, using networks approaches and graph theories as they promise to enhance the understanding of relationships among genes [25, 26].

In particular, the last 15 years, since the introduction of microarrays for gene expression [1] have seen an evolution of approaches trying to exploit, rather than avoid data complexity. A useful frame to read these advancements can be found in [27], where the evolution of a specific application of systems biology, network based drug discovery (NBDD), is described in 3 phases: (i) use of gene expression signatures, to provide for example a prognosis for cancers [28, 29, 30]; (ii) connection between genomic analyses and genome-wide association (GWA) study, using information on DNA variation to reveal the root causes of diseases, finally combined with gene expression or other molecular phenotypic data to determine whether DNA variations that seem to be associated with disease are also associated with expression levels of an individual gene, for example see [31]; (iii) genotype, gene expression, protein-protein interaction, DNAprotein binding and protein complex data integration to construct a probabilistic, causal gene network to predict the main regulators of important biological subnetworks or modules, and from there to identify relevant drug targets [32].

Important applications of systems biology have shown that this approach can actively contribute to generate knowledge and evidence to be further used in medicine. Recently, Chavali et al. performed an analysis of the metabolism of *Leishmania major* [33] a poorly and yet very widespread organism, which causes cutaneous leishmaniasis in mammalian hosts, with an incidence rate of 2 millions per year, leading to roughly 59000 deaths, worldwide. In their work, they characterized a network including more than 500 genes and thousand metabolites and reactions. This model was then used to simulate the lethality of single and double gene deletions, further validated with experimental approaches. Having the ability to characterize the metabolism of this pathogen can promptly provide ways to identify ideal therapeutic targets, i.e. the ones that can readily lead to disrupting the live sustaining activity of the pathogen, with a minimum number of side effects for the host. In general such approaches have strong mathematical roots, which then develop in a specific methodology. In this case flux balance equations were the base of the model, for the reconstruction of the so called S-matrix having in rows metabolites and in columns reactions and including stoichiometric coefficients corresponding to chemical transformation in the network. This approach allows the reconstruction of metabolic networks [34]. Another example is given by the definition of the S-systems ([35]) which allow simplified manipulations of non-linear equations apt at the description of biological interactions. Also, several theoretical approaches were imported from mathematics and systems theory into the broad area of gene network reconstruction based on linearized differential equations [36, 37], boolean [38], bayesian [39] models or association networks [40].

Available methods for the reverse engineering of biological networks can also find applications in human cells and not only in lower eukaryotes with simple genomes. An interesting example comes from the application of the identification of a relevance network in human B cells [41]. In this work, Basso et al. collected different genome-wide expression profiling experiments from more than 300 microarrays samples where normal, tumor and manipulated human B cells had been diversely collected. The existence of different conditions or perturbations is crucial for network reconstruction, as this allows the observation of the system in different states which highlight and explain the flexibility of the system itself. They then applied ARACNE [40], an algorithm for the computation of mutual information (an information theory measure able to identify non linear associations between variables, [42]) to the expression profiles of all genes across the 336 experiments. They were also able to eliminate a remarkable part of false positive associations, thanks to the use of the Data Processing Inequality (DPI), a triangular inequality allowing the removal of indirect connections among variables. With this approach they were able to reconstruct a gene network with expected topology: scale free networks. These types of network have a peculiar, exponential, distribution of the connections departing (or reaching) each node. This means that a large number of nodes has few connections, and a small number of nodes has several connections. These nodes are called *hubs* and they represent the robustness of the network. In fact, their high degree of connectivity (number of links attached to a node) allows the nodes to be reachable even if a large number of connections is distrupted. This structure is very robust in case of random break-down of the connections, while it is very fragile in case attacks to the network are programmed towards the hubs. This structure appears to be quite "natural", i.e. it seems to be the result of the *preferential attachment* principle, quite ubiquitous in nature, that states that nodes that have more connections will continue to see their degree of connectivity rising, since it is more economical and efficient for the communication across the network (as a classical example: an airport with more available destination than others will see new airports routes preferentially connect to it) [43]. Back to the B-cells network, interestingly, among the most highly connected genes, Basso et al. found *cMYC* which in turn connects to known and unknown targets (successively experimentally validated) showing how such an approach is able to identify relevant targets in the control of all B cells related diseases.

These advanced were achieved with a synergic use of high throughput data, algorithmic approaches from a variety of areas (physics, mathematics, computer sciences and so on) and subsequent final validation of the *in silico* findings. With the growing availability of data, this integration will become stronger, and promises to accelerate our understanding of the complex interplay among different layers of molecules (proteins, DNA, RNA).

3.2. Impact on Pharmacology

Pharmacology is the study of the interactions that occur between a living organism and exogenous chemicals that alter normal biochemical function. Although based on very ancient principles, this science has achieved tremendous advances in the last decades with the ability to identify or synthesize the molecules apt at targeting molecules whose abundance or activity was gone awry. This success story was based in the past decades on advanced knowledge of the genes and proteins activity, and on the idea that the identification of THE molecule gone awry was the gold standard to reverse the disrupted process. Despite great successes that have make the pharmacology industry blossom in the past 20 years, there is now a strong change in the rate of discovery of new drugs able to target highly spreading complex diseases. The reason for this difficulty may report to different causes, however, several authors [44, 45, 46] indicate that the main issue may lie in the approach to pharmaceutical research. The ideal one-gene-one-disease-one-drug paradigm, seems to have exahusted its potential, and in this area, as well, the reductionistic approach may have to give the pace to a more systemic approach, similar and following the shift in paradigm that molecular biology is undergoing with the advent of systems biology.

The necessity of this shift, in fact, is rooted in the recent discoveries in the area of molecular biology, and in particular, the latest phenomena connected to the effects of knock-out. It appears in fact that, across a number of model organisms, only up to 19% of the genes knock-out lead to lethality. Systems biology is offering remarkable insights in this direction, showing for example how single versus multiple knock-out can reveal completely different degrees of damages to the organisms (see above, [33]), bringing upfront the necessity of new concepts like disease-causing network vs disease-causing gene. Interestingly, more-over, the lower percentage of genes that are crucial for survival under ideal conditions, increases abruptly when other molecules are added besides the knock-out, indicating that although the redundancy and robustness of the network can cope with the failure of a limited number of nodes, the resistence to multiple aggression is very different. From these concepts the *polypharmacology* approach, that aims at the identification of compounds able to hit specifically 2 or more molecular targets. This can have tremendous impact on cancer and other complex diseases research. In fact, the identification of cancer-cell specific targets is very rare, which means that most of anticancer therapies rely on the differential effect that drug can have on the same vital cell functions, but in cells growing in different ways. Thus the identification of drugs which in combinations would be able to only affect cancer cells would represent a safer approach to cancer. To be efficient, these approaches must rely on a complete catalogue of drugs and targets, on an effective representation of the possible interactions and on an efficient way to navigate across such interactions to identify the most interesting molecules. This problem is tackled by another emerging area of research *Combination Chemical Genetics* (CCG, [47]), aiming at deciphering and quantifying the synergistic activity of small compound on cell's functions. It is clear at this point that these novel application areas (polypharmacology, network pharmacology, CCG) all necessitate of the theory and advances in systems, graphs and information theory, the same areas that are contributing to the development of systems biology.

3.3. Impact on Medicine

The change in the medical area is more subtle, probably less visible, but is also the one with the stronger long term impact. Briefly, the possibility to observe genome-wide variations has triggered a change in the perception of health and cure, leading to the emergence of novel types of medicine and namely paving the way for an actual personalized medicine. This change is rooted in the possibility offered to researchers to observe such comprehensive amount of data that define the *molecular portrait* of an individual. This is the fundamental information on which personalized medicine can operate to quantify information that can explain the complexity of the disease [48]. In fact, before the advent of the *omic* era, life sciences have for most part been strongly rooted in the reductionist and mechanicistic perspective, that tries to break the complexity of the system of interest into small simpler pieces to study and understand these less complex parts [23]. This approach has been successful for decades and centuries; however, as described above, the difficulties in front of complex diseases such as cancers or diabetes, have forced medical and biological researchers to change perspective. Historically, microarrays, being the first *omic* platform, have opened the door to a tangible way of analyzing biological data in a completely different way, allowing scientists from numbers of academic institutions to observe data from a systemic point of view, processing data with a parallelism that was not even thinkable before the advent of such technology. The impact of these concepts is already changing the landscape of treatments by drugs, however, another, maybe unexpected player is entering the game of health care.

In fact, the ability to explore at relative low costs and in relative short times large amount of data continues to expand our range of interests and curiosity. As a results, not only are we able to sequence a growing number of organisms' genomes, but we are also exploring more in details the real extension of our own. In particular, the bacteria we live in constant vicinity with and which perform crucial functions for the correct functioning of all our activities -the human *microbiome*-, consitute a large and growing body of information with a tremendous impact on the re-intepretation of the etiology of metabolic, inflammatory and other diseases [49]. The pioneering work of Nicholson et al. [50], represents a cornerstone in this area, thank to the introduction of several innovative concepts.

First of all the extension of the concept of metabolism in mammals, which must be modified, given the tight interaction of the molecular activity of mammals with the activity of other commensal (gut microbiome) and symbiotic organisms (skin and mouth microorganisms). In fact, the proper description of the activity ongoing at the metabolic level in mammals cannot make use of the traditional concepts of endogenous and xenobiotic compounds produced by the host organism (mammal) and the commensal or symbiotic organisms (microbiome bacteria) respectively. It is indeed more appropriate to define a *Continuum of Metabolism* [50], where purely endogenous and xenobiotic processes are accompanied and interact with *sym-endogenous* processes (process and compounds essential to host biological function and which can be metabolized or further utilized by host, but for which there is no biosynthetic capability of the host genome, like vitamins and essential amino acids) and sym- (metabolites or processes involving co-metabolism by two or more organisms that are commensal or symbiotic, that may not be essential to the host, but that can influence endogenous or other xenobiotic metabolic processes) and trans-xenobiotic (compound of extra-genomic or chemical origin but which are metabolically converted to endogenous species or metabolites that can be utilized directly in endogenous processes) processes.

This leads to the concept of mammals, and humans in particular, as *supra-organisms*. This concept highlights the complex interactions that occur between the control of endogenous metabolic pathways and the metabolism of foreign compounds. Importantly, this work leads to the revisitation of the very concepts of pathways, which cannot only take into account the involvement of molecules from the host organism, but must account for the complex interaction with commensal and symbiotic organisms, as they do interact with the metabolism. In this perspective, this adds a layer of complexity to network pharmacology, as in fact, the proper definition of treatments personalized on individual patients cannot preclude from the study of the supra-human metabolism, adding to the molecullar biology problem the ecology perspective [49].

Although this research area stems from microbiology, its impact on human health via the union of molecular biology and ecological approaches and then to medicine is undeniable. Recent discoveries, in fact, link metabolic diseases such as diabetes, obesity, and hypertension [51, 52, 53, 54] to the activity of the immune system [55].

Medical practice is traditionally, and for good reasons, a conservatory area in which paradigm shifts can happen, and rightly so, given the caution that needs to be taken when changes can affect so directly our lives and well-being. However, hot debate is ongoing in this area as well, challenging the traditional reductionist approach to medicine to embrace systems biology as a base and a framework for innovation. In particular, Ahn et al. [45, 46] presented 2 essays where a picture of the current limitations of the application of reductionism in medicine are discussed. In particular, 4 practices in medicine are highlighted as being particularly limiting at this point: the focus on a singular dominant factor when

investigating the causes for disease, the emphasis on homeostasis, the inexact risk modification approach, and the issues encountered when additive treatments must be supplied
to the patient. The following, and last, section introduces an area in which a large part of
these limitations is taken into account. This is one of the main reason why CAM should be
investigated further, as its synergy with conventional medicine could generate integrative
and powerful medicines.

4. Potential in CAM

This final Section aims at introducing the existing centers of interests around CAM,
the sources of funding, the scientific channels for diffusion, and, with specific focus on
acupuncture, highlight the existence of validated clinical results and present the (poor)
theoretical background. The goal is to collect the existing information and to clarify the
limitations and room for improvement in our knowledge of these techniques and/or on the
properties of self-healing and placebo, with a brief digression on the current misconception
on CAM, possibly responsible for the slow advances in this area.

Conventional and Alternative Medicines (CAM) are defined as "a group of diverse
medical and health care systems, practices, and products that are not generally considered
part of conventional medicine" by the National Center for Complementary and Alternative
Medicine (NCCAM) one of the agencies of the prestigious American National Institute
of Health (NIH). This agency, and several others (National Science Foundation of China
-NSFC-, european institutions funded by 7th Framework Program -FP7[1]) support research
for providing evidence to the use of such therapies. International, peer-reviewed journals,
indexed in PubMed have emerged in the past years, indicating a trend of interest in this direction (for example: Evidence-based Complementary and Alternative Medicine (eCAM)
from Oxford Journals, BMC Complementary and Alternative Medicine), however, CAM
research is still perceived as poorly scientific and merely a matter for "believers".

It may be interesting to perform a parallel with another currently booming area of interest: environmentalism. For years this has been a philosophical attitude, often perceived
a matter for utopian and anachronistic visionaries, naïf to the point of ignoring the im-
possibility to apply the concepts of alternative energy to the economy of the real world.
Oil companies were indicated (not always inappropriately) as the stronger opponents to
alternative energies sources development in particular and to the global environmentally
friendly vision in general, and "believers" were often sectary in their application of the
principles of environmentalism. The parallel between this and the current perception of
CAM is quite striking, with pharmaceutical companies substituting oil companies, with the
same demagogic vision and stereotypes proposed from both sides ("believers" and opponents). Nowadays, environmentalism is embraced in a more balanced way, and is more
and more perceived as an opportunity for growth in number of areas ([56] carried out for
the Directorate-General for Energy and Transport in the European Commission). From research -on the generation of new technologies for efficient use and production of energy; to
economy -given the vast basin of applications, and the consequent generation of new jobs;
to politics -as issues related to the access to fuel and other resources is critical for political

---

[1]HEALTH-2007-2.1.2-7: Traditional Chinese Medicine in post-genomic era

stability-, numbers of human activities are now involved with environmentalism. Briefly, a large new market is now appreciable and appealing to a growing number of entities, and environmentalism has undergone a shift in its perception which was crucial for its effective progression and for the (pro)active involvement of society in this area (for more arguments on that, an interesting perspective is proposed in [57]).

Research in CAM, although largely perceived as non-scientific, economically unpractical and disadvantageous, seems to bear the same potential to improve our quality of life in several very important and practical areas: technology and theory development, with the necessity to improve and design methodologies for evidence-based clinical trials, integration of drugs development and other clinical practices; economy, as pharmaceutical companies, in particular, as described above, need to boost their research approaches; politics, as issues related to the ageing of population requires to deal with growing number of patients affected by chronic diseases which appear to take good advantage from CAM; social, as currently patients spontaneously invest their own money for non-refundable CAM treatments.

The bases on which a shift in the perception of CAM -as an opportunity rather than a threat to the process of scientification of medicine- can occur, are already in place, but need further development. Herman et al. [58] have shown that alternative treatments are cost-effective and can be used in specific cases where they are competitive or outperform conventional therapies. Superiority can be due to similar outcome with less expenses, or similar expenses and less side effects, or prolonged effects or combinations of the above. Although data collection, study perception and preparation require *ad hoc* guidelines and overall better evidence-based practice from the point of view of practitioners, the economic evaluation conducted was subjected to quality review of the clinical studies, which at the time of the economic study (2005) was comparable with the ones in conventional medicine. After all, medicine is only recently becoming a science with the introduction of the concept of *evidence based medicine* [59, 60].

Important advances in the direction of appropriate practice of evidence based medicine are given by the International Conference on Harmonisation of Technical Requirements for Registration of Pharmaceuticals for Human Use (ICH, www.ich.org), which brings together the regulatory authorities of Europe, Japan and the United States and experts from the pharmaceutical industry to discuss scientific and technical issues of product registration, to define recommendations on ways to achieve greater uniformity in the interpretation and application of technical guidelines and requirements for product registration to reduce or nullify the need to duplicate the testing carried out during the research and development of new medicines. In this frame *non-inferiority clinical trials* have been clearly described and defined [61]. These clinical studies are used when palcebo cannot be ethically approved, for example in the case of degenerative diseases, or when historical records or previous study show evidence for existing effective treatment, or relevant to the case under study, when placebo is difficult to produce. For example *sham* acupuncture (using non-acupoints for treatment) does not appear to define a proper placebo for acupuncture, both because patients can recognize the difference nullifying the placebo effect, and because, given the still uncertain origin of acupoints it is still not clear how misplaced needles can affect the efficacy of the treatment. Non-inferiority trials can then be used as they aim at demonstrating that the therapy under study is simply not inferior (i.e. from a statistical point of view, the null hypothesis tested is an inequality) to another assessed treatment.

Although some authors are critical towards this approach [62], the global medical and pharmaceutical community approves it as a reasonable method to preserves patients care, while guaranteeing appropriate statistical validation [63, 64].

Although several clinical study have shown the effectiveness of specific CAM treatments on specific diseases (http://apps.who.int/medicinedocs/en/d /Js4926e/5.html), and cost-effectiveness appears also to be an advantage, it is necessary to provide explanation on the mechanisms of actions of such approaches. In fact, this is a crucial information needed and an active area of research to boost synergies between conventional medicine and CAM, improve the identification of appropriate targets diseases, and overall achieve a better healthcare delivery. The whole CAM area is too broad to be discussed here, this chapter is thus limited to the hypotheses on the mechanisms of action of acupuncture. The reasons are that acupuncture is part of a complete body of knowledge (Chinese Medicine), and that a large number of diseases has been proven and approved by the WHO to be advantageously treated with acupuncture instead of conventional medicine (see again http://apps.who.int/ medicinedocs/en/d/Js4926e/5.html).

Acupuncture is a technique of inserting and manipulating fine needles (or laser or warm moxa or electrostimulated needles) into specific points on the body (acupoints) to relieve pain or for other therapeutic purposes. Acupuncture points are situated along meridians, which represents channels interconnecting acupoints.

There exist diverse theories on the functioning of acupuncture that are accessible in english literature, some sharing basic concepts, and trying to connect the system of meridians and acupoints to known anatomical systems and some trying to describe known anatomical part as coherent systems in the frame of meridians and acupoints.

In a recent article [65], acupuncture has been defined as an approach highly interlinked with the psychosocial context in which the treatment is delivered. Basically, in this theory, attention is turned to the importance of the expectation of the effects of acupuncture, an expectation crucial for the effective outcome of a process which would be otherwise perceived as harmful (needles harm). Briefly, it is stated that the conscious and focused attention that the patient brings to the area of the needle would allow the localized production of molecules (opioids) necessary for healing (pain reduction). In the view of the author this does not reduces acupuncture to a mere placebo, but suggests to deepen the study of the relationship between placebo and acupuncture to shed light on the mode-of-action of acupuncture. Although this theory is supported by some evidence reported by the author in other areas, it seems to reduce the potential of acupuncture to pain relief, although other types of issues have been proven to benefit from such treatments (only as an example, reduction of the side effects of chemotherapy). Also, acupuncture by laser appears to be as effective as needles one, while the consciousness brought to the point by the patients in this case may be somewhat different. Nevertheless, the necessity to deepen our understanding of placebo is highlghted by other authors [66] indicating that the placebo and nocebo concepts represent complex ideas which challenge the very definition of these terms, and may bring important insight into self-healing and the use we make of placebo as a gold standard for clinical studies, as in fact nothing is properly a placebo, since molecular studies indicate the presence of active principles participating in the process.

An earlier theory of acupuncture is based on the work of Melzack et al., [67] which takes advantage of the attempt to unify the mechanism that perceives and transmits pain through the nervous system. This theory is known as the Gate Theory and states that there are nerve fibers that transmit pain to the spinal cord, and other that inhibits the transmission of pain. Both stimuli are integrated in the spinal cord by the *substancia gelatinosa*. According to this theory pain is perceived only if the pain input overrides the inhibition of pain, and it has been used in implantable medical devices for example to relieve back pain in Parkinsonian patients (Medtronic Synergy device). However, this theory also fails to explain how the effects of acupuncture can last for some months after the acupuncture needle has been removed. Moreover, acupuncture is a valuable treatment in a variety of non-painful diseases and the Gate Theory makes no attempt to explain the mechanism of acupuncture in the treatment of these diseases.

Another theory has been recently updated and summarized in [68]. In this work, emphasis is given to the anatomical foundation of the structure of meridians considered to identify a structure bounded by the skin where there are abundant nociceptive receptors of various types that are moreover bound below by another layer of connective tissue with flowing interstitial fluid (including proteins with surface charges and ions) as ground substance, which pressure changes during body movements. These extracellular channels of body fluid provide migratory tracks mainly due to durotaxis (movement of cell motility up or down a rigidity gradient) for mast cells, fibroblasts and other cells (including adult stem cells) able to carry out a number of physiological functions like triggering neurogenic inflammation, vasotone homeostasis, wound repair. In this view, acupoints are functional sites along the meridian channels, this is why acupuncture applied to these sites could improve the efficiency of the above functions forcing for example mast cells to release antimicrobial cytotoxic molecules to destroy invading microorganisms.

C. Shang from Harvard Medical School proposes a different interpretation, although somehow including the theory above, tracking the origin of acupoints back to embryogenesis. In particular, it is based on the idea that every physiological system is developed through a growth control system mediated by organizers (specific groups of stems cells, perduring in adulthood) and growth control boundaries. These organizers respond also to the definition of stem cells niches in adults, groups of cells that control the conservation and regeneration of organs. The growth control signal transduction necessary to this goal is embedded in various physiological functions (hypertrophy, hyperplasia, atrophy, apoptosis and signal transduction pathways involving growth control genes such as proto-oncogenes). One of the models for growth control system suggests that it originates from a network of organizers and separatrices which -because of their origin in the embryo- locate and distribute at extreme points of structural surface (or interface) curvature in the grown (adult) system. Organizers and growth control boundaries (separatrices) have several characteristics: they show macroscopic singularities (discontinuity and abrupt transition) of morphogen gradient field and bioelectric field and small, nonspecific perturbations around such singular points can have long lasting systemic effect. Manipulating these points offers an efficient way of manipulating the growth system. This growth control model also suggests that singular points - organizers and separatrices - boundaries in growth control form an undifferentiated, interconnected cellular network that regulates growth and physiology both during and after embryogenesis. Intriguingly, the ensemble of acupuncture points and meridians appear to match the description of organizers and growth control boundaries respectively. In particular in fact, organizers have high electric conductance, high electric current density and high density of gap junctions; growth control boundaries have high electric conductance and high density of gap junctions, booth characteristiscs shared by acupoints and meridians; singularity has important role in morphogenesis and morphogens and organizers partially retain their regulatory function after embryogenesis. This would explain why nonspecific stimulation at acupoints - potential organizers in adult, could cause extensive growth control effects. This theory also explains another peculiarity of acupuncture, i.e. why the auricular pavillion is so rich in acupoints: given its highly convex structure it is enriched in organizers. Independent reviews on stem cells niches [69, 70] summarizes how the concept of extracellular matrix regulating primitive cells is longstanding [70]. In particular, it appears that "matrix components provide localizing niche elements that can contribute stimulatory, or impose inhibitory, influences on the stem-cell pool. They, like other stimuli in the niche, balance opposing possibilities". Although this represents an interesting hypothesis, the collected information are far from indicating real convergency with the acupuncture theory, and to the best of my knowledge there has not been any experimental independent evidence of the distribution of stem cells niches.

Finally, the best scientifically conducted research comes from the lab of H. Langevin. She has been involved in studies on the anatomical/physiological properties of acupoints and meridians [71]. The most intriguing and striking effect reported comes from the identification of a clear mechano-transduced signal transmitted from the needle rotation to the fibroblasts in the interstitial connective tissue, that is more abundant below the majority of acupoints [72]. Such signal was able to induce changes in subcutaneous tissue fibroblasts, which then involved Rho and Rac signaling mechanisms as well as actomyosin contractility.

It is clear that the variety of theory reflects the lack of molecular bases able to direct the research on the fundamental mechanisms of acupuncture. However, technology can today help to shed light on some of these theory.

Some attempts to study the effects of acupuncture at the genome-wide level have recently been done, for example on animal model affected with asthma [73], or to test the ability of acupuncture to improve survival, differentiation of the bone marrow mesenchymal stem cells [74]. In humans this has been tested on allergic rhinitis [75, 76] and to identify individual differences of acupuncture analgesia [77]. In all cases it was possible to identify specific genes function activation before and after treatment or in comparison with controls. However, in the absence of a specific functional hypothesis to test, these findings, although confirmative of the effects of acupuncture, remain superficial with respect of the modernization, standardization and systematization of acupuncture.

5. Conclusion

This chapter has introduced most of the new high throughput technologies that allow today the analysis of molecular biology from a perspective that encompasses the understanding of a single molecule activity or a single pathway, but tries to get a systemic, genome-wide vision of what is ongoing in a cell. The technological advancement that have permitted this have also influenced the vision and the way in which research is performed in several areas, from biology itself, to pharmacology and medicine. Having summarized these large scale changes, it is possible to envision the application of these technologies and the changes that are affecting and renewing conventional medicine to the area of alternative and complementary medicine. This addresses governmental requests that need to understand and help their citizens willing to pay for such therapies, and pharmacological research and medicine and biology all intimately connected in the query for novel and efficient therapies.

Several challenges need to be faced to apply the tools and methods designed for evidence-based conventional medicine to complementary and alternative medicine. In particular the design of clinical trials requires care, as the identification of placebo alternatives is often not viable, blindness is impossible when comparing any manipulative approach with drugs and randomization appear complex, as often the patients choice for alternative treatment will cause them to leave the trial if randomization does not suit their desire.

However, the definition of non-inferiorirty trials, as well as the study of the effects of such treatment at the molecular level can offer another level of detail, provide some insight into the mechanisms of action of unclear therapies such acupuncture, and from there allow a broader understanding of the applicability and limitations of such treatments.

Importantly, this research challenges the notions of placebo, which appear to be extremely complex and that may deserve more attention as an advantageous and usable mechanisms, rather than an unavoidable noise in clinical studies.

References

[1] Brown PO, Botstein D. Exploring the new world of the genome with DNA microarrays. *Nat Genet.* 1999;21(1):33–37.

[2] Guiducci C, Nardini C. High Parallelism, Portability and Broad Accessibility: Technologies for Genomics. *ACM J Emerg Technol Comput Syst.* 2008;4(1):Article 3.

[3] Ji H, Davis RW. Data quality in genomics and microarrays. *Nature Biotechnology.* 2006;24:1112 – 1113.

[4] Fu X, Fu N, Guo S, Yan Z, Xu Y, Hu H, et al. Estimating accuracy of RNA-Seq and microarrays with proteomics. *BMC Genomics.* 2009;10:161–161.

[5] Bloom JS, Khan Z, Kruglyak L, Singh M, Caudy AA. Measuring differential gene expression by short read sequencing: quantitative comparison to 2-channel gene expression microarrays. *BMC Genomics.* 2009;.

[6] Görg A, Weiss W, J DM. Current two-dimensional electrophoresis technology for proteomics. *Proteomics.* 2004;4(12):3665 – 3685.

[7] Aebersold R, M M.   Mass   spectrometry-based   proteomics.   *Nature.* 2003;422(6928):198–207.

[8] Joung J, Ramm E, Pabo C.   A bacterial two-hybrid selection system for studying protein-DNA and protein-protein interactions. *Proc Natl Acad Sci.* 2000;97(13):73827387.

[9] Walhout AJM, Vidal M. High-Throughput Yeast Two-Hybrid Assays for Large-Scale Protein Interaction Mapping. *Methods.* 2001;24(3):297 – 306.

[10] Esteller M. The necessity of a human epigenome project. *Carcinogenesis.* 2006;27:1121 – 1125.

[11] Dejardin J, Kingston RE. Purification of proteins associated with specific genomic loci. *Cell.* 2009;136:175186.

[12] Maxam AM, Gilbert W. A new method for sequencing DNA. *Proc Natl Acad Sci.* 1977;74(2):560 – 564.

[13] Sanger F, Coulson AR. A rapid method for determining sequences in DNA by primed synthesis with DNA polymerase. *J Mol Biol.* 1975;94(3):441–448.

[14] Holt RA, Jones SJ. The new paradigm of flow cell sequencing. *Genome Res.* 2008 Jun;18(6):839–846.

[15] Shendure J, Ji H. Next-generation DNA sequencing. *Nat Biotechnol.* 2008 Oct;26(10):1135 – 1145.

[16] M R. Pyrosequencing sheds light on DNA sequencing. *Genome Research.* 2001;11(1):3–11.

[17] Shendure J, Porreca GJ, Reppas NB, Lin X, McCutcheon JP, Rosenbaum AM, et al. Accurate multiplex polony sequencing of an evolved bacterial genome. *Science.* 2005 Sep;309(5741):1728–1732.

[18] Wang H, Wang W, ans P S Yu JY. Clustering by pattern similarity in large data sets. *Proceedings of ACM SIGMOD.* 2002;.

[19] Gygi SP, Corthals GL, Zhang Y, Rochon Y, Aebersold R. Evaluation of two-dimensional gel electrophoresis-based proteome analysis technology. *Proc Natl Acad Sci.* 2000;97(17):9390–9395.

[20] Watson JD, Crick FHC. Genetical Implications of the Structure of Deoxyribonucleic Acid. *Nature.* 1953;171:964 – 967.

[21] Watson JD, Crick FHC. Molecular Structure of Nucleic Acids: A Structure for De-oxyribose Nucleic Acid. *Nature.* 1953;17:737 – 738.

[22] Collins FS, Morgan M, Patrinos A. The Human Genome Project: Lessons from Large-Scale Biology. *Science.* 2003;300(5617):286–290.

[23] Hocquette JF. Where are we in genomics? *Journal of Physiology and Pharmacology.* 2005;56(3):37–70.

[24] Quackenbush J. Extracting biology from high-dimensional biological data. *J Exp Biol.* 2007;210(10.1242/jeb.004432):1507 – 1517.

[25] Segal E, Sirlin CB, Ooi C, Adler AS, Gollub J, Chen X, et al. Decoding global gene expression programs in liver cancer by noninvasive imaging. *Nature Biotechnology.* 2007;25(6):675–680.

[26] West M, Blanchette C, Dressman H, Huang E, Ishida S, Spang R, et al. Predicting the clinical status of human breast cancer by using gene expression profiles. *Proc Natl Acad Sci.* 2001;98(20):11462–11467.

[27] Schadt EE, Friend SH, Shaywitz DA. A network view of disease and compound screening. *Nature Reviews Drug Discovery.* 2009;8:286–295.

[28] Lapointe J, Li C, Higgins JP, van de Rijn M, Bair E, Montgomery K, et al. Gene expression profiling identifies clinically relevant subtypes of prostate cancer. *Proc Natl Acad Sci.* 2004;101(3):811–816.

[29] Sørlie T, Tibshirani R, Parker J, Hastie T, Marron JS, Nobel A, et al. Repeated observation of breast tumor subtypes in gene expression data sets. *Proc Natl Acad Sci.* 2003;100(14):8418–8423.

[30] Sørlie T, Perou CM, Tibshirani R, Aas T, Geisler S, Johnsen H, et al. Gene expression patterns of breast carcinomas distinguish tumor subclasses with clinical implications. *Proc Natl Acad Sci.* 2001;98(19):10869–10874.

[31] Morley M, Molony C, Weber T, Devlin J, Ewens K, Spielman R, et al. Genetic analysis of genome-wide variation in human gene expression. *Nature.* 2004;430(7001):743747.

[32] Zhu J, Zhang B, Schadt EE. A systems biology approach to drug discovery. *Adv Genet.* 2008;60:603635.

[33] Chavali A, Whittemore J, Eddy J, Williams K, Papin J. Systems analysis of metabolism in the pathogenic trypanosomatid Leishmania major. *Molecular systems biology.* 2008;4(177).

[34] Palsson BO. *Systems Biology Properties of reconstructed networks.* New York: Cambridge University Press; (2006).

[35] Voit EO. *Canonical Nonlinear Modeling.* New York: VAn Nostrand Reinhold; (1991).

[36] Gardner TS, di Bernardo D, Lorenz D, Collins JJ. Inferring Genetic Networks and Identifying Compound Mode of Action via Expression Profiling. *Science.* 2003;301(5629,):102–105.

[37] Nelander S, Wang W, Nilsson B, She QB, Pratilas C, Rosen N, et al. Models from experiments: combinatorial drug perturbations of cancer cells. *Mol Syst Biol.* 2008;4(216).

[38] Shmulevich I, Dougherty ER, Zhang W. Gene perturbation and intervention in probabilistic Boolean networks. *Bioinformatics.* 2002;18(10):R57–R66.

[39] Yu J, Smith VA, Wang PP, Hartemink AJ, Jarvis ED. Advances to Bayesian network inference for generating causal networks from observational biological data. *Bioinformatics*. 2004;20(18):3594–3603.

[40] Margolin AA, Nemenman I, Basso K, Klein U, Wiggins C, Stolovitzky G, et al.. ARACNE: An Algorithm for the Reconstruction of Gene Regulatory Networks in a Mammalian Cellular Context; 2004. Available from: `doi:10.1186/1471-2105-7-S1-S7`.

[41] Basso K, Margolin AA, Stolovitzky G, Klein U, Dalla-Favera R, Califano A. Reverse engineering of regulatory networks in human B cells. *Nat Genet*. 2005 Apr;37(4):382–390.

[42] Cover TM, Thomas JA. *Elements of Information Theory*. John Wiley and Sons; 2001.

[43] Barab'asi AL, Oltvai ZN. Network Biology: Understanding the cells functional organization. *Nat Rev Genet*. 2004;5:101–113.

[44] Hopkins AL. Network pharmacology: the next paradigm in drug discovery. *Nat Chem Biol*. 2008 Nov;4(11):682–690.

[45] Ahn AC, Tewari M, Poon CS, Phillips RS. The Limits of Reductionism in Medicine: Could Systems Biology Offer an Alternative? *PLoS Medicine*. 2006;3(6):e208.

[46] Ahn AC, Tewari M, Poon CS, Phillips RS. The Clinical Applications of a Systems Approach. *PLoS Medicine*. 2006;3(7):e209.

[47] Lehár J, Stockwell BR, Giaever G, Nislow C. Combination chemical genetics. *Nature Chemical Biology*. 2008;4:674– 681.

[48] West M, Ginsburg GS, Huang AT, Nevins JR. Embracing the complexity of genomic data for personalized medicine. *Genome Res*. 2006;16:559– 566.

[49] Nicholson JK, Holmes E, Wilson ID. Gut microorganisms, mammalian metabolism and personalized health care. *Nature Reviews Microbiology*. 2005;3:431–438.

[50] Nicholson JK, D WI. Understanding 'Global' Systems Biology: Metabonomics and the Continuum of Metabolism. *Nature*. 2003;2:668–675.

[51] Turnbaugh PJ, Ley RE, Mahowald MA, Magrini V, Mardis ER, Gordon JI. An obesity-associated gut microbiome with increased capacity for energy harvest. *Nature*. 2006 Dec;444(7122):1027–1031.

[52] Cani PD, Amar J, Iglesias MA, Poggi M, Knauf C, Bastelica D, et al. Metabolic endotoxemia initiates obesity and insulin resistance. *Diabetes*. 2007 Jul;56(7):1761–1772.

[53] Holmes E, Loo RL, Stamler J, Bictash M, Yap IK, Chan Q, et al. Human metabolic phenotype diversity and its association with diet and blood pressure. *Nature*. 2008 May;453(7193):396–400.

[54] Wen L, Ley RE, Volchkov PY, Stranges PB, Avanesyan L, Stonebraker AC, et al. Innate immunity and intestinal microbiota in the development of Type 1 diabetes. *Nature.* 2008 Oct;455(7216):1109–1113.

[55] Tsuji M, Komatsu N, Kawamoto S, Suzuki K, Kanagawa O, Honjo T, et al. Preferential Generation of Follicular B Helper T Cells from Foxp3+ T Cells in Gut Peyer's Patches. *Science.* 2009;323(5920):1488– 1492.

[56] EmployRES Partners.   EmployRES - *The impact of renewable energy policy on economic growth and employment in the European Union.* 2009;Available from: `http://ec.europa.eu/energy/renewables/studies/renewables_en.htm`

[57] Nordhaus T, Shellenberger M. *Break Through: From the Death of Environmentalism to the Politics of Possibility.* Houghton Mifflin Company; 2007.

[58] Herman P, Craig B, Caspi O.   Is complementary and alternative medicine (CAM) cost-effective? a systematic review. *BMC Complementary and Alternative Medicine.* 2005;5(1):11.

[59] McQueen MJ. Overview of evidence-based medicine: challenges for evidence-based laboratory medicine. *Clin Chem.* 2001;47(8):1536–1546.

[60] Neumayer L, Meterissian S, McMasters K, for the Members of the Evidence Based Reviews in Surgery Group. Canadian Association of General Surgeons and American College of Surgeons Evidence Based Reviews in Surgery. 23. ASCO recommended guidelines for sentinel lymph node biopsy for early-stage breast cancer. Evidence-based medicine. A new approach to teaching the practice of medicine. *Can J Surg.* 2007 Dec;50(6):482–484.

[61] Group IW. E10: Choice of Control Group and Related Issues in Clinical Trials. FDA Federal Register. 2001;66(93):24390–24391.

[62] Snapinn SM.   Noninferiority trials.   *Curr Control Trials Cardiovasc Med.* 2000;1(1):1921.

[63] D'Agostino RS, Massaro J, Sullivan L. Non-inferiority trials: design concepts and issues. *Stat Med.* 2003;22(2):169–86.

[64] D'Agostino RS, Campbell M, Greenhouse J. Non-inferiority trials: continued advancements in concepts and methodology. *Stat Med.* 2006;25(7):1097–1099.

[65] Liu T. Acupuncture: What Underlies Needle Administration? *eCAM.* 2009;6(2):185–193.

[66] Kaptchuk TJ. Powerful Placebo: The Dark Side of the Randomized Controlled Trial. *Lancet.* 1998;351:1722–1725.

[67] Melzack P, Wall PD.   Pain mechanisms: a new theory.   *Science.* 1965;150(3699):971979.

[68] Fung PCW. Probing the mystery of Chinese medicine meridian channels with special emphasis on the connective tissue interstitial fluid system, mechanotransduction, cells durotaxis and mast cell degranulation. *Chinese Medicine.* 2009;4(10).

[69] Moore KA, Lemischka IR. Stem Cells and Their Niches. *Science.* 2006;311(5769):1880– 1885.

[70] Scadden DT. The stem-cell niche as an entity of action. *Nature.* 2006;441(29):1075– 1079.

[71] Langevin HM, Yandow JA. Subcutaneous Tissue Fibroblast Cytoskeletal Remodeling Induced by Acupuncture: Evidence for a Mechanotransduction-Based Mechanism;.

[72] Langevin HM, Bouffard NA, Badger GJ, Churchill DL, Howe AK. Subcutaneous tissue fibroblast cytoskeletal remodeling induced by acupuncture: evidence for a mechanotransduction-based mechanism. *J Cell Physiol.* 2006 Jun;207(3):767–774.

[73] Yin LM, Jiang GH, Wang Y, Wang Y, Liu YY, Jin WR, et al. Use of serial analysis of gene expression to reveal the specific regulation of gene expression profile in asthmatic rats treated by acupuncture. *Journal of Biomedical Science.* 2009;16(46).

[74] Ding Y, Yan Q, Ruan JW, Zhang YQ, Li WJ, Zhang YJ, et al. *Electro-acupuncture promotes survival, differentiation of the bone marrow mesenchymal stem cells as well as functional recovery in the spinal cord-transected rats;.*

[75] Shiue HS, Lee YS, Tsai CN, Hsueh YM, Sheu JR, Chang HH. DNA microarray analysis of the effect on inflammation in patients treated with acupuncture for allergic rhinitis. *J Altern Complement Med.* 2008 Jul;14(6):689–698.

[76] Shiue HS, Lee YS, Tsai CN, Hsueh YM, Sheu JR, Chang HH. Gene Expression Profile of Patients with Phadiatop-Positive and -Negative Allergic Rhinitis Treated with Acupuncture. *J Altern Complement Med.* 2010 Jan;.

[77] Chae Y, Park HJ, Hahm DH, Yi SH, Lee H. Individual Differences of Acupuncture Analgesia in Humans Using cDNA Microarray. *J Physiol Sci.* 2006;56(6):425431.

In: Synthetic and Integrative Biology
Editor: James T. Gevona, pp. 149-197

ISBN: 978-1-60876-678-9
© 2010 Nova Science Publishers, Inc.

Chapter 8

THE CHALLENGE OF COMBINING CELLS, SYNTHETIC MATERIALS AND GROWTH FACTORS TO ENGINEER BONE TISSUE

Melba Navarro and Alexandra Michiardi

Institute for Bioengineering of Catalonia (IBEC),
CIBER-BBN, Barcelona, Spain

Abstract

Tissue engineering has emerged as a response to the problems associated with the substitution of tissues lost due to diseases or trauma. Nowadays, xenografts, allografts or autografts are commonly used to replace the damaged tissue. However, these options involve numerous drawbacks such as rejection, chronic inflammation and severe organ donor shortages. Tissue engineering keeps the promise to overcome these limitations by creating biological substitutes capable of replacing the injured tissue.

Cells, temporary 3D constructs and biochemical signals that trigger tissue regeneration cascades are the three major components for engineering tissues. The adequate combination of these components leads to the successful repair of damaged tissues. In addition to these three main elements, the use and development of bioreactors has come out as an essential tool for the study and achievement of engineered tissues under *in vitro* conditions while mimicking the *in vivo* environment.

Thus, tissue engineering is an interdisciplinary field that applies the principles of engineering and life sciences to develop biological substitutes that restore, maintain, or improve the tissue functions.

This chapter discusses the challenge of creating engineered bone tissues by combining biological and engineering skills. In particular, it will review the issue of stem cell biology, the fabrication methods and artificial materials used for 3D constructs, the principal growth factors used in bone applications and the key role played by bioreactors. More importantly, it will highlight the interdependence of all these parameters and the need for interdisciplinary research for a successful approach.

Introduction

Bone degenerative problems including bone fractures, osteoporosis and bone retrieval due to cancer and other pathologies affecting the musculoskeletal system represent half of all chronic diseases in people over 50 in developed countries. This trend is expected to double in the next 15 years due to the high aging rate in the population. Thus, there is a real need to develop new systems to remedy this situation.

Tissue engineering has emerged as a potential alternative to currently used techniques such as allografts, autografts and xenografts which present several limitations, namely, donor site scarcity, rejection, diseases transfer, harvesting costs and postoperative morbidity [1-3]. Tissue engineering and regenerative medicine are recent research fields that explore how to repair and regenerate tissues and organs using the biological cell signalling pathways and their components such as growth factors and peptide sequences among others, in combination with synthetic scaffolds and stem cells [4].

There are three main approaches described for bone tissue engineering (illustrated in Figure 1), which are: i) guidance of tissue regeneration using engineered 3D porous scaffolds; ii) injection of cells in the implantation place; and/or iii) combination of 3D scaffolds with cells to guide bone regeneration. The first method involves implanting a scaffold at the site of interest and allowing cell ingrowth from surrounding tissues to colonize the scaffold. The second method also known as cell therapy is less invasive. It involves the use of cells optionally genetically manipulated prior to injection or infusion. In the third method, 3D porous scaffolds designed to mimic extracellular matrices are loaded with cells and located in the implantation site.

In practice, organ-specific cells are often seeded into the scaffold *ex vivo* prior to implantation, and with time the cells synthesize a new extracellular matrix as the scaffold degrades simultaneously and eventually produce a new properly functioning tissue [5].

Tissue engineering is constituted of three major components (Figure 2): 1) cells building the new tissue, 2) 3D porous scaffold mimicking the extracellular matrix and guiding tissue regeneration, and 3) specific signalling systems that trigger the healing cascade through the activation of genes responsible for the secretion of products responsible for tissue differentiation. These three components must be properly combined for a successful repair and regeneration of tissues.

Furthermore, the use and development of bioreactors has emerged as an essential tool for the study and attainment of tissues under *in vitro* conditions while mimicking physiological *in vivo* conditions.

Therefore, tissue engineering is a multidisciplinary and interdisciplinary field that requires the combination of knowledge and expertises of chemists, engineers, biologists and physicists among others in order to overcome the multiple demands and challenges inherent to the development of tissue regeneration systems.

More insight about each of these three major components as well as the approaches and strategies used to achieve bone repair and regeneration will be discussed in this chapter.

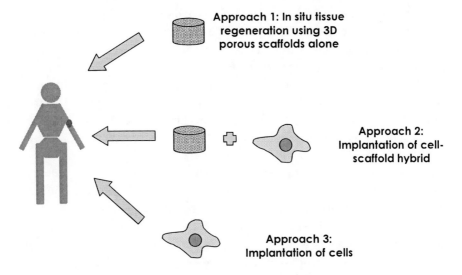

Figure 1. Main approaches to tissue engineering.

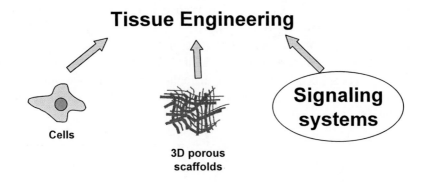

Figure 2. The three major components of tissue engineering.

Cell Biology in Tissue Engineering

The shortage of tissues and organs for transplantation has led to the rapid development of tissue engineering as an alternative to overcome this problem. Some of the tissues found in the body possess cells capable of initiating regeneration or repair after injury. Cell regeneration potential depends on the cell type, nature and location of the injury, the size of the defect to be repaired, and patient's age among other aspects. Nevertheless, most human tissues do not regenerate spontaneously. This is the reason why fabrication of biotissues that mimic the natural ones is so promising.

In vivo bone healing is generally considered to be biologically optimal since the majority of defects in this tissue, experience spontaneous healing with minimal treatment. However, it is known that from the total amount of fractures occurring every year in the United States, 5-10% require further treatment to achieve full healing because of either interposition of soft tissue, improper fracture fixation, bone loss, metabolic disturbances, impairment of blood supply or infection [6]. Moreover, in certain clinical conditions, large pieces of bone must be retrieved to treat benign and malign tumours, osteomyelitis and also bone deficiencies and abnormal loss in the maxillofacial area. In these cases, the use of bone substitutes and systems to enhance tissue regeneration is absolutely required.

Autografts, which are grafts made of tissue obtained from the patient himself, are the gold standard in these situations, because they avoid most problems related to transfection and rejection. However, autologous bone sources are limited and the harvesting process is usually painful and involves risks of infection.

Synthetic substrates as well as the use of allografts that are grafts made of tissue from other donor (usually post-mortem), and xenografts which are grafts of tissue proceeding from other species, have been used in the last years to overcome the drawbacks of autografts. Nevertheless, these three alternatives also present important limitations. Both allografts and xenografts imply the risk of immunological reactions and infections, and in the case of allografts, availability of donors is also a main concern. At present, as an alternative to the before mentioned grafts, synthetic substrates have only been used successfully in small defects in direct contact with bone tissue.

Thus, all these limitations and drawbacks related to the attainment and harvesting of autologous bone have impelled the development of novel alternative techniques including the use of growth factors and stem cells.

Independent of the therapeutic approach to regenerate the diseased or injured tissue, cell sourcing is the first issue to consider in the development of bioengineered tissues. Nowadays, a number of cell sources are being investigated; including adult stem cells, adult differentiated cells, embryonic and fetal stem cells, cells generated by nuclear transportation, and *ex vivo* manipulated cells [7].

The Role of Stem Cells

Stem cells are characterized by three main features i) they are capable of self-renewal ii) they have the ability to give rise to different cell lineages and iii) they are capable of *in vivo* functional regeneration of the tissues to which they give rise [8]. Stem cells biology offers the potential to grow tissues by following a developmental pathway, which means that they have the capability of mimicking the developmental process followed during the formation of an embryo, where cells from a fertilized egg are able to differentiate and form a complex multicellular organism. This ability to differentiate into a variety of cell types is known as potency. Stems cells potency varies depending on their source; cells that are able to produce only one type of cell are unipotent cells, whereas cells able to produce a wide variety of cells are pluripotent. Totipotent cells are those able to differentiate in any cell lineage comprised in the body (stems cells hierarchy is illustrated in Figure 3). This potency ability of stem cells has raised great interest and is considered as a promising resource for tissue engineering applications and transplantation. Besides, the use of stem cells in regenerative medicine has raised great interest given the insights they offer into the understanding of tissue repair and regeneration processes.

Stem cells can be retrieved from both embryonic and adult tissues. Totipotency of embryonic stem cells makes them the only cell source capable to give rise to all sorts of adult cell lineages. Embryonic stem cells can only be collected at very early stages of embryogenesis. Sources of embryonic stem cells are supernumerary embryos produced by in vitro fecundation or embryos created via the nuclear transfer technique. Both the collection and usage of this type of cells deals with important ethical issues. For instance, it must be emphasized that using human embryonic progenitor cells is banned in many countries, although a modification of the so-called bioethical law allows importation of human embryonic cell lines for research purposes.

Adult progenitor or stem cells have a more limited potential than embryonic ones. Indeed, most of them are unipotent, and at present only those collected from bone marrow, brain, and adipose tissue seem to be pluripotent cells [9]. These cells have been isolated from a wide variety of tissues and although they lack tissue-specific characteristics, they can differentiate into specialized cells with a phenotype different from that of the precursor when they are stimulated with the appropriate signals. One of the most important points in the utilization of adult stem cells is that their collection does not involve ethical restrictions.

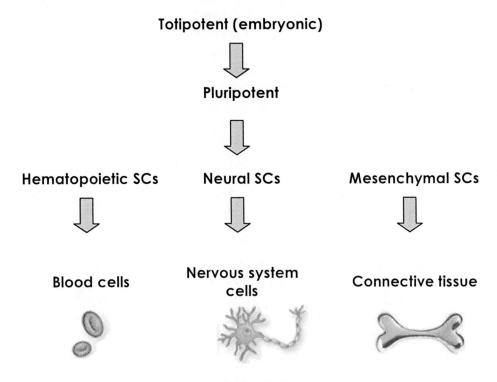

Figure 3. Stem cells hierarchy.

Although it has been demonstrated that adult stem cells are available from different sources such as bone marrow, brain and adipose tissue among others, up to now, only those hematopoietic stem cells which give rise to all the blood cell types including myeloid (monocytes and macrophages, neutrophils, basophils, eosinophils, erythrocytes, megakaryocytes/platelets, dendritic cells) and lymphoid lineages such as T-cells, B-cells and NK-cells, and mesenchymal stem cells collected from the bone marrow have been used for therapeutic applications.

The Promise of Mesenchymal Stem Cells

The term mesenchymal stem cells (MSCs) is commonly used to refer to connective tissue cells in adult tissues such as (myo)fibroblasts, bone, cartilage, fat, tendon, muscles, and nerve tissue. These cells represent a sub-group of precursor cells that sticks to the stem cell features (self-renewal and the ability to give rise to different cell types). Indeed, their ability to differentiate in mature cells and several lineages and generate new tissues has been shown by several authors [10]. MSCs can be isolated from several sources, including bone marrow, fat, umbilical cord blood, and also peripheral blood [11-13] and may differentiate into several tissue cells, including osteoblasts, chondroblasts, myoblasts and adipocytes. Recently, mice models have provided evidence that such cells may differentiate into cardiac myocytes and even neurones.

Interest in the use of mesenchymal stem cells is mainly focused on their abilities to produce various functional tissues. Furthermore, another property known as induction of immune tolerance to grafts or even immunosuppression has been recently attributed to these cells, which makes then even more appealing for tissue engineering applications.

Among the different MSCs sources, bone marrow is the most currently used. Bone marrow is a natural reservoir of skeletal mesenchymal stem cells. These cells contained in the stromal compartment of bone marrow were first identified by Friedenstein and Petrakova [14] who isolated bone-forming progenitor cells from rat marrow. These cells represent a minimal fraction (0.001-0.01%) of the total population of nucleated cells in marrow [10].

From the bone tissue engineering point of view, mesenchymal stem cells have a number of advantages: i) their isolation is easy as it relies primarily on the ability of these cells to adhere to tissue-culture plastic [15]; ii) they have a high proliferative potential [16-18]; iii) the default pathway of MSCs is the osteogenic pathway; iv) bone formation is not correlated to the number of cell passages as long as the human stem cells retain their proliferative potential [15;19]; and v) freezing conditions do not affect the osteogenic potential of MSCs, a condition that greatly facilitates their storage [17].

Besides bone marrow, there are other cell sources with osteogenic potential, namely, periosteum [20-22], trabecular bone [23-25] adipose tissue [26-28], synovium [29], skeletal muscle [30], lung [31] and deciduous teeth [32]. Nonetheless, further studies in clinically relevant animal models are needed to validate the osteogenic potential of stem cells isolated from these alternative sources.

Cell-Based Therapies for Bone Regeneration

In general, therapies based on the use of cells for achieving bone repair include both the use of i) cells without gene modifications and ii) cells genetically engineered, as shown in Figure 4. The first approach involves the implantation of stem cells directly in the place of interest in order to stimulate bone repair. In this case, the choice of the adequate scaffold is crucial. Scaffolds must possess osteoinductive (that induce the formation of new bone) and osteoconductive (that stimulates bone ingrowth) properties to facilitate bone formation. Thus, the cells/scaffold combination must trigger the osteogenic (bone formation) cascade to enhance the regeneration of the bone tissue.

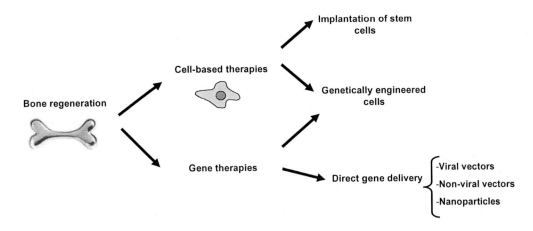

Figure 4. Cell and gene based therapies for bone regeneration.

Generally, both mesenchymal stem cells and muscle-derived stem cells are the most used for bone tissue engineering applications. Mesenchymal stem cells play a key role in cell-based therapies due to their inherent ability to differentiate in several lineages. Osteogenic activation can be triggered in the presence of β-glycerol-phosphate, ascorbic acid-2-phosphate, dexamethasone and fetal bovine serum. When cultured in monolayer in the presence of these supplements the cells acquire an osteoblastic morphology with upregulation of alkaline phosphatase activity and deposition of a calcium-rich mineralized extracellular matrix.

As already mentioned, an alternative source for adult stem cells is the muscle tissue. It has been demonstrated that a population of muscle-derived stem cells (MDSCs) isolated from mouse skeletal muscle produced alkaline phosphatase in a dose dependent manner when stimulated with recombinant human bone morphogenetic proteins 2 and 4 (rhBMP-2 and rhBMP-4). These cells were also able to differentiate toward the osteogenic lineage and, consequently, improved bone healing in calvarial defects in mice [33-35].

The second approach is based in the use of genetically engineered cells for bone regeneration. In the cell-based gene therapy cells are genetically engineered *ex vivo* to express a certain transgene that is then implanted *in vivo*. Cell-based gene delivery is becoming a primary approach in bone tissue engineering. It takes advantage of the ability of adult stem cells to express a transgene that can both affect the cells themselves and recruit host stem cells to achieve bone formation [36].

Gene-Based Therapies for Bone Regeneration

Therapies that involve gene modifications to enhance bone formation consist of two different approaches: a) direct *in vivo* delivery of genes into the injured place, and b) *ex vivo* transduction and subsequent transplantation of cells expressing the osteoinductive factor (Figure 4). The selection of the gene delivery approach depends on several factors, including the particular gene of interest, indication targeted, desired duration of gene expression, and delivery vector.

MSCs can also be genetically engineered to express a desired gene. In the case of bone tissue engineering cells are genetically modified to express an osteogenic gene, which induces them to form bone *in vivo*. The efficiency of using stem cell-based gene therapy for bone formation has been demonstrated in many studies [26;37-41].

It is important to mention that if stem cell-based gene therapy is used, the number of MSCs necessary for implantation can be reduced. Each engineered cell will produce the specific therapeutic protein, leading to the recruitment of additional MSCs from host tissues and subsequent differentiation into bone cells.

The effectivity of the cell-gene-based techniques using engineered MSCs to generate bone tissue has been evaluated using micro–computed tomography and molecular analyses of gene and protein expression [36;42].

Most gene therapy studies in the field of bone tissue engineering focus on the Bone Morphogenetic Proteins (BMP) family (that will be described in detail further in this chapter). However, some studies have also involved the use of other genes that induce osteogenic differentiation.

The delivery of genes into MSCs can be done by different methods; most of them involve the use of viral vectors (modified viruses for gene delivery), such as adenovirus and retrovirus. These vectors are potentially hazardous because of the risks of insertional mutagenesis or potential evoking of the immune system. Until recently, there was no nonviral alternative for these vectors because all conventional nonviral vectors failed in efficiently transfecting (introducing genes into cells) MSCs. In this sense, the electroporation method, which is based in the increase in permeability of the cell membrane due to an externally applied electrical field has been suggested as an alternative to viral vectors. It has been successfully modified and used to transfect bone marrow–derived MSCs without the need of a viral vector [43]. To demonstrate the efficacy of the electroporation strategy, MSCs were nucleofected with BMP-2 and BMP-9 plasmids and then implanted ectopically. Bone formation was evident after 4 weeks, proving that *ex vivo* nonviral gene delivery into adult bone marrow–derived stem cells is a viable alternative to viral methods of transduction [38]. Nevertheless, further studies should be conducted to determine more deeply the ability of electroporated cells to regenerate a critical-size defect in an animal model.

Another promising method for transfecting cells without the usage of viral vectors is the use of polymer nanoparticles for the entrapment and delivery of genetic material. This issue will be discussed later in this chapter.

In order to enhance bone formation effectively, genes involved in the osteogenesis process must be known. Genetically engineered MSCs can also be used to find novel candidate therapeutic genes for bone repair. To this end, different studies based on gene arrays followed by a clustering analysis are used to generate a database of genes that play a major role in the bone formation process that is induced by genetically modified MSCs.

Scaffolds: Synthetic 3D Structures for Bone Tissue Engineering

Bone is a complex tissue with multiple cell phenotypes, distinct tissue types, high vascularisation and plays a very demanding mechanical role. Therefore, the attainment of systems that substitute original bone is an extremely difficult task.

Bone transplantation is one of the most successful methods to restore bone functionality in bone defects and injuries. In particular, trabecular bone autografts are the gold standard in bone transplantation. The high porosity of trabecular bone allows the tissue ingrowth and vascularisation of the graft within few weeks and new bone formation within months. Thus, the ideal bone substitute should resemble trabecular bone's architecture, biochemistry and mechanical properties [44].

Cells count on a natural scaffold which consists of various macromolecules and is known as extracellular matrix (ECM). The ECM is a combination of specific proteins that are secreted by cells to form a complex network. This network is a supporting framework where cells grow and differentiate giving the form and shape of the desired tissue. The ECM provides the proper environment within which migratory cells can move and interact with one another and stationary cells are anchored. Cell-matrix interactions are paramount to initiate and mediate biological events that control cell growth, migration, differentiation, survival, tissue organization, and matrix remodelling among others. ECM also plays a structural role. For instance, in the case of connective tissues, ECM is the "stress bearing" element. Most of the mechanical stresses undergone by this type of tissue are borne by the ECM. The function of the tissue engineering scaffold is to act as a synthetic ECM mimicking its properties for support of cell growth and tissue development.

Scaffolds are short -term matrices for bone growth and provide a specific environment and architecture for tissue development. The material composition as well as structural characteristics such as porosity, interconnectivity and pore size and distribution among others are crucial for the success of tissue engineering approaches based on the usage of acellular constructs [45;46].

Temporary synthetic 3D porous constructs that stimulate cells attachment, in-growth, proliferation and differentiation into functional osteoblastic cells are currently being explored as provisional support for the formation of the new tissue. Materials used in the elaboration of these scaffolds are placed within the context of the third generation of biomaterials, which deals with the development of new materials able to stimulate specific cellular responses at the molecular level [47].

Ideal scaffolds that mimic autologous bone grafts must possess three key properties: osteoconductivity, osteoinductivity and osteogenicity. Bone substitute materials usually possess two of these key characteristics.

Besides these three properties, porous structures aimed to tissue engineering applications need to fulfil the following criteria [48;49]:

- The material must be biocompatible and its degradation by-products non-cytotoxic.
- The scaffold must be biodegradable and should resorb at the same rate as the tissue is repaired.
- The scaffold must possess a highly interconnected porous network, formed by a combination of macro and micro pores that enable a proper tissue ingrowth, vascularization and nutrient delivery.
- The mechanical properties of the scaffold must be appropriate to regenerate bone tissue in load bearing sites. Moreover, the material must keep its structural integrity during the first stages of the new bone formation.

Other wanted properties are an adaptable shape to the defect size and geometry as also radioopaque qualities to allow radiographic differentiation between the implanted material and the new formed bone [50].

Thus, biomaterials used as tissue engineering scaffolds must combine both biodegradability and bioactivity properties among other aspects in order to success. Surface functionalization with peptide sequences that mimic the extracellular matrix components, delivery of biochemical factors, and control of cell behaviour through mechanotransduction in order to trigger specific cell responses are some of the approaches that are currently under study in order to complete the three key properties and add osteoinductive characteristics to the materials [51-53].

Scaffolds' porosity must include a wide variety of pore sizes. Microporosity with pores less than 10 μm is needed for capillary ingrowth and to promote protein adhesion and consequently cell-matrix interactions such as cell adhesion and proliferation. Macroporosity with pore sizes ranging between 150 and 900 μm allows for nutrient supply and waste removal of cells grown on the scaffold [54;55]. In spite of the controversy about the optimum pore size, in general, an average pore size around 100-350 μm is considered adequate [56]. Pore diameters over 100μm are necessary for cell ingrowth and diameters over 200μm are required for osteoconduction.

Various materials have been used to produce scaffolds that meet the requirements mentioned above. The most important are natural and synthetic biodegradable polymers as well as ceramics.

Polymeric Scaffolds

Both natural and synthetic polymers have been used in the development of new 3D scaffolds for bone tissue engineering. Natural polymers can be of both plant and animal origin. These polymers usually offer the advantage of biological recognition; however, they may also include pathogenic impurities and in general offer low reproducibility.

In contrast, synthetic polymers offer high reproducibility and the possibility of large-scale production. In particular synthetic biodegradable polymers have raised special attention because they enable a better control of their physico-chemical properties and also because they have been successfully used in clinical applications. Polylactic acid (PLA), polyglycolic acid (PGA) and polycaprolactone (PCL) are the most studied polymers for bone tissue engineering purposes.

Commonly Used Biodegradable Polymers

Polylactic Acid

One of the most widely used synthetic polymeric materials is polylactic acid (PLA). PLA, which structure is shown in Figure 5, is a biocompatible, thermoplastic, resorbable aliphatic polyester from the poly(α-hydroxyacid) family, it is FDA (Food and Drug Administration) approved, and has been used clinically as sutures, bone fracture fixation devices and as drug release systems. PLA is produced by the ring-opening polymerization of lactide; a cyclic diester. The polymerization requires heat and a metallic or an organometallic catalyst. Stannous octoate is the most commonly used catalyst because it is also FDA approved.

PLA is a chiral molecule, and thus exists as two stereoisomers or enantiomers: L-lactide and D-lactide

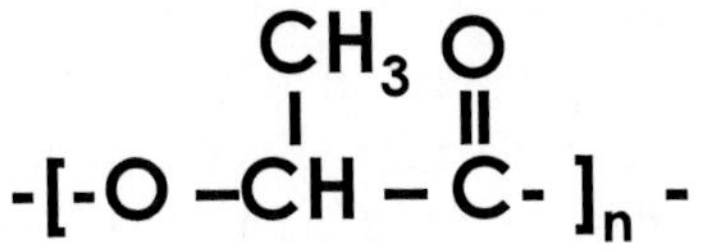

$$-[-O-CH-\overset{\overset{\displaystyle CH_3}{|}}{\underset{}{C}}-]_n-$$

Figure 5. Polylactic acid (PLA) structure.

PLA can be polymerized into four morphologically distinct forms: poly-DD-LA, poly-LL-LA (also known as PLLA), poly-DL-LA (also known as PDLA) and poly-meso-LA. PLLA is a semicrystalline polymer, with a glass transition temperature (Tg) ranging between 50-65°C, and a melting temperature (Tm) between 170-190°C. PDLA is an amorphous polymer with a Tg ranging between 50-60°C. As with most of the polymers, crystallinity, Tg and molecular weight are factors that modulate PLA's mechanical and degradation properties. PLLA is the most frequently employed of the polylactic polymers because it yields the L-lactide acid upon hydrolytic degradation which is the naturally occurring steroisomer of lactic acid [57].

PLA degrades by random bulk cleavage of its ester bonds. This process is auto-catalyzed by the ends of the carboxylic chains that are produced during the ester hydrolysis. The autocatalytic cleavage of the PLA ester bonds has important effects on the degradation behaviour of PLA implants. The cleavage of the ester bonds in PLA releases lactic acid which tends to acidify the milieu of the PLA implant and may be toxic to the surrounding tissues [58]. This is one of the main drawbacks of PLA implants and its application as a tissue engineering material.

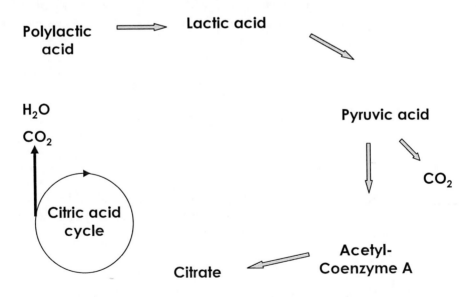

Figure 6. Schematic description of the metabolic degradation of polylactic acid.

Degradation by-products (lactic acid) are finally eliminated as CO_2 and H_2O [59]. First, polylactic acid degrades into lactic acid which in turn gives pyruvic acid. In the presence of sufficient oxygen, pyruvic acid is converted into carbon dioxide, CO_2, and acetyl-coenzime A. This coenzyme is the main input to the citric acid or tricarboxilic acid cycle; a series of chemical reactions of central importance to all living cells. Within the citric acid cycle, acetyl-coenzyme A reacts with oxaloacetate to produce citrate which is the first and the last product of the cycle. A schematic description of the process is shown in Figure 6.

Polyglycolic Acid

Polyglycolic acid (PGA) is the simplest linear aliphatic polyester. PGA was used to develop the first totally synthetic absorbable suture that has been patented as DEXON® since the 1960s by Davis and Geck [60;61]. Glycolide monomer is synthesized from the dimerization of glycolic acid. As in the case of PLA, PGA is obtained by ring-opening polymerization of the cyclic diesters catalized by antimony, zinc or lead. PGA is highly crystalline (45-55%) with a high melting point ranging between 220 and 225°C and a glass transition temperature between 35 and 40°C [61]. The chemical structures of PLA and PGA are similar except that the PLA has a methyl pendant group (see Figures 5 and 7). This structural difference confers PGA a higher hydrophilicity in comparison to PLA. This fact contributes to significant differences in their degradation kinetics; PGA degrades much faster than PLA. While PGA degrades in few weeks [62;63], PLA can remain stable for over 1 year or more depending on its degree of crystallinity [64].

As in the case of PLA, PGA degradation begins with random hydrolysis in an aqueous environment. *In vivo*, however, enzymes are thought to enhance the initial degradation. The hydrolytic degradation *in vivo* may take place via non-specific esterases and carboxyl peptidases that produce glycolic acid monomers which are converted enzymatically into glycine, which can be used in protein synthesis, or into pyruvate that enters the tricarboxylic acid (TCA) cycle yielding energy, water and carbon dioxide. Besides, glycolic acid is partially excreted in urine.

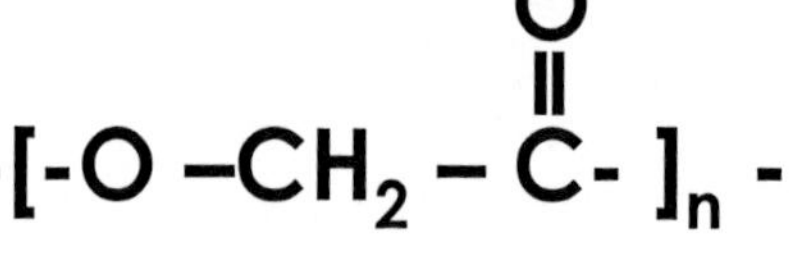

$$-[-O-CH_2-\overset{\displaystyle O}{\overset{\displaystyle \|}{C}}-]_n-$$

Figure 7. Polyglycolic acid (PGA) structure.

Glycolide has been copolymerized with other monomers to reduce its stiffness and modulate its degradation rate. The most common copolymer is the poly(lactic-co-glycolic) acid.

Polycaprolactone

Poly(ε-caprolactone) (PCL): PCL is an aliphatic polyester that has also been widely studied as degradable biomaterial (Figure 8). The ring opening polymerization of ε-caprolactone yields a semicrystalline polymer with a low melting point of 59-64°C and a exceptionally low glass-transition temperature around -60°C. Thus, this polymer is always in a rubbery state at room temperature. PCL can also be degraded by a hydrolytic mechanism under physiologic conditions. The degradation by-products of this polymer are metabolized intracellularly following a pathway similar to that of the poly(α-hydroxy acids). The homopolymer has a degradation time of the order of two years. Thus, it possesses a significant slower degradation rate in comparison with PLA and PGA. Different polymer blends have been investigated to combine the advantages of various polymers. For instance, PCL's degradation rate can be tailored by combining it with other polymers, such as DL-lactide which increases PCL degradation rate, or glycolide that reduces stiffness compared to pure PCL and is being sold as a suture [65].

In general, hydrolysis of these biodegradable polymers depends on several aspects such as their molecular weight, surface area/weight radio, porosity and monomer concentration, geometric isomerism and conformation and crystallinity. The pH of the aqueous medium is also crucial as highly acidic or basic media strongly affects the chemical structure of these polymers accelerating there degradation rate [63;66;67].

One of the strategies to obtain scaffolds that are both biodegradable and bioactive is the combination of organic and inorganic phases in a composite material. Biodegradable composite scaffolds combining biodegradability and bioactivity offer unique advantages in the bone tissue engineering field. The incorporation of an inorganic phase into the bioabsorbable polymer matrix modifies the mechanical behaviour of the porous structure [68], enhances the scaffold bioactivity and also modifies the degradation pattern of the polymer[69], [49]. Furthermore, the incorporation of a second inorganic phase into the polymeric matrix may buffer poly(α-hydroxy acids)'s acidic degradation by-products.

$$-[-\overset{\overset{\textstyle O}{\|}}{C}-(CH_2)_5-O-]_n-$$

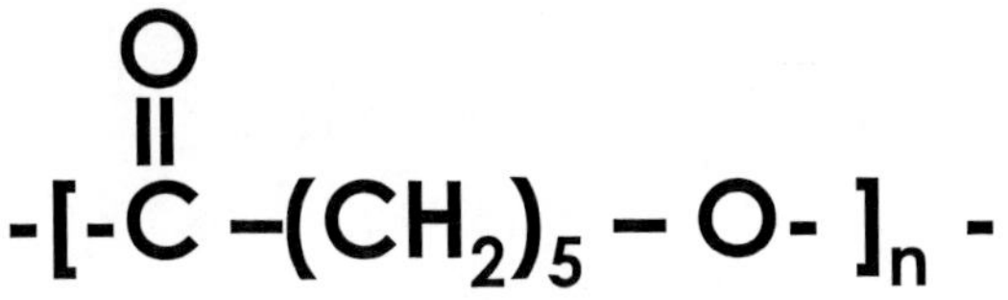

Figure 8. Poly(ϵ-caprolactone) (PCL) structure.

Elaboration Techniques

Numerous elaboration techniques and approaches to the development of 3D scaffolds that combine biodegradability and bioactivity are currently under study. Each elaboration technique provides specific and different structural characteristics to the final scaffold. Therefore, the choice of the technique depends on the requirements of the final application. Some of the most promising techniques for the elaboration of such scaffolds are gel casting, solvent casting and particulate leaching, laminated object manufacturing (LOM), phase separation, gas saturation, fibre bonding and membrane lamination among others [70]. Scaffolds' micro and macrostructure depends strongly on the processing technique.

Solvent Casting and Particulate Leaching

The solvent casting and particulate leaching method was developed by Mikos et al [71] amongst others for polylactic and polyglycolic acid polymers, and several authors have used the method to manufacture composite scaffolds [72-74]. It consists of dissolving a polymer in a solvent and then adding particles of a leachable porogen: salt particles, glucose, paraffin spheres, etc. The mixture forms a thick paste which is left to dry in air or under vacuum until the solvent has evaporated completely. The porogen is leached out afterwards leaving behind a network of interconnected pores. In the case of composites, the second phase is added with the porogen and remains within the structure after the porogen is leached out. Additionally, a thermal treatment can be used to modulate the crystallinity of the polymer by melting the polymer and controlling the cooling rate. The advantages of the solvent casting method are that it is a simple and fairly reproducible method which does not require sophisticated instruments. The disadvantages include thickness limitations intrinsic to the particulate leaching process, limited mechanical properties, and some authors question the homogeneity and interconnection of the pores in the scaffolds, as well as the presence of residual porogen and solvent [75].

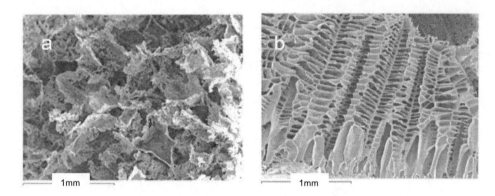

Figure 9. Polylactic acid scaffolds elaborated by the a) solvent casting and b) phase separation techniques.

Phase Separation

Thermally induced phase separation was first applied to PLA scaffolds by Schugens et al [76], several authors have applied this technique to composite scaffolds [48;77;78]. It consists of inducing a solid-liquid or liquid-liquid phase separation. This is done by dissolving the polymer in a solvent and quenching the solution at a certain temperature. The rapid cooling process, known as quenching induces a phase separation into a polymer-rich phase and a polymer-poor phase. The solvent must then be removed from the phase separated solutions either by freeze-drying, or by solvent extraction. The solvent leaves behind a microstructural foam. The main advantage of the phase separation method is that pore morphology and orientation can be tailored by altering the thermodynamic and kinetic parameters of the processing. Its disadvantages include the use of potentially toxic solvents and a high degree of anisotropy of the porosity. The latter may actually be beneficial for certain biomedical applications such as nerve regeneration [77;79]. Figure 9 shows the morphology of polylactic scaffolds elaborated using two different techniques, solvent casting followed by particulate leaching (Figure 9a) and the phase separation method (Figure 9b).

Gas Foaming

The gas foaming process is used to fabricate highly porous foams without the use of organic solvents [88-90]. Organic solvents may leave residues behind which can have toxic effects *in vitro* and may cause inflammation *in vivo*. The process consists of saturating the polymer mix with gas at high temperatures and pressures. Then, a thermodynamic instability is created by quickly decreasing the temperature and pressure which stimulates the nucleation and growth of pores of gas within the polymer. Gas-foaming yields high porosities (up to 93%) and varying the temperature, pressure, and rates of parameter reductions can modulate pore sizes. The main disadvantage is due to the poor interconnectivity of the porosity, and the fact that surfaces are mostly nonporous.

Fibre Bonding

The fibre bonding method was first developed by Cima et al [80] who produced scaffolds made of polyglycolic (PGA) acid polymer. They took advantage of the fact that PGA was available as sutures and thus in the shape of long fibres. Mikos et al [71] improved the structural stability of the constructs developing a fibre bonding technique in which the PGA fibres joined at their cross-linking points by "sintering" above their melting point temperature. The main advantage of this technique is the very high surface area/volume ratio which makes them ideal for tissue engineering applications.

Electrospinning

The electrospinning is a simple and cost-effective process that uses an electric field to control the formation and deposition of polymer fibres on a substrate. Sheets and cylindrical shapes can be fabricated with this technique. This method can produce fibres with diameters between several microns down to 100nm or even less. This is of great interest in the development of tissue engineering scaffolds since these fibres can mimic ECM's proteins structure. Electrospinning is able to produce both random and oriented networks which are also a requirement when mimicking natural tissues.

Rapid Prototyping

Rapid prototyping, also known as solid free-form fabrication allow the production of complex scaffolds from 3D databases. All rapid prototyping techniques are based on the same principle of building 3D models layer by layer.

Their main advantage is the possibility of creating intricate 3D shapes and guaranteeing pore interconnectivity. One of the most consolidated techniques, and probably the oldest, is 3D printing. In this case, a thin layer of polymer powder is spread over a platform and a liquid binder is printed onto the layer. The following layer is created by lowering the platform and applying another layer of polymer powder. Thus, the previous layer is joined to the present layer by the binder creating a three-dimensional shape. The operation parameters can be controlled exactly via a computer-assisted design program and the process takes place at room temperature. Some other techniques include the following:

- Stereo-lithography: photo-polymerization by a low-power highly focused UV laser.
- Selective laser sintering: laser sintering of polymer powders.
- Fuse deposition Modelling: extrusion of the polymer, the polymers is usually standard and medical grade, elastomer, polycarbonate, polyphenilsulfone.
- Solid ground curing: similar to stereolithography: but entire layers are cured at time thanks to the use of photomasks.
- Ink-jet printing: 3D binding of polymer powders by a binderfluid; usually needs post process infiltration.

The main limitation of these techniques is their resolution limit (50-300 μm depending on the technique) which makes it difficult to design scaffolds with fine microstructures [81].

Ceramic Scaffolds

Some ceramics and glasses have been used for the elaboration of porous scaffolds. As in the case of polymers, a high degree of macro, micro and nanoporosities is needed. In addition, the degradation rate of the biomaterial and the regeneration rate of the tissue must be equilibrated in order to enable a proper bone turn-over process [82].

Ceramics

Calcium phosphate ceramics have been studied over many years and are currently used for clinical applications. In particular hydroxyapatite ($Ca_{10}(PO_4)_6(OH)_2$, HA) and tricalcium phosphate (especially β-TCP) that have similarities with the chemistry and crystallography of the mineral phase of bone. These calcium phosphates are known as biocompatible, bioactive and osteoconductive and are usually used both in compact and porous forms as well as granules. The filling of bone defects with these materials aims at stimulating a faster and stable healing process. Especially, hydroxyapatite (HA) has been and is used extensively as a substitute in bone grafts, because the crystalline phase of natural bone is basically HA. Moreover, HA as well as other calcium phosphate ceramics possesses bioactive properties and show excellent abilities to bond to bone.

HA possesses a low degradation rate, which is a hurdle for tissue engineering applications. To overcome this problem, HA is usually combined with β-TCP that possesses a faster degradation rate. This combination of materials is also known as biphasic calcium phosphates [83].

Other types of ceramics used in bone repair include porous calcium metaphosphate ($[Ca(PO_3)_2]n$) blocks [69] and natural coral.

Though these artificial calcium phosphate ceramics can possess osteoconductive and, osteogenic properties, they clearly have no osteoinductive effects on regenerating bone [84]. Their combination with bone morphogenetic proteins (BMP), mesenchymal stem cells from bone marrow, and angiogenesis inductive factors may solve this drawback [85]. Other strategy involves the use of chitosan foams covered with calcium phosphate slurries to obtain scaffolds with the advantages of the osteoinductive properties of chitosan together with the osteoconductive properties of calcium phosphates.

Current research is focused in the development of nanocrystalline structures resembling bone mineral phase crystals, organic-inorganic composites, the use of fibres and microspheres for the elaboration of porous structures, 3D amorphous calcium phosphate scaffolds, HA , tuned porosity microstructures [86] and hierarchically organized structures [87].

Calcium phosphate cements foams have been used as templates for *in situ* regeneration with very promising results. Calcium phosphate cements based on β-TCP have been foamed using albumen and other foaming agents showing positive *in vivo* results. Scaffolds with porosities around 75% and spherical pores ranging between 100-500 μm can be obtained using this technique [88;89].

Glasses and Glass-Ceramics

Biological glasses both bioactive and bioabsorbable, as well as some calcium phosphate glass-ceramics have been also used for the fabrication of 3D porous scaffolds for bone tissue engineering.

Bioactive glasses such as the well known Bioglass were first developed by Hench et al [90]. They discovered that certain glass compositions had the capacity to form a tight bone bonding. Bioactive glasses based on SiO_4 as network former are able to create a calcium deficient carbonated phosphate surface layer that allows the formation of the chemical bond to bone. The formation of this surface layer and posterior binding to bone is known as bioactivity. This bioactivity that is also present in some calcium phosphate ceramics such as HA is induced by interfacial and cell mediated reactions in the aqueous medium [91].

The formation of a tight bond to the bone tissue guarantees a good fixation between the scaffold and the surrounding tissue. Bioactive glasses have demonstrated to support enzyme activity, vascularization, osteoblast adhesion, growth and differentiation. In addition, they have also shown to induce the differentiation of mesenchymal cells into osteoblasts, which is of great importance in cellular tissue engineering applications [48;92;93].

The degradation by-products of these bioactive SiO_4 based glasses have been analysed. According to the obtained results, dissolution products from bioactive glasses upregulate the gene expression that control osteogenesis and the production of growth factors [91]. Besides, it has been shown that the presence of silicon in ceramic materials and glasses play a key role in bone mineralization and gene activation. These findings are of great impact for bone tissue engineering since they can stimulate materials' osteoinductivity.

Glasses bioactivity and osteoconductivity together with their osteogenic properties make them promising materials for bone tissue engineering applications.

Phosphate glasses also represent an interesting option as materials for tissue engineering applications given that their chemistry can be modulated in order to obtain glasses chemically similar to the bone mineral phase. Furthermore they have demonstrated to present a controlled solubility [94].In fact, their solubility can be modulated with the addition of highly charged and small radius modifying ions [95]. Additionaly, previous studies have revealed the biocompatibility of these glasses. *In vitro* cultures have shown that these formulations elicit no cytotoxicity [96]. In particular glasses in the system P_2O_5-CaO-Na_2O-TiO_2 have shown to accelerate the early differentiation of osteoblastic cells *in vitro* [96]

Different methods for the elaboration of these 3D vitreous or ceramic constructs have been proposed such as the introduction of diverse kinds of porosifiers, foaming agents and emulsifiers, the solid free form fabrication technique, the impregnation of a skeleton of porous polyurethane foam with ceramic emulsions, sol-gel and gel-casting techniques among others [89;97-101]. Among this variety of processes for fabrication of porous materials, the replication technique (also called the polymersponge method) produces porous ceramic structures that are most similar to those of spongy bone [102].

The replication method consists in impregnating a body of porous polymer foam with slurry containing the ceramic or glass powder, water and some optional additives. The polymer foam is the responsible of the porosity, interconnectivity degree and pores size. Once the foam has been impregnated with the slurry, it is exposed to a heat treatment that allows the ceramic densification and elimination of the organic foam. HA and bioactive glass scaffolds have been fabricated by means of the replication method [103;104].

Incorporation of porosifiers implies the use of organic compounds that can be pyrolitically removed leaving behind pores. The size and shape of the pores depends on the nature of the porosifier agent. Ceramic granules or particles are mixed with the porosifier agent and pressed forming the green body that will be subsequently heated in order to eliminate the organic matter and to sinter the ceramic material.

The sol-gel process involves the preparation of a mixture of distilled water, some alkoxide precursors and salts, and a catalyst for hydrolysis. Once hydrolysis is completed, aliquots of sol are foamed with the addition of surfactants and vigorous agitation. In this case, porosity strongly depends on the concentration of surfactant. After the foaming process is finished the gelation process is also completed and the constructs proceed to the aging and drying processes to remove solvents, and finally the thermal stabilisation process takes place to allow partial densification of the matrix [105].

Incorporation of foaming agents such as hydrogen peroxide (H_2O_2) or albumin has been also studied. In this case, a calcium phosphate ceramic powder or glass particles slurry is formed together with the foaming agent solution. Afterwards, the foamed mixture is heated up to remove the foaming agent and sinter the ceramic or glass particles. Figure 10 displays the fracture surface of two porous glass-ceramic materials foamed with albumin (Figure 10a) and hydrogen peroxide (Figure 10b). There is a clear difference in pores amount morphology, size and distribution depending on the elaboration method.

In addition, new strategies to generate highly complex three-dimensional (3D) ceramic-based scaffolds arise from RP technologies that have been adapted to the specific demands concerning materials and processing [106;107].

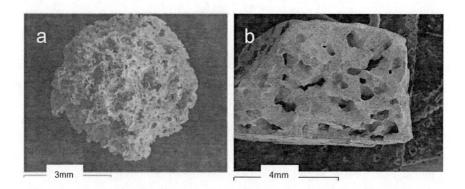

Figure 10. Calcium phosphate glass-ceramic scaffolds elaborated from $CaO-P_2O_5-Na_2O-TiO_2$ glasses using two different foaming agents, a) albumin and b) H_2O_2

Metallic Scaffolds

Although metallic materials are not biodegradable, they have also been used in the development of porous structures for bone tissue engineering. The development of porous metallic foams for bone tissue engineering and drug delivery applications has been mostly focused on the used of titanium and titanium alloys. Nevertheless, elaboration of metallic foams using Ta and Mg has also been reported [108].

Titanium and its alloys are highly resistant to corrosion due to the formation of an adhesive TiO_2 oxide layer at their surface; possess a relative low elastic modulus in comparison with other metals used for biomedical applications, and is able to become tightly integrated into bone.

Although numerous studies have been performed on the fabrication processes and design of metallic foams [109;110], their biological response has not been characterized properly and information dealing with the *in vitro* or *in vivo* behaviour of these metallic porous scaffolds is still scarce. However, there are some studies that report good biological behaviour, for instance titanium foams tested *in vitro* with human osteoblasts have shown to efficiently support osteoblast colonization and differentiation into mature bone cells [111]. Other studies have reported titanium fibre meshes (86% porosity and a 250 ☐m average pore size) that have been used for the *ex vivo* culture of rat bone marrow stromal cells, under static conditions and dynamic conditions (flow perfusion bioreactor), and subsequent implantation in cranial defects in rats [112]. Furthermore, these scaffolds have also found application as delivery systems for transforming growth factor β1 (TGF-β1) and have been used in rabbit cranial defects [113].

The main hurdles associated to these scaffolds is that they are not resorbable and hence their permanent implantation in the body can trigger risks of toxicity caused by the accumulation of metal ions due to corrosion [114], premature failure due to poor wear properties, and higher elastic modulus compared with bone, leading to heterogeneous stress distributions.

Research on shape memory metallic foams is currently carried out. In particular NiTi alloys are under studied, as to reduce stress shielding (removal of bone normal stresses due to the presence of high elastic modulus implants) and increase wear resistance of conventional porous titanium scaffolds. At the moment, only some *in vitro* preliminary studies have been carried out with osteoblastic and endothelial cells to evaluate these materials' cytocompatibility [115].

Surface Functionalization to Improve Cell-Material Interactions

Since most synthetic materials lack osteoinductivity properties, those must be supplied by other sources. It is known that cell response is highly affected by the physicochemical features of the material surface. Thus, tailoring surface characteristics such as surface charges, energy, topography and chemical composition among others may balance this shortage of osteoinductive signals. This chapter will only focus on the chemical approach, specifically on functionalization of surfaces with biomolecules since it is one of the most promising alternatives to provide chemical signals that activate and stimulate cellular events at the molecular level.

Cell adhesion is mediated by protein-cell interactions based on the biological recognition of protein sequences by transmembrane cell receptors known as integrins. In the case of cell adhesion, the most important peptide sequence is RGD (Arginine-Glycine-Aspartic acid) that is found in many ECM proteins and enhances cell attachment. Some of the most commonly employed strategies are the functionalization of biomaterial surfaces using proteins and peptides that mimic the ECM chemistry, in particular RGD sequences [116;117], and the addition of growth factors into the scaffolds composition for a controlled delivery to the surrounding cells. For this last approach, various growth factors have already been used: fibroblast growth factor (FGF), platelet-derived growth factor, insulin growth factor, transforming growth factor (TGF), bone morphogenetic proteins (BMP), interleukins and interferons [118] (described in detail later in this chapter).

Other functionalization techniques include dip-coating and more sophisticated techniques like the immobilization of biomolecules via self assembled monolayers (SAMs) or grafting from techniques among others.

Dip-coating consists in the impregnation of the material with a solution containing the desired biomolecule. This method is based on the physisorbtion of the molecules to the materials surface. The superficially absorbed molecules are released rapidly within the biological environment. In this case, control over release kinetics is difficult to accomplish.

Surface modification with specific molecular motifs by means of their immobilization via SAMs or via grafted polymer brushes has also been explored.

Self assembled monolayers are surfaces consisting of a single layer of molecules on a substrate. They can be prepared simply by adding a solution of the desired molecule onto the substrate and washing off the excess. The most common example of SAM is an alkane thiol on gold. An alkane with a thiol head group will stick to the gold surface due to the sulphur affinity to gold, and form an ordered assembly with the alkyl chains packing together due to van der Waals forces. SAMs are good platforms for mimicking cell membrane and for immobilizing biomolecules involved in the different cell functioning processes.

Polymer brushes were shown to be a versatile setting for the immobilization of peptide sequences that influence cell behaviour [119;120]. Biointerfaces based on the use of binded polymer chains have several advantages over SAMs: polymer brushes provide multiple binding sites for biomolecules, their flexible nature allows reorganization of the functionalities upon the adhesion of cells and, most importantly, and they can be synthesized very easily and on a variety of substrates [121].

For example, in the case of the cell adhesion process, it not only depends on the receptor/ligand or integrin/RGD interactions but also on the formation of receptor's clusters to form cell focal adhesion points. The flexibility and mobility of peptide sequences coupled to polymer brushes promote the formation of such clusters.

More specific and sophisticated methods for surface functionalization and for modulating cell behaviour are presently being developed. It is predictable that the short term trends in biomaterials intended for tissue engineering applications will involve growing efforts from biochemistry and cell biology fields.

The Use of Growth Factors in Bone Tissue Engineering

In vivo, mammalian cells can communicate in several different ways to coordinate their activities. One of these principal ways is the secretion of soluble signals, called growth factors (GF), by a signalling cell. These growth factors are biochemical signals sent to a target cell in order to guide its biological behaviour [119]. These signals, which are indeed small proteins on the order of 15 to 20 kDa in size, are known as cytokines or chemokines whether they affect cell proliferation and differentiation or cell migration respectively. Numerous studies allowed unravelling the crucial role of a variety of growth factors secreted by different cells that are involved in the formation process of different tissues. The knowledge acquired from these studies has been the starting point of the application of growth factors in tissue engineering (TE) systems. Presently, there is compelling evidence available to indicate that the incorporation of growth factors into in vitro tissue engineering systems has a dramatic effect on tissue generation. The formation, growth and functionality of tissues obtained from cells seeded on 3D constructs are enhanced when exposed to a microenvironment where growth factors are present. More importantly, without a delivery carrier, the growth factor is not able to influence bone regeneration significantly. The direct injection of the growth factor is not efficient enough to enhance tissue regeneration [120].

Requirements for Successful Delivery of Growth Factors

The rationale for using GF into TE systems is to provide the cells with the adequate signals that will guide them toward an appropriate biological response which will lead to the formation of a functional tissue. Therefore, the incorporation of growth factors into a 3D porous scaffold should allow their release and delivery to cells in a timely and prolonged manner that matches biological needs. For a successful delivery, parameters such as i) loading capacity of the matrix, ii) drug distribution into it, iii) binding affinity with it, iv) release kinetics and v) drug stability over a long period of time must be considered. An optimized delivery system for bone application should deliver efficient doses of osteogenic agents while reducing as much as possible the amount of introduced growth factor. This is both for questions of economic viability and safety to avoid potential high-doses side effects. In addition, the biological activity of the growth factors must be preserved during their loading into the delivery carrier.

Different Strategies for Growth Factor Incorporation into a Carrier Material

Growth factors can be either attached to the scaffold or entrapped into it. The attachment of growth factors is mainly performed onto preformed scaffolds, whereas the entrapment generally involves the mixing of the scaffold material (most often polymeric material) with the growth factors during the scaffold fabrication step. Growth factors can be attached through covalent attachment via chemical cross-linking between the growth factors and the material scaffold [121;122], or by simple physical adsorption via ionic complexes formation generally achieved by soaking the scaffold into a growth factor-containing solution (with opposite charges to that of the scaffold) [123].

If the incorporation into the carrier material is done during the fabrication process, the challenge is to avoid denaturing the growth factors because of organic solvents use or other harsh conditions during processing. The use of supercritical fluids to fabricate scaffolds enables to overcome these problems preserving the biological activity of the loaded growth factors [124]. This technique generally consists of dissolving the polymer/growth factor complex in supercritical CO_2, and of expanding it rapidly in a low temperature and pressure environment [125]. In addition, growth factors can be mixed directly with polymeric or ceramic materials using the different techniques of scaffold fabrication detailed anteriorly, such as solvent casting/particulate leaching or electrospinning methods.

The fabrication of microspheres or microparticules is a common way for entrapping growth factors for a controlled delivery [123;126-130]. Microspheres as drug carriers have the advantages of sustained or controlled release, passive or active drug targeting to specific tissues, which will notably reduce the side effects of drugs and improve their bioavailability [131]. Therefore, microspheres as drug delivery system have drawn much attention in pharmaceutical field and have been successfully applied in some clinical trials. These microspheres can either be incorporated into a scaffold, by homogeneous mixing, or be fused to form a scaffold.

The encapsulation of growth factors into microspheres, or alternatively plasmid DNA of growth factors [132], can be performed by different techniques. Either they can be incorporated after the fabrication of the microspheres, via soaking, similarly to the attachment onto scaffold, or they can be entrapped into the microspheres during their fabrication process. For this latter method, various strategies have been used. Two popular methods involving solvent extraction are commonly used, namely double-emulsion and single-emulsion methods.

The double-emulsion method is based on the formation of a double water/oil/water emulsion (W/O/W) [129;130;133-135]. In this method, an aqueous solution of the growth factors is dispersed in a polymer-containing organic solution, forming the primary water-in-oil emulsion (W/O). This primary W/O emulsion is then dispersed via continuous mechanical agitation into a stabilizer-containing aqueous solution, forming a secondary oil-in-water emulsion (O/W). After evaporation of the organic solvent contained in the emulsion droplets, the microspehres loaded with growth factors are obtained. In the single-emulsion technique, the growth factors are directly dispersed into the organic solution of the polymer, forming a unique oil-in-water emulsion [136].

Another technique that can be used for encapsulation into microspheres is based on the phase separation of two water-soluble polymers in an all-aqueous system and subsequent emulsified condensation polymerization [126;127;137].

A simplified diagram representing the different strategies available for the incorporation of growth factors into a matrix is shown in Figure 11.

Depending on the incorporation method (attachment or entrapment) and on the nature of the carrier material (microspheres, hydrogels or 3D matrices), the release rate of the growth factors will vary, and should be tailored as a function of the requirements of the application.

Principal Growth Factors Used in Bone Tissue Engineering

The principal growth factors used in bone tissue engineering are i) Transforming Growth Factor β (TGF-β1), ii) Bone Morphogenetic Proteins (BMP-2, BMP-6, BMP-7, and BMP-9), iii) Insulin-like Growth Factor (IGF-1), iv) Fibroblast Growth Factor (FGF-2), and v) Vascular endothelial Growth Factor (VEGF).

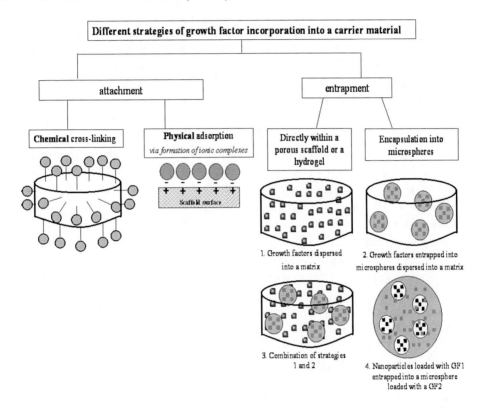

Figure 11. Different strategies for growth factors incorporation (for details, please refer to the text).

Transforming Growth Factor β (TGFβ)

TGFβ is a superfamily of about forty polypeptidic growth factors. They are pleiotropic factors which share similarities in their structure and play a major role in developmental biology. TGFβ are classified into two groups. The first one includes the bone morphogenetic proteins (BMP) and the growth differentiation factors (GDF), while the second one is constituted by TGFβ, activin and nodal [138]. These factors are broadly expressed throughout the body and regulate many cellular pathophysiological processes including cell fate, cell proliferation, cell senescence and tissue repair.

Among the three isoforms of TGFβ that have been described so far, the most interesting one for bone tissue engineering is TGFβ1. It modulates the bone healing process and regulates fracture repair in humans. Moreover, it is locally produced during bone development and regeneration [139-142]. It has been shown to increase the expression of many genes associated with osteoblast activity and to activate osteoblast progenitors [143]. In addition, some other studies showed that TGFβ1 increases alkaline phosphatase activity, collagen, and osteocalcin production by human osteoblasts [144]. TGFβ1-mediated stimulation of *in vivo* and *in vitro* bone formation is linked with an increase in Type I collagen, fibronectin and osteonectin production [142;145;146].

Bone Morphogenetic Proteins (bmps)

BMPs have been implicated in a variety of functions [147-149]. They not only induce the formation of both cartilage and bone, but also play a role in a number of non-osteogenic developmental processes. BMP may be the most widely used inductive factor in bone tissue engineering applications. They play an important role in embryonic development. Since their discovery in the 60s by Urist [149], at least 20 types of BMPs have been identified and characterized in humans. BMP signal transduction is induced via interaction with the heterodimeric complex of two transmembrane serine/threonine kinase receptors. Although the molecular mechanisms underlying osteoblastic differentiation remain to be identified, BMPs play an important role in regulating osteoblast differentiation and subsequent bone formation. The BMPs with greatest osteogenic capacity are BMP-2, -4, -5, -6, -7, and-9 [147].

BMPs mainly act as a differentiation stimulating factor to direct endochondral ossification and chondrogenesis of mesenchymal stem cells. Recombinant forms (i.e. cloned) of BMPs, particularly BMP-2, BMP-4 and BMP-7, have the ability to heal critical sized bone defects in rodents, dogs, sheep and non-human primates when combined with a carrier of collagen, guanidine-extracted demineralized bone matrix, hydroxyapatite or biodegradable polymers. Of these, recombinant human rhBMP-2 and rhBMP-7 (or osteogenic protein-1, BMP-7) are now commercially available. Other BMP-containing osteoinductive materials are currently being evaluated in animal and clinical studies.

Insulin-Like Growth Factor (IGF)

IGF is a strong stimulant of proliferation and chemotactic migration of many cell populations, and it is involved in bone metabolism [138;150]. The correlation between local IGF expression and new bone formation and mineralization has been reported in many studies. It seems that IGF regulates bone formation through a different mechanism that of BMPs [148].

Fibroblast Growth Factor (FGF)

FGF2, or basic FGF, is part of a family of at least 19 structurally related growth factors. This family has been implicated in a variety of normal and pathologic processes such as repair processes in neural, cartilage, and soft tissue injury among others [151]. FGF2 is also a potent mitogenic factor and, with its receptors, can be found in essentially all tissues of the body [152;153]. In bone, FGF2 is produced intracellularly by osteoblasts, and can be found both in their nucleus and nucleoli, and secreted into the surrounding matrix, hence regulating cell function at the transcriptional level [154-157]. FGF2 has been shown to induce osteoblast expression of TGFβ1 [158] and TGFβ2 [159]. Fibroblast growth factors play a critical role in bone growth [160] and development affecting both chondrogenesis and osteogenesis. During the process of intramembranous ossification, which leads to the formation of the flat bones of the skull, unregulated FGF signaling can produce premature suture closure or craniosynostosis and other craniofacial deformities. Indeed, many human craniosynostosis disorders have been linked to activating mutations in FGF receptors (FGFR) 1 and 2 [161].

As a consequence, FGF-2 has been actively studied as a stimulant of bone healing [148]. Although several lines of evidence indicate that FGFs regulate both proliferation and differentiation in osteoblasts [162], the effects of FGF remain unclear. Apparently, conflicting reports on the exact nature of these effects exist in the literature. This is probably due to differential effects of FGF depending on the stage of osteoblast maturation [159;163]: whereas there has been general agreement that FGF stimulates the proliferation of osteoblasts in vitro, FGF appears to inhibit expression of differentiation markers such as phosphatase alkaline (ALP) and osteocalcin (OC) in human and rat calvarial cells [162], but increases the levels of ALP, OC, and differentiation of osteogenic precursors in the bone marrow [163]. The mechanism by which FGF signaling increases proliferation in immature osteoblasts, and paradoxically inhibits DNA synthesis and increases apoptosis in differentiating cells is not clear at the moment.

Table 1. Summary of different types of incorporation technique of different growth factors used in bone tissue engineering applications and of the carrier materials used to incorporate them

Carrier material	Matrix Type	Growth Factor	Incorporation technique	References
PEG	Hydrogel	bFGF	Crosslinking	[121]
Gelatin	Microsphere	TGFβ1	Soaking	[172]
Chitosan-based	Hydrogel	rhBMP	Mixing before processing	[173]
PLA	Porous scaffold	VEGF	Supercritical processing	[174]
PLA	Porous scaffold	BMP2	Supercritical processing	[175]
Silk fibroin	Porous scaffold	BMP2	Electrospinning	[176]
PLGA	Microspheres	BMP2	Double-emulsion	[133]
PLGA	Microspheres	TGFβ1	Double-emulsion	[135]
PLGA/PEG	Microspheres	VEGF	Single-emulsion	[136]
Collagen	Sponge	BMP2	Soaking	[177;178]
Alginate	Hydrogel	BMP2, TGFb3	Soaking	[179]
Dextran-co-gelatin	Microspheres	IGF1	Soaking	[180]
Dextran-co-gelatin	Microspheres	BMP2	Phase-separation Double-phase emulsion	[126]
Gelatin	Hydrogel	TGFβ1	Soaking	[181]
Gelatin	Hydrogel	BMP2	Soaking	[182]
Gelatin	Hydrogel	TGF, IGF	Soaking	[183]

Vascular Endothelial Growth Factor (VEGF)

Vascularisation is a crucial issue in bone tissue engineering [164]. The formation of blood vessels is primordial for the transport of oxygen, nutrients and growth factors into the newly formed tissue, and hence for the viability of the organ. During bone development and fracture healing, vascularisation is observed before bone formation. In intramembranous bone formation, osteoblasts arise from mesenchymal precursors and differentiate into mature osteoblasts. At the transition of preosteoblasts to osteoblasts extensive vascularisation is observed. In endochondral bone formation a cartilage scaffold is formed, which is subsequently replaced by bone. In the latter process bone formation is also accompanied by invasion of blood vessels [165]. Cross-talk between endothelial cells and chondrocytes or osteoblasts has been demonstrated in cocultures [166;167]. In these cultures, endothelial cells stimulated the differentiation of chondrocytes and osteoblasts through production of endothelial-derived growth factors [167;168], whereas osteoblasts stimulated the proliferation of endothelial cells [167]. In addition, it has been demonstrated that BMPs induce the production of VEGF by osteoblasts, which then stimulates angiogenesis. Therefore, BMP-induced VEGF production in osteoblastic cells play a role in the coupling of bone formation and angiogenesis by acting as a chemoattractant for neighboring endothelial cells.

VEGF stimulates proliferation and migration of endothelial cells, which then assemble to form tubular blood vessels. Although the main function of VEGF is related to vasculature, some studies pointed out its implication in the recruitment, survival and activity of bone forming cells [169]. It has been shown that VEGF stimulated the migration and differentiation of primary human osteoblasts [170;171]. In addition, it seems that VEGF is a mediator of different other osteoinductive factors such as TGF-β1, IGF and FGF-2, which in turn regulate the expression pattern of VEGF. Although VEGF is somewhat implicated in the bone formation process, its application in bone tissue engineering is mainly related to its capacity to promote angiogenesis. The combined use of VEGF with other growth factors could synergistically enhance bone formation and fracture healing.

Table 1 presents a summary of some of the recent works that deal with the incorporation of growth factors into a synthetic or natural matrix as a delivery carrier for tissue engineering applications, and particularly for bone tissue engineering.

Bioreactors: Mimicking in vivo Physiological Conditions

Bioreactor Definition

Mammalian tissues have complex three-dimensional and organized structures that give them their specific functionality. Therefore, it is now evident that 2D culturing systems are not appropriate for mimicking tissue regeneration process in vitro, and that 3D systems are a prerequisite for the success of the TE strategy. However, a key question in 3D culture is the maintenance of specific cell phenotype and functions for a long period of time. The development of *in vitro* systems that mimic as close as possible the physiological conditions of the cells cultured, such as nutrients and metabolic environment among others, is therefore crucial. For that purpose, devices known as bioreactors have been developed, and it is presently accepted that they are essential for a controlled fabrication of reproducible engineered constructs.

Bioreactors are *in vitro* culture vessels that provide a controlled environment, which generally include physical, biochemical and mechanical signals (e.g. pH, temperature, pressure, fluidic and mechanical stimuli, nutrient supply and waste removal), to a 3D hybrid cell-scaffold construct in order to achieve the development and/or the physical conditioning and testing of a functional tissue. In addition, new designs of these devices are presently under development as to allow a real-time monitoring of cellular behaviour in response to specific stimuli applied to the hybrid construct. Real-time evaluation will provide essential information on the formation process of 3D tissues, which is a primordial issue if large scale industrial applications are meant.

Bioreactor Principal Functions: Requisites and Limitations

Four of the most common functions of bioreactors are i) the establishment of a spatially uniform cell distribution throughout the 3D construct, ii) the maintenance of desired concentrations of gas (particularly O_2 and CO_2) and nutrients in the culture medium, iii) the supply of efficient mass transfer to the growing tissue and iv) the exposure of the growing tissue to mechanical stimuli.

The first function regards the cell seeding procedure of the 3D scaffold, which is the first crucial step of bioreactor cultivation of engineered tissues [184]. Cell seeding can be done previously to the introduction of the 3D constructs inside the bioreactor, in a different in vitro vessel, or directly inside the same bioreactor where the construct will be kept for tissue generation. This will basically depend on the bioreactor design.

Cell seeding might play a critical role in determining the progression of tissue formation [185]. A successful cell seeding is achieved with:

(i) A high percentage of attached cells from the initial solution. High efficiency of seeding is important to maximize cell utilization (particularly interesting when working with stem cells) and to achieve high cell densities into scaffolds after seeding. High cell density has been associated with enhanced tissue formation in 3D constructs, including increased bone mineralization [186].

(ii) A high kinetic rate to minimize the time in suspension for anchorage-dependent and shear-sensitive cells, and hence to limit the number of death cells.

(iii) A high and spatially uniform distribution of attached cells for rapid and uniform tissue growth. The initial distribution of cells within the scaffold after seeding has been related to the distribution of tissue that is subsequently formed. This suggests that uniform cell-seeding could be the basic parameter for uniform tissue generation [186-189]. Even with a small 3D construct, it can be a significant challenge to distribute a high density of cells efficiently and uniformly throughout the scaffold volume [190].

In spite of several studies that pointed out low seeding efficiencies [186;189;191-193] and non-uniform cell distributions within scaffolds [186;189;192;194-199], static loading remains the most common technique for cell seeding. Significantly higher efficiencies and uniformities can be obtained by dynamic loading. This will be described in detail in the corresponding part of the different bioreactor designs that allows dynamic seeding (please refer to the state-of-the-art paragraph).

The second key point in a properly-designed bioreactor is the controlled delivery of nutrients and gas to the cells, which is typically a mass-transfer issue [200]. Some of the design challenges to be considered here are:

1. the achievement of adequate flux of oxygen at physiological concentration. The oxygen has to be delivered at the same rate it is being consumed, however it has a low solubility in culture media. Low concentration of oxygen leads to cell death whereas high concentration of oxygen can inhibit cell functions and produce cytotoxic free radicals [186]. Moreover, the oxygen flux has to be proportional to the number of cells and therefore should increase with culture time. Oxygen is commonly delivered in two different ways: i) via fluid flow, where the oxygen concentration and flow rate are the variable parameters to achieve adequate amount of oxygen delivery or ii) *in situ* over an oxygenation membrane. In the first case, heterogeneous delivery can derived from significant differences in oxygen concentration between the inlet and outlet stream. On the other hand, the oxygenation membrane is a better way to achieve uniform delivery of oxygen.
2. a uniform flow distribution.
3. the provision of cyto and chemokines and other important molecules (growth factors, proteins, etc.) that must be properly balanced at the same time as oxygen and nutrients are delivered.

As important as delivery, removal of wastes such as carbon dioxide and urea is essential for an optimum process. However, the monitoring of urea concentration in reactors is rarely done, partly due to the unavailability of on-line sensors.

Each one of these key issues has to be tailored as a function of the dimensional and functional requirements of the tissue to be engineered. Mathematical models based on mass transfer theory can be applied for an accurate design as a function of the cellular needs [200;201].

As mentioned earlier, fluid flow is an important aspect of bioreactor's design. With a properly controlled fluid flow, uniform cell seeding (through perfusion systems), nutrients and gas delivery, efficient mass transfer and even mechanical stimuli can be achieved. However, uniform fluid flow can be difficult to achieve with some bioreactor designs, which can lead to an inhomogeneous tissue distribution and growth over the 3D construct. In addition, taking into account the complexity of interconnected porous structures inside a 3D scaffold, it can be difficult to achieve flow uniformity throughout the whole 3D structure. However, this is only relevant when uniform seeding has been previously achieved throughout the 3D scaffold.

Moreover, the flow-induced shear stress applied to the cells inside the scaffold is another crucial issue that has to be rigorously controlled. It is widely accepted that shear stress has a determinant impact on tissue function and viability, and there is a maximal value of sustainable shear stress for every type of cells [201]. An adequate shear stress value can promote cell growth, whereas higher values can provoke cell damage and necrosis of the tissues. In addition, it has been suggested that a homogeneous pore distribution in a 3D scaffold could enable a more precise control over shear stress [202]. However, deeper studies have to be carried out as to gain knowledge on shear stress thresholds to be used in the bioreactor as a function of cell type.

State-of-the-Art of Principal Bioreactor Designs

Presently, there are few models of bioreactors commercially available. Most of these devices are only suitable for experimental studies and not for clinical applications due to their small size and hence to the small size of the engineered tissue. Generally, researchers into TE and bioreactor fields develop their own in-house reactors depending on what kind of experimental studies they want to perform.

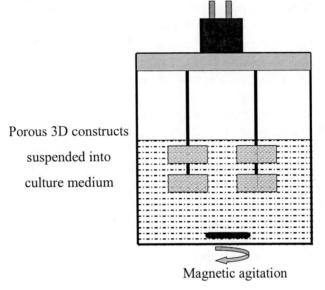

Porous 3D constructs suspended into culture medium

Magnetic agitation

Figure 12. Simplified view of a typical stirred-tank bioreactor.

In this part, some of the most commonly used working principles applied to bioreactor designs are presented as to give the reader a general idea on the state-of-the-art of bioreactor development.

First Generation Bioreactors

1. Petri dishes that were orbitally mixed were firstly used because they enhanced tissue growth comparing with static dishes [197;203]. However, the thickest bone tissue reported in such reactors were of 0.5 mm [204], which is not big enough to serve as a graft for tissue replacement (it should be at least a few millimetres).
2. Stirred-tank reactor:

In this case, mixing of oxygen and nutrients within the culture medium is achieved by magnetic agitation of the fluid into the flask, in which the scaffolds seeded with the cells are suspended (Figure 12).

The first advantage of this type of reactors for cell seeding is that they enable significantly higher efficiencies and uniformities of cell seeding compared to static loading, due to the convective transport of the cells into the scaffold [197]. However, some studies have pointed out low seeding efficiencies [189;205] and heterogeneous distributions of cells [194;198], with a higher density of cells on the outer surface of the scaffold [185] when using stirred-tank reactors. This is possibly due to ineffective convection of cells inside the scaffolds.

Rotating-Wall Vessel Reactor

Three common models can be found in the literature:

1. The Slow Turning Lateral Vessel (STLV, Figure 13a), that consists in two concentric cylinders. One inner cylinder that is generally static and provides gas exchange through a gas exchange membrane; and one outer cylinder that rotates at a determined speed as to maintain the constructs motionless in a state of continuous free-fall (the gravitational, centrifugal and drag forces applied to the scaffold are balanced.)
2. The Rotating Wall Perfused Vessel (RWPV, Figure 13b) is similar to the STLV except that it also includes a recirculation system that allows periodic medium exchange and hence a better control of nutrients and other molecules delivery.
3. The High Aspect Ratio Vessel (HARV, Figure 13c), which principle of operation is similar to both previous reactors. However, its particular design allows reducing the rotational speed of the cylinder, and it includes a larger gas exchange membrane to enhance gas exchange.

The hydrodynamic environment present in these rotating vessel bioreactors seems to be more advantageous for growing engineered tissues than simply stirred-tanks [184].

Perfusion Reactor

Two configurations of perfusion bioreactor can be encountered:

1. The perfusion column (Figure 14a), in which the same fluid flow goes through more than one 3D construct.
2. The perfusion chamber (Figure 14b), in which the medium flows directly through the pores of a unique scaffold.

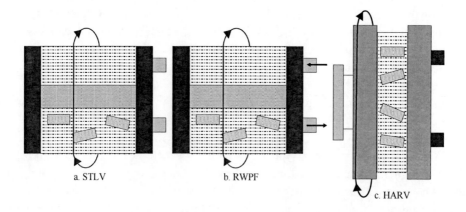

a. STLV   b. RWPF   c. HARV

Figure 13. Three types of rotating-wall vessel bioreactors. a/ the Slow Turning Lateral Vessel; b/ the Rotating-Wall Perfused Vessel; c/ The High Aspect Ratio Vessel (see text for details).

In both configurations, there is a continuous medium recirculation. The fluid can be forced to pass through the porous constructs either by a pumping system (Figure 14b) or an up-and-down motion of the scaffold through the fluid (Figure 14c) [206].

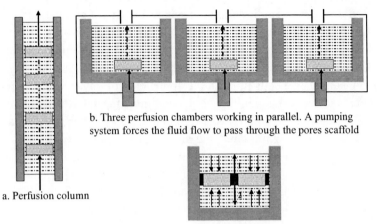

b. Three perfusion chambers working in parallel. A pumping system forces the fluid flow to pass through the pores scaffold

a. Perfusion column

c. Example of perfusion chamber in which an up-and-down motion (1 and 2) is applied to the scaffolds into the fluid as to force the fluid to pass through the pores of the constructs

Figure 14. Example of bioreactors based on a perfusion system. a/ perfusion column reactor; b/ perfusion chamber-based bioreactor; c/ similar to b/ but with different fluid flow system.

In that kind of bioreactors, the dynamic seeding process leads to high efficiency and homogeneous cell distribution. Continuous recirculation of fresh medium enables maintaining physiological concentrations of nutrients and paracrine factors, as well as reducing the accumulation of toxic metabolic products. These factors play undoubtedly a major role in the enhancement of osteogenesis of bone engineered constructs. Several studies have shown that perfusion systems enable to enhance cell viability, alkaline phosphatase activity and osteocalcin production by osteoblastic cells comparing with conventional systems [207;208] as well as mineralized matrix deposition by bone cells [209;210]. However, the flow rate of the medium must be carefully optimized to be the good balance between "too high" and "too low" fluid flows. From one hand, removal of newly synthesized extracellular matrix components off the construct and harmful effects of high shear stresses can derive from high fluid flows and hence have to be avoided. On the other hand, inappropriate mass transfer of nutrients and waste products can be a consequence of low fluid flows.

Rotating-wall vessel reactors and perfusion reactors have efficient designs as to allow excellent transport properties through the scaffold. However, they still need improvement to better control mechanical stimuli; although it is true that the benefits observed for perfusion systems on osteogenesis are partly due to the flow-induced shear stress derived from these systems. For that purpose, a new generation of bioreactors are under development. This is a generation of devices that enable the application of different controllable mechanical loads onto the hybrid construct (cell-seeded scaffold), and that is discussed below.

Bioreactor with Mechanical Stimulation

The increasing interest in bioreactors that include mechanical stimuli control over the 3D constructs derives from several studies that unravelled the direct effect of mechanical forces on biosynthetic cell activity. Other studies provide evidence that differentiation of multi-potent cells along specific lineages could be directed by the application of specific mechanical forces applied. For example, it has been demonstrated that human bone marrow stromal cells (hBMSCs), in the absence of specific ligament growth and regulatory factors, could differentiate into ligament-like cells through the application of physiologically relevant cyclic multi-dimensional mechanical strain [211]. In addition, mechanical stimulation of Bone Marrow Stem Cells induced increased levels of alkaline phosphatase activity, alkaline phosphatase and osteopontin gene expression and mineralized matrix production [212].. However, the nature and intensity of the mechanical forces that are stimulatory for a specific engineered tissue are still unclear and need to be investigated more deeply. Moreover, a modulation of the applied mechanical stimuli is another requirement derived from the variable "needs" of the growing tissue depending on its developmental stage.

Bioreactors including a mechanical system able to apply controllable dynamic compression, and multidimensional strains (simultaneous compression and torsion) to the growing tissue housed within the bioreactor have already been studied [190;213]. In addition to be used for enhancing biosynthetic cell activity for in vitro tissue regeneration, these kinds of bioreactors could be valuable tools for the study of pathophysiological effects of physical forces on developing tissues, and of the effects of physiological forces the engineered tissue will have to bear after implantation in the body.

Future Perspective

Despite bioreactors are widely viewed as essential for the controlled fabrication of reproducible functional engineered tissues, the recent advances made in the field are generally limited to research-scale production. Mass transfer issue still remains one of the major limitations before bioreactors enable the production of engineered tissues with relevant size for clinical applications [214]. This problem could be overcome with the development of innovative designs of circulatory systems that mimic *in vivo* vascularisation of tissues, which is mainly dependant on scaffold production methodologies. One of the solutions proposed to achieve a microfluidic circulatory system is the incorporation of microchannels into the 3D scaffold [215;216], or the promotion of scaffold vascularisation by means of co-culturing vascular cells with the specific cells of the tissue to be generated. This could require the fabrication of different microenvironments inside the 3D constructs as to allow both vascular cells and other specific cells to grow and differentiate. However, the success of the tissue engineering strategy via bioreactor-mediated in vitro culture of hybrid constructs (cell-seeded scaffold) not only depends on innovative bioreactor development but also on multiple interdependent parameters that together form a complex chain which final goal is to achieve mass-production of reproducible functional engineered tissues for clinical routine (Figure 15).

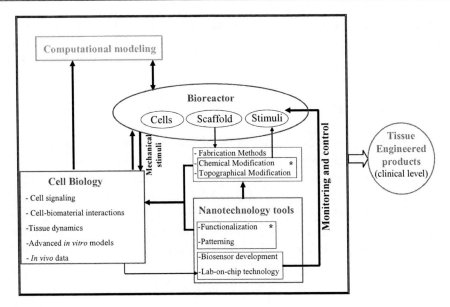

Figure 15. Interdependence of multiple scientific research fields that play a major role in the development of tissue engineered products (see text for details).

Conclusion

As mentioned in the introduction, the tissue engineering approach is an interdisciplinary issue that relies on three basic components which are i) human cells, ii) 3D porous scaffold for supporting cell growth and tissue development, and iii) stimuli aimed at creating a favourable environment for in vitro tissue generation, and which include physical, chemical and mechanical cues for cells (Figure 2). Acquisition of new data and knowledge in cell biology (including cell-biomaterial interactions, cell signalling and tissue dynamics), scaffold development (including innovative methods of production, surface chemical and topographical modification methods and new materials study) and the effect of chemical, physical and mechanical stimuli on tissue growth and development is primordial for bioreactor technology development. Bioreactor technology advances are in turn a crucial factor to enable progress in these different research fields. The passage of laboratory-scale to industrial-scale engineered tissue products is therefore a complex and interdisciplinary issue that could be described by highlighting four interdependent research fields, as described in Figure 15:

1. Bioreactor Design and Development

Bioreactors are considered as tools for studying the effect of cell microenvironment, including mechanical stimulation, on the formation of tissues. For that purpose, a tightly controlled-environment and accurate real-time monitoring is required. This can be achieved through biosensor development and lab-on-chip technology (see Nanotechnology paragraph). The integration of these devices into bioreactors would enable the monitoring and detection of specific cellular processes and the automatic regulation of culture conditions by feedback loops, which would improve tissue regeneration considerably. However, progress in cell biology is essential to identify specific cellular processes that would be considered excellent indicators of the tissue formation process and hence that would be interesting to monitor.

2. Cell Biology Research

Deeper knowledge is still needed regarding cell-biomaterial interactions. How physicochemical parameters, and particularly nanotopography and chemical cues, influence cell-signalling and hence biological response and tissue regeneration remains unclear. For this purpose, advanced in vitro models need to be developed. Microarray technology, nanopatterning and surface functionalization of biomaterials (see Nanotechnology paragraph) appear to be among the most promising tools for elucidating cell biological pathways and hence allowing the design and optimization of biomaterials to serve as a construct for cell culture.

3. Computational Modelling

Future bioreactor designs will undoubtedly integrate considerations from computational modelling, including fluid mechanics for a specific design, as well as mechanics of the scaffold material and tissue dynamics. This last issue is more difficult to address because it requires the development of multi-level and multi-scale computational modelling to capture spatio-temporal dynamics of tissue [214]. These models would enable predicting the development of the engineered tissue [190]. Therefore, it would be possible to define accurately the physical, chemical and mechanical parameters that are to be imposed on the bioreactor system to create a favourable microenvironement at each stage of tissue development. In addition, it would also allow the planning of timely surgery. However, the implementation of these computational models requires the well-characterized and validated experimental data to produce the underlying rules of the model. These experimental data could be obtained by means of in vitro and *in vivo* cell experiments.

4. Nanotechnology

The application of nanotechnology tools to the development of structures at the molecular level enables the study and the improvement of the interactions between material surfaces and biological entities. Nanotechnologies provide the possibility to produce surfaces, structures and materials with nanoscale features that can mimic the natural environment of cells, to promote certain functions, such as cell adhesion, cell mobility and cell differentiation. Biomaterial surface modifications by means of nanostructuration techniques and chemical functionalisation, particularly self-assembly, are some examples of the application of nanotechnology tools to regenerative medicine [217]. The use of nanotechnology in tissue engineering also seems to be promising for the development of nanodevices, such as nanobiosensors, that could be incorporated on laboratory-on-a-chip (Lab-on-Chip) in order to detect biological, chemical, mechanical or electrical reactions as indicative of specific biological response taking place in the bioreactor. Examples of nanosensors that could be included in bioreactors would be pH sensors or oxygen sensors that use nanotechnology for locally discrete measurements or molecule-release sensors (such as a calcium or potassium detector).

In summary, the prospect of regenerating damaged or non-functional tissues by using an off-the-shelf synthetic product is far from being achieved and economically-viable in the near future. However, this perspective would definitely and radically impact and change medical science. Within this context, fundamental interdisciplinary research needs to be carried out to provide a comprehensive control over specific microenvironmental factors in 3D cultures as to achieve an economically viable approach to obtain reproducible and functional tissue grafts at industrial-scale.

References

[1]   Banwart, JC; Asher, MA; Hassanein, RS. Iliac Crest Bone-Graft Harvest Donor Site Morbidity - A Statistical Evaluation. *Spine.*, 1995, 20(9), 1055-1060.

[2]   Fernyhough, JC; Schimandle, JJ; Weigel, MC; Edwards, CC; Levine, AM. Chronic Donor Site Pain Complicating Bone-Graft Harvesting from the Posterior Iliac Crest for Spinal-Fusion. *Spine.*, 1992, 17(12), 1474-1480.

[3]   Goulet, JA; Senunas, LE; DeSilva, GL; Greenfield, MLVH. Autogenous iliac crest bone graft - Complications and functional assessment. *Clinical Orthopaedics and Related Research.*, 1997, (339), 76-81.

[4]   Hardouin, P; Anselme, K; Flautre, B; Bianchi, F; Bascoulenguet, G; Bouxin, B. Tissue engineering and skeletal diseases. *Joint Bone Spine.*, 2000, 67(5), 419-424.

[5]   Kuo, CK; Tuan, RS. Tissue Engineering with Mesenchymal Stem Cells. *IEEE Engineering in Medicine and Biology Magazine.*, 2003, September/October, 51.

[6]   Logeart-Avramoglou, D; Anagnostou, F; Bizios, R; Petite, H. Engineering Bone:Challenges and Obstacles. *Tissue Engineering Review Series.*, 2005, 9(1), 72-84.

[7]   Sipe, JD. Tissue engineering and reparative medicine. Reparative Medicine: *Growing Tissues and Organs.*, 2002, 961, 1-9.

[8]   Verfaillie, CM. Adult stem cells: assessing the case for pluripotency. *Trends in Cell Biology.*, 2002, 12(11), 502-508.

[9]   Stoltz, JF; Bensoussan, D; Decot, V; Netter, P; Ciree, A; Gillet, P. Cell and tissue engineering and clinical applications: An overview. *Bio-Medical Materials and Engineering.*, 2006, 16(4), S3-S18.

[10]   Pittenger, MF; Mackay, AM; Beck, SC; Jaiswal, RK; Douglas, R; Mosca, JD; et al. Multilineage potential of adult human mesenchymal stem cells. *Science.*, 1999, 284(5411), 143-147.

[11]   Chim, H; Schantz, JT. Human circulating peripheral blood mononuclear cells for calvarial bone tissue engineering. *Plastic and Reconstructive Surgery.*, 2006, 117(2), 468-478.

[12]   Fuchs, JR; Hannouche, D; Terada, S; Zand, S; Vacanti, JP; Fauza, DO. Cartilage engineering from ovine umbilical cord blood mesenchymal progenitor cells. *Stem Cells.*, 2005, 23(7), 958-964.

[13] Kern, S; Eichler, H; Stoeve, J; Kluter, H; Bieback, K. Comparative analysis of mesenchymal stem cells from bone marrow, umbilical cord blood, or adipose tissue. *Stem Cells.*, 2006, 24(5), 1294-1301.

[14] Friedenstein, A; Petrakova, KV. Osteogenesis in transplants of bone marrow cells. The Journal of Embryological Exp*erimental Morphology.* 1966, 16, 381-390.

[15] Goshima, J; Goldberg, VM; Caplan, AI. Osteogenic Potential of Culture-Expanded Rat Marrow-Cells As Assayed Invivo with Porous Calcium-Phosphate Ceramic. *Biomaterials.*, 1991, 12(2), 253-258.

[16] Haynesworth, SE; Goshima, J; Goldberg, VM; Caplan, AI. Characterization of Cells with Osteogenic Potential from Human Marrow. *Bone.*, 1992, 13(1), 81-88.

[17] Bruder, SP; Jaiswal, N; Haynesworth, SE. Growth kinetics, self-renewal, and the osteogenic potential of purified human mesenchymal stem cells during extensive subcultivation and following cryopreservation. *Journal of Cellular Biochemistry.*, 1997, 64(2), 278-294.

[18] Jaiswal, N; Haynesworth, SE; Caplan, AI; Bruder, SP. Osteogenic differentiation of purified, culture-expanded human mesenchymal stem cells *in vitro. Journal of Cellular Biochemistry.*, 1997, 64(2), 295-312.

[19] Krebsbach, PH; Kuznetsov, SA; Satomura, K; Emmons, RVB; Rowe, DW; Robey, PG. Bone formation *in vivo*: Comparison of osteogenesis by transplanted mouse and human marrow stromal fibroblasts. *Transplantation.*, 1997, 63(8), 1059-1069.

[20] Fukumoto, T; Sperling, JW; Sanyal, A; Fitzsimmons, JS; Reinholz, GG; Conover, CA; et al. Combined effects of insulin-like growth factor-1 and transforming growth factor-beta 1 on periosteal mesenchymal cells during chondrogenesis *in vitro. Osteoarthritis and Cartilage.*, 2003, 11(1), 55-64.

[21] Nakahara, H; Bruder, SP; Haynesworth, SE; Holecek, JJ; Baber, MA; Goldberg, VM; et al. Bone and Cartilage Formation in Diffusion-Chambers by Subcultured Cells Derived from the Periosteum. *Bone.*, 1990, 11(3), 181-188.

[22] Zarnett, R; Salter, RB. Periosteal Neochondrogenesis for Biologically Resurfacing Joints - Its Cellular-Origin. *Canadian Journal of Surgery.*, 1989, 32(3), 171-174.

[23] Noth, U; Osyczka, AM; Tuli, R; Hickok, NJ; Danielson, KG; Tuan, RS. Multilineage mesenchymal differentiation potential of human trabecular bone-derived cells. *Journal of Orthopaedic Research.*, 2002, 20(5), 1060-1069.

[24] Sottile, V; Halleux, C; Bassilana, F; Keller, H; Seuwen, K. Stem cell characteristics of human trabecular bone-derived cells. *Bone.*, 2002, 30(5), 699-704.

[25] Tuli, R; Seghatoleslami, MR; Tuli, S; Wang, ML; Hozack, WJ; Manner, PA; et al. A simple, high-yield method for obtaining multipotential mesenchymal progenitor cells from trabecular bone. *Molecular Biotechnology.*, 2003, 23(1), 37-49.

[26] Dragoo, JL; Choi, JY; Lieberman, JR; Huang, J; Zuk, PA; Zhang, J; et al. Bone induction by BMP-2 transduced stem cells derived from human fat. *Journal of Orthopaedic Research.*, 2003, 21(4), 622-629.

[27] Gronthos, S; Franklin, DM; Leddy, HA; Robey, PG; Storms, RW; Gimble, JM. Surface protein characterization of human adipose tissue-derived stromal cells. *Journal of Cellular Physiology.*, 2001, 189(1), 54-63.

[28] Wickham, MQ; Erickson, GR; Gimble, JM; Vail, TP; Guilak, F. Multipotent stromal cells derived from the infrapatellar fat pad of the knee. *Clinical Orthopaedics and Related Research.*, 2003, (412), 196-212.

[29] De Bari, C; Dell'Accio, F; Tylzanowski, P; Luyten, FP. Multipotent mesenchymal stem cells from adult human synovial membrane. *Arthritis and Rheumatism.*, 2001, 44(8), 1928-1942.

[30] Jankowski, RJ; Deasy, BM; Huard, J. Muscle-derived stem cells. *Gene Therapy.*, 2002, 9(10), 642-647.

[31] Noort, WA; Kruisselbrink, AB; in't Anker, PS; Kruger, M; van Bezooijen, RL; de Paus, RA; et al. Mesenchymal stem cells promote engraftment of human umbilical cord blood-derived CD34(+) cells in NOD/SCID mice. *Experimental Hematology.*, 2002, 30(8), 870-878.

[32] Miura, M; Gronthos, S; Zhao, MR; Lu, B; Fisher, LW; Robey, PG; et al. SHED: *Stem cells from human exfoliated deciduous teeth.* Proceedings of the National Academy of Sciences of the United States of America, 2003, 100(10), 5807-5812.

[33] Lee, JY; Musgrave, D; Pelinkovic, D; Fukushima, K; Cummins, J; Usas A; et al. Effect of bone morphogenetic protein-2-expressing muscle-derived cells on healing of critical-sized bone defects in mice. *Journal of Bone and Joint Surgery-American Volume.* 2001, 83A(7), 1032-1039.

[34] Peng, HR; Wright, V; Usas, A; Gearhart, B; Shen, HC; Cummins, J; et al. Synergistic enhancement of bone formation and healing by stem cell-expressed VEGF and bone morphogenetic protein-4. *Journal of Clinical Investigation.*, 2002, 110(6), 751-759.

[35] Wright, VJ; Peng, HR; Usas, A; Young, B; Gearhart, B; Cummins, J; et al. BMP4-expressing muscle-derived stem cells differentiate into osteogenic lineage and improve bone healing in immunocompetent mice. *Molecular Therapy.*, 2002, 6(2), 169-178.

[36] Gazit, D; Turgeman, G; Kelley, P; Wang, E; Jalenak, M; Zilberman, Y; et al. Engineered pluripotent mesenchymal cells integrate and differentiate in regenerating bone: A novel cell-mediated gene therapy. *Journal of Gene Medicine.*, 1999, 1(2), 121-133.

[37] Lieberman, JR; Daluiski, A; Stevenson, S; Wu, L; McAllister, P; Lee, YP; et al. The effect of regional gene therapy with bone morphogenetic protein-2-producing bone-marrow cells on the repair of segmental femoral defects in rats. *Journal of Bone and Joint Surgery-American Volume.*, 1999, 81A(7), 905-917.

[38] Aslan, H; Zilberman, Y; Arbeli, V; Sheyn, D; Matan, Y; Liebergall, M; et al. Nucleofection-based *ex vivo* nonviral gene delivery to human stem cells as a platform for tissue regeneration. *Tissue Engineering.*, 2006, 12(4), 877-889.

[39] Aslan, H; Zilberman, Y; Kandel, L; Liebergall, M; Oskouian, RJ; Gazit, D; et al. Osteogenic differentiation of noncultured immunoisolated bone marrow-derived CD105(+) cells. *Stem Cells.*, 2006, 24(7), 1728-1737.

[40] Moutsatsos, IK; Turgeman, G; Zhou, SH; Kurkalli, BG; Pelled, G; Tzur, L; et al. Exogenously regulated stem cell-mediated gene therapy for bone regeneration. *Molecular Therapy.*, 2001, 3(4), 449-461.

[41] Peterson, B; Zhang, J; Iglesias, R; Kabo, M; Hedrick, M; Benhaim, P; et al. Healing of critically sized femoral defects, using genetically modified mesenchymal stem cells from human adipose tissue. *Tissue Engineering.* 2005, 11(1-2), 120-129.

[42] Gafni, Y; Pelled, G; Zilberman, Y; Turgeman, G; Apparailly, F; Yotvat, H; et al. Gene therapy platform for bone regeneration using an exogenously regulated, AAV-2-based gene expression system. *Molecular Therapy.*, 2004, 9(4), 587-595.

[43] Aluigi, M; Fogli, M; Curti, A; Isidori, A; Gruppioni, E; Chiodoni, C; et al. Nucleofection is an efficient nonviral transfection technique for human bone marrow-derived mesenchymal stem cells. *Stem Cells.,* 2006, 24(2), 454-461.

[44] Yaszemski, MJ; Payne, RG; Hayes, WC; Langer, R; Mikos, AG. Evolution of bone transplantation: Molecular, cellular and tissue strategies to engineer human bone. *Biomaterials.,* 1996, 17(2), 175-185.

[45] Meinel, L; Hofmann, S; Karageorgiou, V; Zichner, L; Langer, R; Kaplan, D; et al. Engineering cartilage-like tissue using human mesenchymal stem cells and silk protein scaffolds. *Biotechnology and Bioengineering.,* 2004, 88(3), 379-391.

[46] Sharma, B; Elisseeff, JH. Engineering structurally organized cartilage and bone tissues. *Annals of Biomedical Engineering.,* 2004, 32(1), 148-159.

[47] Hench, LL; Polak, JM. Third-generation biomedical materials. *Science.,* 2002, 295(5557), 1014-+.

[48] Roether, JA; Gough, JE; Boccaccini, AR; Hench, LL; Maquet, V; Jerome, R. Novel bioresorbable and bioactive composites based on bioactive glass and polylactide foams for bone tissue engineering. *Journal of Materials Science-Materials in Medicine.,* 2002, 13(12), 1207-1214.

[49] Spaans, CJ; Belgraver, VW; Rienstra, O; de Groot, JH; Veth, RPH; Pennings, AJ. Solvent-free fabrication of micro-porous polyurethane amide and polyurethane-urea scaffolds for repair and replacement of the knee-joint meniscus. *Biomaterials.,* 2000, 21(23), 2453-2460.

[50] Bruder, SP; Fox, BS. Tissue engineering of bone - Cell based strategies. *Clinical Orthopaedics and Related Research.,* 1999, (367), S68-S83.

[51] Temenoff, JS; Mikos, AG. Review: tissue engineering for regeneration of articular cartilage. *Biomaterials.,* 2000, 21(5), 431-440.

[52] Salgado, AJ; Coutinho, OP; Reis, RL. Bone tissue engineering: State of the art and future trends. *Macromolecular Bioscience.,* 2004, 4(8), 743-765.

[53] Olivier, V; Faucheux, N; Hardouin, P. Biomaterial challenges and approaches to stem cell use in bone reconstructive surgery. *Drug Discovery Today.,* 2004, 9(18), 803-811.

[54] Pachence, JM; Kohn, J. Biodegradable Polymers. In: R; Langer, RP; Lanza, JP; Vacanti, editors. *Principles of Tissue Engineering*. San Diego: *Academic Press*, 2000, 263-274.

[55] Vonrecum, HA; Cleek, RL; Eskin, SG; Mikos, AG. Degradation of Polydispersed Poly(L-Lactic Acid) to Modulate Lactic-Acid Release. *Biomaterials.,* 1995, 16(6), 441-447.

[56] Grizzi, I; Garreau, H; Li, S; Vert, M. Hydrolytic Degradation of Devices Based on Poly(Dl-Lactic Acid) Size-Dependence. *Biomaterials.,* 1995, 16(4), 305-311.

[57] Kohn, J; Langer, R. Bioresorbable and bioerodible materials. In: BD; Ratner, FJ; Schoen, JE; Lemons, editors. *Biomaterials Science*. New York: *Academic Press*, 1996, 64-72.

[58] Shalaby, SW; Johnson, RA. Synthetic absorbable polyesters. In: Shalaby SW; editor. Biomedical biopolymers. *Designed to degrade systems*. New York: Hanser, 1994, 1-34.

[59] Chu, CC. The Invitro Degradation of Poly(Glycolic Acid) Sutures - Effect of Ph. *Journal of Biomedical Materials Research.,* 1981, 15(6), 795-804.

[60] Chu, CC. An Invitro Study of the Effect of Buffer on the Degradation of Poly(Glycolic Acid) Sutures. *Journal of Biomedical Materials Research.,* 1981, 15(1), 19-27.

[61] Vert, M; Li, SM; Garreau, H. Attempts to Map the Structure and Degradation Characteristics of Aliphatic Polyesters Derived from Lactic and Glycolic Acids. *Journal of Biomaterials Science-Polymer Edition.*, 1994, 6(7), 639-649.

[62] Achindler, A; Jeffcoat, R; Kimmel, GL; Pitt, CG; Wall, ME; Zwiedinger, R. Biodegradable polymers for sustained druf delivery. *Contemporary Topics in Polymer Science.*, 1977, 11, 711-719.

[63] Vert, M; Chabot, F; Leray, J; Christel, P. Stereoregular Bioresorbable Polyesters for Orthopedic-Surgery. *Makromolekulare Chemie-Macromolecular Chemistry and Physics.*, 1981, 30-41.

[64] Nakamura, T; Hitomi, S; Watanabe, S; Shimizu, Y; Jamshidi, K; Hyon, SH; et al. Bioabsorption of Polylactides with Different Molecular-Properties. *Journal of Biomedical Materials Research.*, 1989, 23(10), 1115-1130.

[65] Navarro, M; Ginebra, MP; Planell, JA; Zeppetelli, S; Ambrosio, L. Development and cell response of a new biodegradable composite scaffold for guided bone regeneration. *Journal of Materials Science-Materials in Medicine.*, 2004, 15(4), 419-422.

[66] Navarro, M; Ginebra, MP; Planell, JA; Barrias, CC; Barbosa, MA. *In vitro* degradation behavior of a novel bioresorbable composite material based on PLA and a soluble CaP glass. *Acta Biomaterialia.*, 2005, 1(4), 411-419.

[67] Yang, S; Leong, K; Du, Z; Chua, C. The design of scaffolds for tissue engineering. Part I. Traditional factors. *Tissue Engineering.*, 2001, 7, 679-689.

[68] Mikos, AG; Bao, Y; Cima, LG; Ingber, DE; Vacanti, JP; Langer, R. Preparation of Poly(Glycolic Acid) Bonded Fiber Structures for Cell Attachment and Transplantation. *Journal of Biomedical Materials Research.*, 1993, 27(2), 183-189.

[69] Kasuga, T; Maeda, H; Kato, K; Nogami, M; Hata, K; Ueda, M. Preparation of poly(lactic acid) composites containing calcium carbonate (vaterite). *Biomaterials.*, 2003, 24(19), 3247-3253.

[70] Marra, KG; Szem, JW; Kumta, PN; DiMilla, PA; Weiss, LE. *In vitro* analysis of biodegradable polymer blend/hydroxyapatite composites for bone tissue engineering. *Journal of Biomedical Materials Research.*, 1999, 47(3), 324-335.

[71] Liu, Q; De Wijn, JR; van Blitterswijk, CA. Composite biomaterials with chemical bonding between hydroxyapatite filler particles and PEG/PBT copolymer matrix. *Journal of Biomedical Materials Research.*, 1998, 40(3), 490-497.

[72] Nam, YS; Park, TG. Porous biodegradable polymeric scaffolds prepared by thermally induced phase separation. *Journal of Biomedical Materials Research.*, 1999, 47(1), 8-17.

[73] Schugens, C; Maquet, V; Grandfils, C; Jerome, R; Teyssie, P. Polylactide macroporous biodegradable implants for cell transplantation .2. Preparation of polylactide foams by liquid-liquid phase separation. *Journal of Biomedical Materials Research.*, 1996, 30(4), 449-461.

[74] Ma, PX; Zhang, RY. Microtubular architecture of biodegradable polymer scaffolds. *Journal of Biomedical Materials Research.*, 2001, 56(4), 469-477.

[75] Zhang, RY; Ma, PX. Poly(alpha-hydroxyl acids) hydroxyapatite porous composites for bone-tissue engineering. I. Preparation and morphology. *Journal of Biomedical Materials Research.*, 1999, 44(4), 446-455.

[76] Boccaccini, AR; Notingher, I; Maquet, V; Jerome, R. Bioresorbable and bioactive composite materials based on polylactide foams filled with and coated by Bioglass (R)

particles for tissue engineering applications. *Journal of Materials Science-Materials in Medicine.*, 2003, 14(5), 443-450.

[77]   Cima, LG; Langer, R; Vacanti, JP. Polymers for Tissue and Organ-Culture. *Journal of Bioactive and Compatible Polymers.*, 1991, 6(3), 232-240.

[78]   Hutmacher, DW; Sittinger, M; Risbud, MV. Scaffold-based tissue engineering: rationale for computer-aided design and solid free-form fabrication systems. *Trends in Biotechnology,* 2004, 22(7), 354-362.

[79]   Artzi, Z; Weinreb, M; Givol, N; Rohrer, MD; Nemcovsky, CE; Prasad, HS; et al. Biomaterial resorption rate and healing site morphology of inorganic bovine bone and beta-tricalcium phosphate in the canine: A 24-month longitudinal histologic study and morphometric analysis. *International Journal of Oral & Maxillofacial Implants.*, 2004, 19(3), 357-368.

[80]   Legeros, RZ; Lin, S; Rohanizadeh, R; Mijares, D; Legeros, JP. Biphasic calcium phosphate bioceramics: preparation, properties and applications. *Journal of Materials Science-Materials in Medicine.*, 2003, 14(3), 201-209.

[81]   Bauer, TW; Muschler, GF. Bone graft materials-An overview of the basic science. *Clinical Orthopaedics and Related Research.*, 2000, (371), 10-27.

[82]   Yoshikawa, H; Myoui, A. Bone tissue engineering with porous hydroxyapatite ceramics. *Journal of Artificial Organs.*, 2005, 8, 131-136.

[83]   Tampieri, A; Celotti, G; Sprio, S; Delcogliano, A; Franzese, S. Porosity-graded hydroxyapatite ceramics to replace natural bone. *Biomaterials.*, 2001, 22(11), 1365-1370.

[84]   Furuichi, K; Oaki, Y; Ichimiya, H; Komotori, J; Imai, H. Preparation of hierarchically organized calcium phosphate-organic polymer composites by calcification of hydrogel. *Science and Technology of Advanced Materials.*, 2006, 7(2), 219-225.

[85]   Almirall, A; Larrecq, G; Delgado, JA; Martinez, S; Planell, JA; Ginebra, MP. Fabrication of low temperature macroporous hydroxyapatite scaffolds by foaming and hydrolysis of an alpha-TCP paste. *Biomaterials.*, 2004, 25(17), 3671-3680.

[86]   Gong, WL; Abdelouas, A; Lutze, W. Porous bioactive glass and glass-ceramics made by reaction sintering under pressure. *Journal of Biomedical Materials Research.*, 2001, 54(3), 320-327.

[87]   Hench, LL; Splinter, RJ; Allen, WC. Bonding mechanisms at the interface of ceramic prosthetic materials. *Journal of Biomedical Materials Research.*, 1971, 2, 117-141.

[88]   Hench, LL. *Bioceramics. Journal of the American Ceramic Society.*, 1998, 81(7), 1705-1728.

[89]   Lu, HH; Tang, A; Oh, SC; Spalazzi, JP; Dionisio, K. Compositional effects on the formation of a calcium phosphate layer and the response of osteoblast-like cells on polymer-bioactive glass composites. *Biomaterials.*, 2005, 26(32), 6323-6334.

[90]   Gatti, AM; Valdre, G; Andersson, OH. Analysis of the In-Vivo Reactions of A Bioactive Glass in Soft and Hard-Tissue. *Biomaterials.*, 1994, 15(3), 208-212.

[91]   Xynos, ID; Edgar, AJ; Buttery, LDK; Hench, LL; Polak, JM. Ionic products of bioactive glass dissolution increase proliferation of human osteoblasts and induce insulin-like growth factor II mRNA expression and protein synthesis. *Biochemical and Biophysical Research Communications.*, 2000, 276(2), 461-465.

[92] Navarro, M; Ginebra, MP; Clement, J; Martinez, S; Avila, G; Planell, JA. Physicochemical degradation of titania-stabilized soluble phosphate glasses for medical applications. *Journal of the American Ceramic Society.*, 2003, 86(8), 1345-1352.

[93] Navarro, M; Ginebra, MP; Planell, JA. Cellular response to calcium phosphate glasses with controlled solubility. *Journal of Biomedical Materials Research Part A*, 2003, 67A(3), 1009-1015.

[94] Dean-Mo, L. Fabrication of hydroxyapatite ceramic with controlled porosity. *Journal of Materials Science-Materials in Medicine.*, 1997, (8), 227.

[95] Sepulveda, P. Gelcasting foams for porous ceramics. *American Ceramic Society Bulletin.*, 1997, 76(10), 61-65.

[96] Tuck, C; Evans, JRG. Porous ceramics prepared from aqueous foams. *Journal of Materials Science Letters.*, 1999, 18(13), 1003-1005.

[97] Tian, JT; Tian, JM. Preparation of porous hydroxyapatite. *Journal of Materials Science.*, 2001, 36(12), 3061-3066.

[98] Jones, JR; Hench, LL. Factors affecting the structure and properties of bioactive foam scaffolds for tissue engineering. *Journal of Biomedical Materials Research Part B-Applied Biomaterials,* 2004, 68B(1), 36-44.

[99] Gibson, LJ; Ashby, MF. *Cellular solids: structure and properties.* 2nd ed. Oxford: Pergamon, 1999.

[100] Callcut, S; Knowles, JC. Correlation between structure and compressive strength in a reticulated glass-reinforced hydroxyapatite foam. *Journal of Materials Science-Materials in Medicine.*, 2002, 13(5), 485-489.

[101] Kim, HW; Knowles, JC; Kim, HE. Hydroxyapatite porous scaffold engineered with biological polymer hybrid coating for antibiotic Vancomycin release. *Journal of Materials Science-Materials in Medicine.*, 2005, 16(3), 189-195.

[102] Sepulveda, P; Jones, JR; Hench, LL. Bioactive sol-gel foams for tissue repair. *Journal of Biomedical Materials Research.*, 2002, 59, 340-348.

[103] Seitz, H; Rieder, W; Irsen, S; Leukers, B; Tille, C. Three-dimensional printing of porous ceramic scaffolds for bone tissue engineering. *Journal of Biomedical Materials Research Part B-Applied Biomaterials.*, 2005, 74B(2), 782-788.

[104] Pfister, A; Landers, SR; Laib, A; Hubner, U; Schmelzeisen, R. Biofunctional Rapid Prototyping for Tissue-Engineering Applications: 3D Bioplotting versus 3D Printing. *Journal of Polymer Science: Part A:Polymer Chemistry.*, 2004, 42, 624-638.

[105] Levine, BR; Sporer, S; Poggie, RA; Della Valle, CJ; Jacobs, JJ. Experimental and clinical performance of porous tantalum in orthopedic surgery. *Biomaterials.*, 2006, 27(27), 4671-4681.

[106] Banhart, J. Manufacture; characterisation and application of cellular metals and metal foams. *Progress in Materials Science.*, 2001, 46(6), 559-5U3.

[107] Korner, C; Singer, RF. Processing of metal foams - Challenges and opportunities. *Advanced Engineering Materials.*, 2000, 2(4), 159-165.

[108] St Pierre, JP; Gauthier, M; Lefebvre, LP; Tabrizian, M. Three-dimensional growth of differentiating MC3T3-E1 pre-osteoblasts on porous titanium scaffolds. *Biomaterials.*, 2005, 26(35), 7319-7328.

[109] Sikavitsas, VI; van den Dolder, J; Bancroft, GN; Jansen, JA; Mikos, AG. Influence of the *in vitro* culture period on the *in vivo* performance of cell/titanium bone tissue-

engineered constructs using a rat cranial critical size defect model. *Journal of Biomedical Materials Research Part A.,* 2003, 67A(3), 944-951.

[110] Vehof, JWM; Haus, MTU; de Ruijter, AE; Spauwen, PHM; Jansen, JA. Bone formation in Transforming Growth Factor beta-I-loaded titanium fiber mesh implants. *Clinical   Oral   Implants   Research.,   2002,   13(1),* 94-102.

[111] Rubin, JP; Yaremchuk, MJ. Complications and toxicities of implantable biomaterials used in facial reconstructive and aesthetic surgery: A comprehensive review of the literature. *Plastic and Reconstructive Surgery.,* 1997, 100(5), 1336-1353.

[112] Gu, YW; Li, H; Tay, BY; Lim, CS; Yong, MS; Khor, KA. *In vitro* bioactivity and osteoblast response of porous NiTi synthesized by SHS using nanocrystalline Ni-Ti reaction agent. *Journal of Biomedical Materials Research Part A.,* 2006, 78A(2), 316-323.

[113] Garcia, AJ; Ducheyne, P; Boettiger, D. Cell adhesion strength increases linearly with adsorbed fibronectin surface density. *Tissue Engineering.,* 1997, 3(2), 197-206.

[114] Hersel, U; Dahmen, C; Kessler, H. RGD modified polymers: biomaterials for stimulated cell adhesion and beyond. *Biomaterials,* 2003, 24(24), 4385-4415.

[115] Ripamonti, U; Tasker, JR. Advances in biotechnology for tissue engineering of bone. *Curr. Pharm. Biotech.,* 2000, 1, 47-55.

[116] Tugulu, S; Silacci, P; Stergiopulos, N; Klok, HA. RGD - Functionalized polymer brushes as substrates for the integrin specific adhesion of human umbilical vein endothelial cells. *Biomaterials.,* 2007, 28(16), 2536-2546.

[117] Singh, N; Cui, XF; Boland, T; Husson, SM. The role of independently variable grafting density and layer thickness of polymer nanolayers on peptide adsorption and cell adhesion. *Biomaterials.,* 2007, 28(5), 763-771.

[118] Zhao, B; Brittain, WJ. Polymer brushes: surface-immobilized macromolecules. *Progress in Polymer Science,* 2000, 25(5), 677-710.

[119] Palsson, BO; Sangeeta, NB. Coordination of cellular-fate processes. *Tissue Engineering.* USA: Pearson Prentice Hall, 2004, 105-130.

[120] Hong, L; Tabata, Y; Miyamoto, S; Yamamoto, M; Yamada, K; Hashimoto, N; et al. Bone regeneration at rabbit skull defects treated with transforming growth factor-beta 1 incorporated into hydrogels with different levels of biodegradability. *Journal of Neurosurgery.,* 2000, 92(2), 315-325.

[121] Delong, SA; Moon, JJ; West, JL. Covalently immobilized gradients of bFGF on hydrogel scaffolds for directed cell migration. *Biomaterials.,* 2005, 26(16), 3227-3234.

[122] Mann, BK; Schmedlen, RH; West, JL. Tethered-TGF-beta increases extracellular matrix production of vascular smooth muscle cells. *Biomaterials.,* 2001, 22(5), 439-444.

[123] Holland, TA; Tabata, Y; Mikos, AG. *In vitro* release of transforming growth factor-beta 1 from gelatin microparticles encapsulated in biodegradable, injectable oligo(poly(ethylene glycol) fumarate) hydrogels. *Journal of controlled release.,* 2003, 91(3), 299-313.

[124] Sokolsky-Papkov, M; Agashi, K; Olaye, A; Shakesheff, K; Domb, AJ. Polymer carriers for drug delivery in tissue engineering. *Advanced Drug Delivery Reviews.,* 2007, 59(4-5), 187-206.

[125] Vasita, R; Katti, DS. Growth factor-delivery systems for tissue engineering: a materials perspective. *Expert Review of Medical Devices.*, 2006, 3(1), 29-47.

[126] Chen, FM; Wu, ZF; Wang, QT; Wu, H; Zhang, YJ; Nie, X; et al. Preparation of recombinant human bone morphogenetic protein-2 loaded dextran-based microspheres and their characteristics. *Acta Pharmacologica Sinica.*, 2005, 26(9), 1093-1103.

[127] Chen, FM; Zhao, YM; Sun, HH; Jin, T; Wang, QT; Zhou, W; et al. Novel glycidyl methacrylated dextran (Dex-GMA)/gelatin hydrogel scaffolds containing microspheres loaded with bone morphogenetic proteins: Formulation and characteristics. *Journal of controlled release.*, 2007, 118(1), 65-77.

[128] Green, DW; Leveque, I; Walsh, D; Howard, D; Yang, XB; Partridge, K; et al. Biomineralized polysaccharide capsules for encapsulation, organization, and delivery of human cell types and growth factors. *Advanced Functional Materials.*, 2005, 15(6), 917-923.

[129] Meinel, L; Illi, OE; Zapf, J; Malfanti, M; Merkle, HP; Gander, B. Stabilizing insulin-like growth factor-I in poly(D,L-lactide-co-glycolide) microspheres. *Journal of controlled release.*, 2001, 70(1-2), 193-202.

[130] Wei, GB; Pettway, GJ; McCauley, LK; Ma, PX. The release profiles and bioactivity of parathyroid hormone from poly(lactic-co-glycolic acid) microspheres. *Biomaterials.*, 2004, 25(2), 345-352.

[131] Chen, FM; Wu, ZF; Sun, HH; Wu, H; Xin, SN; Wang, QT; et al. Release of bioactive BMP from dextran-derived microspheres: A novel delivery concept. *International Journal of Pharmaceutics.*, 2006, 307(1), 23-32.

[132] Storrie, H; Mooney, DJ. Sustained delivery of plasmid DNA from polymeric scaffolds for tissue engineering. *Advanced Drug Delivery Reviews.*, 2006, 58(4), 500-514.

[133] Hiraoka, Y; Yamashiro, H; Yasuda, K; Kimura, Y; Inamoto, T; Tabata Y. In situ regeneration of adipose tissue in rat fat pad by combining a collagen scaffold with gelatin microspheres containing basic fibroblast growth factor. *Tissue Engineering.*, 2006, 12(6), 1475-1487.

[134] Nakahara, T; Nakamura, T; Kobayashi, E; Inoue, M; Shigeno, K; Tabata, Y; et al. Novel approach to regeneration of periodontal tissues based on in situ tissue engineering: Effects of controlled release of basic fibroblast growth factor from a sandwich membrane. *Tissue Engineering.*, 2003, 9(1), 153-162.

[135] Tabata, Y; Ikada, Y; Morimoto, K; Katsumata, H; Yabuta, T; Iwanaga, K; et al. Surfactant-free preparation of biodegradable hydrogel microspheres for protein release. *Journal of Bioactive and Compatible Polymers.*, 1999, 14(5), 371-384.

[136] King, TW; Patrick, CW. Development and *in vitro* characterization of vascular endothelial growth factor (VEGF)-loaded poly(DL-lactic-co-glycolic acid)/poly(ethylene glycol) microspheres using a solid encapsulation/single emulsion/solvent extraction technique. *Journal of Biomedical Materials Research.*, 2000, 51(3), 383-390.

[137] Stenekes, RJH; Franssen, O; van Bommel, EMG; Crommelin, DJA; Hennink, We. The preparation of dextran microspheres in an all-aqueous system: Effect of the formulation parameters on particle characteristics. *Pharmaceutical Research.*, 1998, 15(4), 557-561.

[138] Puceat, M. TGF beta in the differentiation of embryonic stem cells. *Cardiovascular Research.*, 2007, 74(2), 256-261.

[139] Andrew, JG; Hoyland, J; Andrew, SM; Freemont, AJ; Marsh, D. Demonstration of Tgf-Beta-1 Messenger-Rna by Insitu Hybridization in Normal Human Fracture-Healing. *Calcified Tissue International.*, 1993, 52(2), 74-78.

[140] Duneas, N; Crooks, J; Ripamonti, U. Transforming growth factor-beta 1: Induction of bone morphogenetic protein genes expression during endochondral bone formation in the baboon, and synergistic interaction with osteogenic protein-1 (BMP-7). *Growth Factors.*, 1998, 15(4), 259-+.

[141] McKinney, L; Hollinger, JO. A bone regeneration study: Transforming growth factor-beta(1) and its delivery. *Journal of Craniofacial Surgery.*, 1996, 7(1), 36-45.

[142] Rosier, RN; O'Keefe, RJ; Hicks, DG. The potential role of transforming growth factor beta in fracture healing. *Clinical Orthopaedics and Related Research.*, 1998, (355), S294-S300.

[143] Mohan, S; Baylink, DJ. Bone-Growth Factors. *Clinical Orthopaedics and Related Research.*, 1991, (263), 30-48.

[144] Lilli, C; Marinucci, L; Stabellini, G; Belcastro, S; Becchetti, E; Balducci, C; et al. Biomembranes enriched with TGF beta(1) favor bone matrix protein expression by human osteoblasts *in vitro*. *Journal of Biomedical Materials Research.*, 2002, 63(5), 577-582.

[145] Centrella, M; Horowitz, MC; Wozney, JM; Mccarthy, TL. Transforming Growth-Factor-Beta Gene Family Members and Bone. *Endocrine Reviews.*, 1994, 15(1), 27-39.

[146] Erlebacher, A; Filvaroff, EH; Ye, JQ; Derynck, R. Osteoblastic responses to TGF-beta during bone remodeling. *Molecular Biology of the Cell.*, 1998, 9(7), 1903-1918.

[147] Gautschi, OP; Frey, SP; Zellweger, R. Bone morphogenetic proteins in clinical applications. *Anz. Journal of Surgery.*, 2007, 77(8), 626-631.

[148] Lee, SH; Shin, H. Matrices and scaffolds for delivery of bioactive molecules in bone and cartilage tissue engineering. *Advanced Drug Delivery Reviews*, 2007, 59(4-5), 339-359.

[149] Xiao, YT; Xiang, LX; Shao, JZ. Bone morphogenetic protein. *Biochemical and Biophysical Research Communications.*, 2007, 362(3), 550-553.

[150] Werner, H; Katz, J. The emerging role of the insulin-like growth factors in oral biology. *Journal of Dental Research.*, 2004, 83(11), 832-836.

[151] Xu, JS; Liu, ZH; Ornitz, DM. Temporal and spatial gradients of Fgf8 and Fgf17 regulate proliferation and differentiation of midline cerebellar structures. *Development.*, 2000, 127(9), 1833-1843.

[152] Baird, A; Walicke, PA. Fibroblast Growth-Factors. *British Medical Bulletin.*, 1989, 45(2), 438-452.

[153] Nimni, ME. Polypeptide growth factors: targeted delivery systems. *Biomaterials.*, 1997, 18(18), 1201-1225.

[154] Bodo, M; Carinci, F; Baroni, T; Becchetti, E; Bellucci, C; Giammarioli, M; et al. Interleukin pattern of Apert fibroblasts *in vitro*. *European Journal of Cell Biology.*, 1998, 75(4), 383-388.

[155] Hurley, MM; Abreu, C; Gronowicz, G; Kawaguchi, H; Lorenzo, J. Expression and Regulation of Basic Fibroblast Growth-Factor Messenger-Rna Levels in Mouse Osteoblastic Mc3T3-E1 Cells. *Journal of Biological Chemistry.*, 1994, 269(12), 9392-9396.

[156] Katoh, R; Urist, MR. Surface-Adhesion and Attachment Factors in Bone Morphogenetic Protein-Induced Chondrogenesis In-Vitro. *Clinical Orthopaedics and Related Research.*, 1993, (295), 295-304.

[157] Yamaguchi, TP; Rossant, J. Fibroblast Growth-Factors in Mammalian Development. *Current Opinion in Genetics & Development.*, 1995, 5(4), 485-491.

[158] Noda, M; Vogel, R. Fibroblast Growth-Factor Enhances Type-Beta-1 Transforming Growth-Factor Gene-Expression in Osteoblast-Like Cells. *Journal of Cell Biology.*, 1989, 109(5), 2529-2535.

[159] Debiais, F; Hott, M; Graulet, AM; Marie, PJ. The effects of fibroblast growth factor-2 on human neonatal calvaria osteoblastic cells are differentiation stage specific. *Journal of Bone and Mineral Research.*, 1998, 13(4), 645-654.

[160] Yu, K; Xu, JS; Liu, ZH; Sosic, D; Shao, JS; Olson, EN; et al. Conditional inactivation of FGF receptor 2 reveals an essential role for FGF signaling in the regulation of osteoblast function and bone growth. *Development.*, 2003, 130(13), 3063-3074.

[161] Moursi, AM; Winnard, PL; Winnard, AV; Rubenstrunk, JM; Mooney, MP. Fibroblast growth factor 2 induces increased calvarial osteoblast proliferation and cranial suture fusion. *Cleft Palate-Craniofacial Journal.*, 2002, 39(5), 487-496.

[162] Mansukhani, A; Bellosta, P; Sahni, M; Basilico, C. Signaling by fibroblast growth factors (FGF) and fibroblast growth factor receptor 2 (FGFR2)-activating mutations blocks mineralization and induces apoptosis in osteoblasts. *Journal of Cell Biology.*, 2000, 149(6), 1297-1308.

[163] Pitaru, S; Kotevemeth, S; Noff, D; Kaffuler, S; Savion, N. Effect of Basic Fibroblast Growth-Factor on the Growth and Differentiation of Adult Stromal Bone-Marrow Cells-Enhanced Development of Mineralized Bone-Like Tissue in Culture. *Journal of Bone and Mineral Research.*, 1993, 8(8), 919-929.

[164] Deckers, MML; van Bezooijen, RL; van der Horst, G; Hoogendam, J; van der Bent, C; Papapoulos, SE; et al. Bone morphogenetic proteins stimulate angiogenesis through osteoblast-derived vascular endothelial growth factor A. *Endocrinology.*, 2002, 143(4), 1545-1553.

[165] Erlebacher, A; Filvaroff, EH; Gitelman, SE; Derynck, R. Toward, A. Molecular Understanding of Skeletal Development. *Cell.*, 1995, 80(3), 371-378.

[166] Bittner, K; Vischer, P; Bartholmes, P; Bruckner, P. Role of the subchondral vascular system in endochondral ossification: Endothelial cells specifically derepress late differentiation in resting chondrocytes *in vitro*. *Experimental Cell Research.*, 1998, 238(2), 491-497.

[167] Wang, DS; Miura, M; Demura, H; Sato, K. Anabolic effects of 1,25-dihydroxyvitamin D-3 on osteoblasts are enhanced by vascular endothelial growth factor produced by osteoblasts and by growth factors produced by endothelial cells. *Endocrinology.*, 1997, 138(7), 2953-2962.

[168] Kasperk, CH; Borcsok, I; Schairer, HU; Schneider, U; Nawroth, PP; Niethard, FU; et al. Endothelin-1 is a potent regulator of human bone cell metabolism *in vitro*. *Calcified Tissue International.*, 1997, 60(4), 368-374.

[169] Hsiong, SX; Mooney, DJ. Regeneration of vascularized bone. *Periodontology.*, 2000, 2006, 41, 109-122.

[170] Mayr-Wohlfart, U; Waltenberger, J; Hausser, H; Kessler, S; Gunther KP; Dehio, C; et al. Vascular endothelial growth factor stimulates chemotactic migration of primary human osteoblasts. *Bone.*, 2002, 30(3), 472-477.

[171] Orlandini, M; Spreafico, A; Bardelli, M; Rocchigiani, M; Salameh, A; Nucciotti, S; et al. Vascular endothelial growth factor-D activates VEGFR-3 expressed in osteoblasts inducing their differentiation. *Journal of Biological Chemistry.*, 2006, 281(26), 17961-17967.

[172] Park, H; Temenoff, JS; Holland, TA; Tabata, Y; Mikos, AG. Delivery of TGF-beta 1 and chondrocytes via injectable, biodegradable hydrogels for cartilage tissue engineering applications. *Biomaterials.*, 2005, 26(34), 7095-7103.

[173] Chenite, A; Chaput, C; Wang, D; Combes, C; Buschmann, MD; Hoemann, CD; et al. Novel injectable neutral solutions of chitosan form biodegradable gels in situ. *Biomaterials.*, 2000, 21(21), 2155-2161.

[174] Kanczler, JM; Barry, J; Ginty, P; Howdle, SM; Shakesheff, KM; Oreffo, ROC. Supercritical carbon dioxide generated vascular endothelial growth factor encapsulated poly(DL-lactic acid) scaffolds induce angiogenesis *in vitro*. *Biochemical and Biophysical Research Communications.*, 2007, 352(1), 135-141.

[175] Yang, XBB; Whitaker, MJ; Sebald, W; Clarke, N; Howdle, SM; Shakesheff, KM; et al. Human osteoprogenitor bone formation using encapsulated bone morphogenetic protein 2 in porous polymer scaffolds. *Tissue Engineering.*, 2004, 10(7-8), 1037-1045.

[176] Li, CM; Vepari, C; Jin, HJ; Kim, HJ; Kaplan, DL. Electrospun silk-BMP-2 scaffolds for bone tissue engineering. *Biomaterials.*, 2006, 27(16), 3115-3124.

[177] Welch, RD; Jones, AL; Bucholz, RW; Reinert, CM; Tjia, JS; Pierce, WA; et al. Effect of recombinant human bone morphogenetic protein-2 on fracture healing in a goal tibial fracture model. *Journal of Bone and Mineral Research.*, 1998, 13(9), 1483-1490.

[178] Hsu, HP; Zanella, JM; Peckham, SM; Spector, M. Comparing ectopic bone growth induced by rhBMP-2 on an absorbable collagen sponge in rat and rabbit models. *Journal of Orthopaedic Research.*, 2006, 24(8), 1660-1669.

[179] Simmons, CA; Alsberg, E; Hsiong, S; Kim, WJ; Mooney, DJ. Dual growth factor delivery and controlled scaffold degradation enhance *in vivo* bone formation by transplanted bone marrow stromal cells. *Bone.*, 2004, 35(2), 562-569.

[180] Chen, FM; Zhao, YM; Wu, H; Deng, ZH; Wang, QT; Zhou, W; et al. Enhancement of periodontal tissue regeneration by locally controlled delivery of insulin-like growth factor-I from dextran-co-gelatin microspheres. *Journal of controlled release.* 2006, 114(2), 209-222.

[181] Ehrhart, NP; Hong, L; Morgan, AL; Eurell, JA; Jamison, RD. Effect of transforming growth factor-beta 1 on bone regeneration in critical-sized bone defects after irradiation of host tissues. *American Journal of Veterinary Research.*, 2005, 66(6), 1039-1045.

[182] Yamamoto, M; Takahashi, Y; Tabata, Y. Enhanced bone regeneration at a segmental bone defect by controlled release of bone morphogenetic protein-2 from a biodegradable hydrogel. *Tissue Engineering.*, 2006, 12(5), 1305-1311.

[183] Srouji, S; Rachmiel, A; Blumenfeld, I; Livne, E. Mandibular defect repair by TGF-beta and IGF-1 released from a biodegradable osteoconductive hydrogel. *Journal of Cranio-Maxillofacial Surgery.*, 2005, 33(2), 79-84.

[184] Freed, LE; Vunjak-Navakovic, G. Tissue Engineering Bioreactors. In: RH; Lanza, R; Langer, J; Vacanti, editors. *Principles of Tissue Engineering.* USA: *Academic Press,* 2000, 143-156.

[185] Vunjak-Novakovic, G; Obradovic, B; Martin, I; Bursac, PM; Langer, R; Freed, LE. Dynamic cell seeding of polymer scaffolds for cartilage tissue engineering. *Biotechnology Progress.,* 1998, 14(2), 193-202.

[186] Holy, CE; Shoichet, MS; Davies, JE. Engineering three-dimensional bone tissue *in vitro* using biodegradable scaffolds: Investigating initial cell-seeding density and culture period. *Journal of Biomedical Materials Research.,* 2000, 51(3), 376-382.

[187] Ishaug-Riley, SL; Crane-Kruger, GM; Yaszemski, MJ; Mikos, AG. Three-dimensional culture of rat calvarial osteoblasts in porous biodegradable polymers. *Biomaterials.,* 1998, 19(15), 1405-1412.

[188] Freed, LE; Hollander, AP; Martin, I; Barry, JR; Langer, R; Vunjak-Novakovic, G. Chondrogenesis in a cell-polymer-bioreactor system. *Experimental Cell Research.,* 1998, 240(1), 58-65.

[189] Kim, BS; Putnam, AJ; Kulik, TJ; Mooney, DJ. Optimizing seeding and culture methods to engineer smooth muscle tissue on biodegradable polymer matrices. *Biotechnology and Bioengineering.,* 1998, 57(1), 46-54.

[190] Martin, I; Wendt, D; Heberer, M. The role of bioreactors in tissue engineering. *Trends in Biotechnology.,* 2004, 22(2), 80-86.

[191] Bruinink, A; Siragusano, D; Ettel, G; Brandsberg, T; Brandsberg, F; Petitmermet, M; et al. The stiffness of bone marrow cell-knit composites is increased during mechanical load. *Biomaterials.,* 2001, 22(23), 3169-3178.

[192] Li, Y; Ma, T; Kniss, DA; Lasky, LC; Yang, ST. Effects of filtration seeding on cell density, spatial distribution, and proliferation in nonwoven fibrous matrices. *Biotechnology Progress.,* 2001, 17(5), 935-944.

[193] Xiao, YL; Riesle, J; Van Blitterswijk, CA. Static and dynamic fibroblast seeding and cultivation in porous PEO/PBT scaffolds. *Journal of Materials Science-Materials in Medicine.,* 1999, 10(12), 773-777.

[194] Burg, KJL; Delnomdedieu, M; Beiler, RJ; Culberson, CR; Greene, KG; Halberstadt, CR; et al. Application of magnetic resonance microscopy to tissue engineering: A polylactide model. *Journal of Biomedical Materials Research.,* 2002, 61(3), 380-390.

[195] Glicklis, R; Shapiro, L; Agbaria, R; Merchuk, JC; Cohen, S. Hepatocyte behavior within three-dimensional porous alginate scaffolds. *Biotechnology and Bioengineering.,* 2000, 67(3), 344-353.

[196] Nehrer, S; Breinan, HA; Ramappa, A; Young, G; Shortkroff, S; Louie, LK; et al. Matrix collagen type and pore size influence behaviour of seeded canine chondrocytes. *Biomaterials.,* 1997, 18(11), 769-776.

[197] VunjakNovakovic, G; Freed, LE; Biron, RJ; Langer, R. Effects of mixing on the composition and morphology of tissue-engineered cartilage. *Aiche Journal.,* 1996, 42(3), 850-860.

[198] Wendt, D; Marsano, A; Jakob, M; Heberer, M; Martin, I. Oscillating perfusion of cell suspensions through three-dimensional scaffolds enhances cell seeding efficiency and uniformity. *Biotechnology and Bioengineering.,* 2003, 84(2), 205-214.

[199] Xie, YB; Yang, ST; Kniss, DA. Three-dimensional cell-scaffold constructs promote efficient gene transfection: Implications for cell-based gene therapy. *Tissue Engineering.*, 2001, 7(5), 585-598.

[200] Palsson, BO; Sangeeta, NB. Scaling up for *ex vivo* cultivation. *Tissue Engineering.* USA: Pearson Prentice Hall, 2004, 223-243.

[201] Martin, Y; Vermette, P. Bioreactors for tissue mass culture: Design, characterization, and recent advances. *Biomaterials.*, 2005, 26(35), 7481-7503.

[202] Raimondi, MT; Boschetti, F; Falcone, L; Fiore, GB; Remuzzi, A; Marinoni, E; et al. Mechanobiology of engineered cartilage cultured under a quantified fluid-dynamic environment. *Biomechanics and Modeling in Mechanobiology.*, 2002, 1(1), 69-82.

[203] Freed, LE; Marquis, JC; VunjakNovakovic, G; Emmanual, J; Langer, R. Composition of Cell-Polymer Cartilage Implants. *Biotechnology and Bioengineering.*, 1994, 43(7), 605-614.

[204] Martin, I; Padera, RF; Vunjak-Novakovic, G; Freed, LE. *In vitro* differentiation of chick embryo bone marrow stromal cells into cartilaginous and bone-like tissues. *Journal of Orthopaedic Research.*, 1998, 16(2), 181-189.

[205] Carrier, RL; Papadaki, M; Rupnick, M; Schoen, FJ; Bursac, N; Langer, R; et al. Cardiac tissue engineering: Cell seeding, cultivation parameters, and tissue construct characterization. *Biotechnology and Bioengineering.*, 1999, 64(5), 580-589.

[206] Timmins, NE; Scherberich, A; Fruh, JA; Heberer, M; Martin, I; Jakob, M. Three-dimensional cell culture and tissue engineering in a T-CUP (Tissue Culture Under Perfusion). *Tissue Engineering.*, 2007, 13(8), 2021-2028.

[207] Cartmell, SH; Porter, BD; Garcia, AJ; Guldberg, RE. Effects of medium perfusion rate on cell-seeded three-dimensional bone constructs *in vitro*. *Tissue Engineering.*, 2003, 9(6), 1197-1203.

[208] Wang, YC; Uemura, T; Dong, R; Kojima, H; Tanaka, J; Tateishi, T. Application of perfusion culture system improves *in vitro* and *in vivo* osteogenesis of bone marrow-derived osteoblastic cells in porous ceramic materials. *Tissue Engineering.*, 2003, 9(6), 1205-1214.

[209] Bancroft, GN; Sikavitsast, VI; van den Dolder, J; Sheffield, TL; Ambrose, CG; Jansen, JA; et al. Fluid flow increases mineralized matrix deposition in 3D perfusion culture of marrow stromal osteloblasts in a dose-dependent manner. *Proceedings of the National Academy of Sciences of the United States of America.*, 2002, 99(20), 12600-12605.

[210] Goldstein, AS; Juarez, TM; Helmke, CD; Gustin, MC; Mikos, AG. Effect of convection on osteoblastic cell growth and function in biodegradable polymer foam scaffolds. *Biomaterials.*, 2001, 22(11), 1279-1288.

[211] Altman, G; Horan, R; Martin, I; Farhadi, J; Stark, P; Volloch, V; et al. Cell differentiation by mechanical stress. *FASEB J.*, 2002, 16(2), 270-272.

[212] Mauney, JR; Sjostorm, S; Blumberg, J; Horan, R; O'Leary, JP; Vunjak-Novakovic, G; et al. Mechanical stimulation promotes osteogenic differentiation of human bone marrow stromal cells on 3-D partially demineralized bone scaffolds *in vitro*. *Calcified Tissue International.*, 2004, 74(5), 458-468.

[213] Altman, GH; Lu, HH; Horan, RL; Calabro, T; Ryder, D; Kaplan, DL; et al. Advanced bioreactor with controlled application of multi-dimensional strain for tissue engineering. *Journal of Biomechanical Engineering-Transactions of the Asme.*, 2002, 124(6), 742-749.

[214] Pancrazio, JJ; Wang, F; Kelley, CA. Enabling tools for tissue engineering. *Biosensors & Bioelectronics.*, 2007, 22(12), 2803-2811.

[215] Bettinger, CJ; Weinberg, EJ; Kulig, KM; Vacanti, JP; Wang, YD; Borenstein, JT; et al. Three-dimensional microfluidic tissue-engineering scaffolds using a flexible biodegradable polymer. *Advanced Materials.*, 2006, 18(2), 165-+.

[216] Leclerc, E; Furukawa, KS; Miyata, F; Sakai, Y; Ushida, T; Fujii, T. Fabrication of microstructures in photosensitive biodegradable polymers for tissue engineering applications. *Biomaterials.*, 2004, 25(19), 4683-4690.

[217] Engel, E; Michiardi, A; Navarro, M; Lacroix, D; Planell, JA. Nanotechnology in regenerative medicine: the materials side. *Trends in Biotechnology.* 2007, In press.

In: Synthetic and Integrative Biology
Editor: James T. Gevona, pp. 199-213

ISBN: 978-1-60876-678-9
© 2010 Nova Science Publishers, Inc.

Chapter 9

CONTRIBUTIONS OF SYNTHETIC BIOLOGY TO THE FIELD OF THE ORIGIN OF LIFE

Pier Luigi Luisi

Department of Biology, University of Rome3
V.le G. Marconi 446, Rome 00146, Italy

Abstract

Three examples of this "chemical synthetic biology" approach are given in this article. The first example deals with the synthesis of proteins that do not exist in nature, and dubbed as "the never born proteins" (NBPs). This research is related to the question why and how the protein structures existing in our world have been selected out, with the underlying question whether they have something very particular from the structural or thermodynamic point of view (for example, folding). The NBPs are produced in the laboratory by the modern molecular biology technique, the phage display, so as to produce a very large library of proteins having no homology with known proteins.

The second example of chemical synthetic biology has also to do with the laboratory synthesis of proteins, but, this time, adopting a prebiotic synthetic procedure, i.e., the fragment condensation of short peptides, where short means that they have a length that can be obtained by prebiotic methods.

The scheme is illustrated and discussed, being based on the fragment condensation catalyzed by peptides endowed with proteolitic activity. Selection during chain growth is determined by solubility under the contingent environmental conditions, i.e., the peptides which result insoluble are eliminated from further growth. The scheme is tested preliminarily with a synthetic chemical fragment-condensation method and brings to the synthesis of a 44-residueslong protein, which has no homology with known proteins, and which has a stable tertiary folding.

Finally, the third example, dubbed as "the minimal cell project". Here, the aim is to synthesize a cell model having the minimal and sufficient number of components to be defined as living. For this purpose, liposomes are used as shell membranes, and attempts are made to introduce in the interior a minimal genome. Several groups all around the world are active in this field, and significant results have been obtained, which are reviewed in this article. For example, protein expression has been obtained inside liposomes, generally with the green fluorescent protein. Our last attempts are with a minimal genome consisting of 37 enzymes, a set which is able to express proteins using the ribosomal machinery.

These minimal cells are not yet capable of self-reproduction, and this and other shortcomings within the project are critically reviewed.

Introduction

The field of the origin of life is based on the common understanding that life on Earth originated from the inanimate matter, starting from simple organic compounds that, due to a slow accumulation of material, evolved towards more and more complex molecular systems provided by more and more specialized functions. Eventually, this process culminated in the formation of closed compartments that could make copies of themselves: the first protocells. After the successful experiments of Stanley Miller over 50 years ago, the chemists are still busy trying to show that the formation of important biochemicals could have been possible under prebiotic conditions. Until now, important pieces are missing in the puzzle, for example the biogenesis of specific macromolecular sequences, like the enzymes, or RNA. The RNA world scenario is still the most popular for the origin of life, as it assumes that a family of self-replicating RNA was the original machinery to start all- but the question where does the sophisticated RNA species originated from, remains an elusive question, and usually elegantly ignored by several authors in this camp.

People in the general field of the origin of life are involved in all these particular questions, and other which are still unsolved-like the origin of the genetic code, or the structure of the early cells. But also the philosophical framework of the ladder leading to the first cellular forms is still a matter of debate. In particular, looking at the prebiotic molecular evolution that goes from simple organic molecules to the early living cells, two main theories are opposing each other: one says that the origin of life was an inescapable event, an outcome that had to be realized once given the prebiotic conditions. This is the view that assumes a kind of absolute determinism in the pathway leading to life, where each step is causally determined by the previous one and determines the next one, in a sequence which inescapably leads to the living cellular form. Christian de Duve, Herbert Morowitz, Stuart Kaufmann, and others appear to favor this view. The opposite front is kept by people like Stephen Jay Gould, and most of the contemporary students in the field, who, in the footstep of classic Monod, accept the view that contingency is the main factor which led to life starting from the simple organic molecules and their basic interactions. Contingency is the modern and more fashionable version of old "chance", and sees that a certain outcome is given by the concomitance of factors which are independent from one another, happens simultaneously causing a certain thing to happen. And since the relative statistical weight of each of these factors is unknown or unpredictable, the outcome will be considered as a chance event, although each of the factors may be per se non un-deterministic. Thus the disappearance of the dinosaurs 60 millions years ago, due the impact with an asteroid, is a typical contingency event, and also the Cambrian revolution, according to Gould, was due to a series of factors with no causal dependability to each other. Change only one of these factors, and the event would not have happened-or happened in a quite different way.

In the things of nature, contingency and determinism go the hand in the hand, as there is no one without the other: the appearance of wings may be due to contingency, but then the extension of the wing in a given bird must obey the natural laws for permitting the flight; and *viceversa*, each contingency event must be born from a thermodynamic asset. However, in considering the origin of life, the two viewpoints appear drastically opposite to each other. Il life due to an inescapable event, or is due to contingency?

This appears to be a philosophical controversy, with experimentalists having little to say about. However, in this paper I will make the point that certain aspects of synthetic biology may permit to tackle this question from an experimental point of view. Synthetic biology is the field that is concerned with the laboratory production of alternative forms of life, or alternative biological structures, alternative in the sense that are not present in extant life. Is the old question: why this and not that, why did nature operate towards a certain compound or structure, and not towards a different one? Why DNA has ribose instead of glucose, why do we have 20 amino acids instead of 10, etc. And synthetic biology may answer by synthesizing DNA with glucose, by making proteins with 10 amino-acids, and studying the corresponding properties. In this way, we may learn why nature followed a certain pathway instead of another one.

In this paper I will give three examples of synthetic biology performed in our laboratory, that go in the direction "why this and not that". In this sense, the following part is based on a recent paper of ours with the title "Chemical synthetic biology" [1] where the term chemical indicates that the new alternative structures are not the products of genetic manipulation, but rather of chemical ingenuity.

1. The Never Born Proteins

The starting point is the numerology of proteins, in particular the well-known consideration that the proteins existing in nature make only an infinitesimal fraction of the theoretically possible structures.

This paradox has been emphasized by various authors, also by Christian de Duve in his latest book [2]. There are many ways to express this. For example, one can say that the ratio between the theoretically possible proteins having a chain with 100 residues, and the actual number of all existing proteins (probably something around 10^{14}), comes close to the ratio between the space of the universe and the space of a single H-atom; or, using a more earthly example, close to the ratio between the all sand of Sahara and one single grain of sand [3]. These astronomic figures may appear deprived of practical physical meaning.

However, they convey a very simple, well graspable concept, i.e., that our life is based on a very limited number of structures; and this, in turn, elicits a very relevant question: how and why have these few structures been selected out?

To give an answer, we go back to our controversy between determinism and contingency, as mentioned in the introduction. Thus, one first possible answer is that "our" proteins have something very special that made the selection possible-that there has been a deterministic, obligatory pathway that determined the selection of our proteins instead of others. For example, they might be the only ones to be stable; or water soluble; or those which have very particular viscosity and/or rheological properties. In all these cases, they would have been selected because of their particular physical properties. This is part of the aforementioned general view according to which life is an inescapable outcome of the laws of nature, and that, therefore, all prerequisites for making life, including the basic macromolecular structures, are determined.

In this sense, an author who should be particularly kept in mind is Christian de Duve, who in his book [2] stated:

"It is self-evident that the universe was pregnant with life and the biosphere with man. Otherwise, we would not be here. Or else, our presence can be explained only by a miracle..."

This is basically the view that the origin of life was an obligatory, inevitable process, and if one literally takes this view, then one has to conclude that the proteins must have been chosen in the right way so as to make life possible. One cannot, in fact, assume the inevitability of life and then let contingency shape the structure of proteins as chance structures.

The alternative point of view is that our proteins have no extraordinary physical properties at all; they have been selected among an enormous number of possibilities of quite similar compounds by a process of contingency, (which is the term that now replaces "chance") , and it happened that they were capable of fostering cellular life. Cast the dice again, and the probability that exactly our 10^{14} or so proteins come out again is at all effects practically zero, (this is the probability of fishing our precisely that "grain of sand") -so that life as it is now may not have started. According to the contingency view, basically "our" life would be a serendipitous property of these casually determined structures.

The view of contingency in evolution and life is advocated, among many others, most notably by Stephen J. Gould [4] and J. Monod [5].

The Experimental Project

The basic idea of the project is to test whether "our" proteins have really something particular with respect to the proteins that have never existed. How can one conduct this project? Simply by synthesizing proteins that do not exist in nature, and comparing them with our proteins. It is a project of chemical synthetic biology, as outlined in the Introduction, aimed at producing a quite different grain of sand– and asking then the question, whether our proteins are really so different and peculiar with respect to those synthetic biology products – in terms of stability, solubility, or folding. Actually, folding is a particularly important and stringent criterion, as the prerequisite for the biological activity of proteins is their globular folding, which is a consequence of the primary structure.

Such a project has been initiated at the Federal Institute of Technology in Zurich, Switzerland, to be pursued by my group transferred to the University of Rome3, Italy, in particular, by Cristiano Chiarabelli and Davide de Lucrezia. The first set of papers describing these results about the 5never born proteins6 (NBPs) has been recently published [6-9].

The principle to produce NBPs is simple: if one makes a long string (say 150 bases in our first project) of DNA purely randomly, the probability of hitting an existing sequence in our Earth is practically zero (it corresponds to a number equivalent to the ratio between one grain of sand and the entire Sahara). If you then let this DNA being processed by standard recombinant DNA and in vivo expression techniques, you will obtain a 50-residues long polypeptide that does not exist on Earth, and when this polypeptide is globularly folded, you have already obtained a NBP.

In practice, what we do is to obtain a large library of DNA by the so-called phage-display method. We obtain first from commercial sources a library of totally random DNA sequences with the desired length (150 base pairs in our case). The random DNA segment is then inserted within a phage genome so that the corresponding random protein is linked to a capside protein. The production of the phage library actually needs the infection of cells that provide the machinery for the synthesis of viral proteins. Those proteins will be displayed on the capside of the phage (one per phage), and they are (in the N-termini portion) totally random, de novo proteins. In our case, the sequence of the NBPs is not completely random, since a tripetide sequence has been inserted in the middle of the random sequence with the aim of selection (vide infra).

In this way, by a first run, a library of ca. 10^9 of 50-residues-long polypeptides was obtained. The first questions at this point were: i) are they really all "never born proteins", i.e., more specifically, are they really absent in the protein data bank collected until now? and: ii) what will be the fraction of globularly folded polypeptides, i.e., of globular proteins? It is also clear that, for practical reasons, one cannot study all 10^9 clones; one can only refer to a selected sampling of it, chosen, however, without any preconceived bias so that the statistical relevance of their properties still hold.

Let us begin with the question about being "never born". The 79 sequences which were selected at random were compared with known protein sequences, and no similarity was found, although a permissive criterion was adopted for the comparative analysis [7].

In conclusion, then, the proteins so synthesized can indeed be considered as nonextant, which permits the terminology of "never born proteins" (NBPs). Of course, it is possible that some of these sequences may have been proposed in the course of molecular evolution, and then gone lost; or that some of them are present in some unexplored plants or micro-organisms of our Earth. But, in first and good approximation, they are not present in any living form we know.

The other question (about folding) has been tackled based on the well-accepted observation that folded proteins are not easily digestible by proteases. The strategy involved the insertion of the overmentioned tripetide PRG (proline-arginine-glycine), substrate for the proteolytic enzyme thrombin, in the otherwise totally random protein sequence (i.e., the DNA library was designed in order to have three non-random codons in the middle of the sequence). In this way, each of the new proteins had the potentiality of being digested by the enzyme, with the expectation, however, that globularly folded NBPs would be protected from digestion. With this idea in mind, the 79 randomly selected clones were incubated in a medium in the presence of thrombin. The larger part of the population was rapidly hydrolyzed, but ca. 20% of the population was highly resistant to the action of thrombin.

Although our criterion of folding should be considered at this point is an approximate one, 20% is a surprisingly high figure. It suggests that folding is indeed a general property, something that arises naturally, even for proteins of medium length. The characterization of some of those folded proteins has begun, and the circular dichroic properties in the far UV region of two of them, labeled preliminarily as A and B, are shown (for the primary sequence, see the original reference [7]). It is apparent from the data of figure 1 that, in both, a significant percentage of periodic structure, a-helix in particular, is present, and, furthermore, very interestingly, the globular folding is thermo-reversible, indicating that is under thermodynamic control.

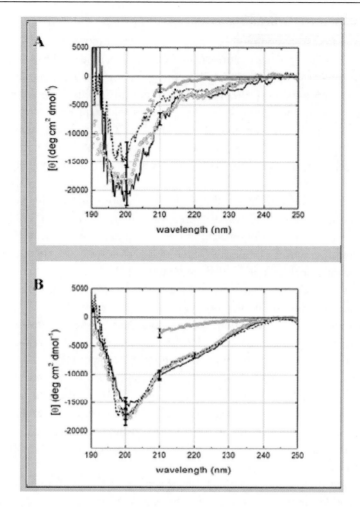

Figure 1. CD Spectrum of two "never born proteins". Note the significant content of secondary structure and the reversibility of the folding with temperature. For a detailed description of these CD experiments, see [7].

In figure 2, the computed folding of these two proteins are illustrated, according to the analysis carried out by Dr. Fabio Polticelli in Roma3. Although the computational method used (Rosetta) is the most reliable of present day's literature, such three-dimensional drawings cannot be considered yet as the definitive structure; for the actual structure, one should await for NMR or X-ray data.

We have now about one dozen of such computed structures, and, although one should wait before attempting generalizations, it appears rather safe at this point to state that folding and thermodynamic stability are not properties that are restricted to our extant proteins, and that, on the contrary, they appear to be rather common features of randomly created polypeptides.

On the basis of this, one is tempted to propose that "our" proteins do not belong to a class of polypeptides with privileged physical properties. And, by inference, one could say that this kind of data, once confirmed by a larger number of cases, permit to brake a lance in favor of the scenario of contingency.

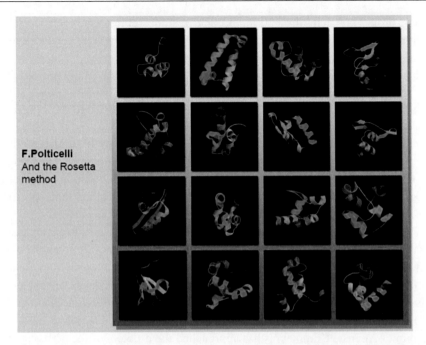

F.Policelli
And the Rosetta
method

Figure 2. The structure prediction of some of the o "never born proteins" by the Rosetta method. As explained in the text, the predicted structures appear to be qualitatively in agreement with the spectroscopic data of CD and fluorescence in the two cases where the NBP have been characterized.

Of course, the NBPs may also have bio-technological importance, and may be also very interesting from the structural point of view: could they, for example, display novel catalytic and structural features that have not been observed in "our" proteins? The answer to these question must await for much more data.

The Case of Never Born RNAs

There is an important addition to be made to the above synthetic-biology program: the synthesis of NBPs is automatically accompanied by the synthesis of the corresponding m-RNAs. This permits to tackle the question whether and to what extent such totally random RNAs are going to be folded.

We have conducted an analysis of several randomly chosen "never born RNAs" [8,9], and found indeed an extensive folding, which we could partly classify in different classes by utilizing an ad hoc developed method of analysis, based on a nuclease enzyme (S1) coupled with a temperature gradient (the "Foster assay"; see [8,9]). Particularly interesting was the observation of an RNA structure which did not unfold at temperatures as high as 60 c. This led us to the hypothesis that thermo-resistant RNA structures may not be so rare.

Now, we are developing the work on NBPs and corresponding RNAs in two directions: one is the characterization of the already made NBPs: we would like to obtain a large number of NBP structures so as to have a statistically significant display.

The other direction of work is to prepare another library of NBPs, this time with a length of 20 residues. In this case, we will be mostly looking for primitive forms of catalysis, which, given the small size, is not expected to be exceptional, but relevant for the origin of life (see the following project). A length of 20 amino acid residues corresponds to a corresponding RNA length of 60 nucleotides, and this is a particularly interesting size, i.e., close to most of the ribozymes' sizes.

2. Synthesis of Polypeptides under Simulated Prebiotic Evolution

The previous Section addresses the question of the frequency of foldable chains in a library of totally random de novo polypeptides, whereby such chains have been obtained by modern molecular biology techniques. Therefore, one of the main questions about the origin of macromolecules remains open: how have multiple copies of identical long specific chains been produced under prebiotic conditions?

Again, that the polypeptides came from long nucleic acids is not an answer, as the question would then be referred to the etiology of specific sequences of polynucleotides.

In fact, if one searches in the literature for the prebiotic syntheses (Merrifield method excluded) of relatively long co-oligopeptides (say at least 30 residues, so that they partly begin to assume a stable folding), one finds almost nothing. Some references are collected in [3].

The group of Auguste Commeyras has approached the problem of the prebiotic formation of peptides by using the condensation of N-carboxy anhydrides (NCA) [10,11], a method that, according to the authors, is prebiotic; but also in this case the critical question of the production of multiple identical copies of long (30 residues or more) co-oligopeptides could not yet be achieved.

How then can one conceive a co-polymerization scheme which produces, for example, lysozyme- kind of molecules? This question forms the basis of our next chemical synthetic-biology project.

The Underlying Model

We need first a work hypothesis for the formation of multiple copies of identical long co-oligopeptide chains. The basic idea is that such a chain elongation proceeds by successive fragment condensation of prebiotically formed short co-oligopetides (i.e., peptide-bond formation, i.e., the reverse reaction of the peptide bond hydrolysis) as reviewed in [3]. In particular, the synthesis of short peptides is realized by the prebiotic NCA condensation. A key assumption is that, in this random library, some peptides may arise, which possess proteolitic activity. Further, one assumes that fragment condensation may be induced by the catalytic action of such peptides.

How realistic are these two assumptions? It has been already reported that even simple peptides may be endowed with proteolytic activity. For example, His –Ser appears to be capable of cleaving peptide and nucleic acid bonds [12]; and even Gly– Gly [13] appears to posses some catalytic activity. One may then consider to start from a prebiotic library of, say, decapeptides (this length is quite possible with the NCA method) and proceed with fragment condensation induced by catalytically active peptides.

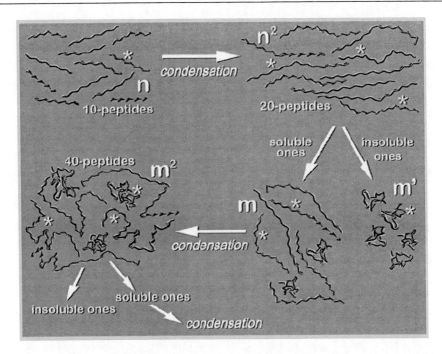

Figure 3. The fragment condensation scheme under simulated prebiotic environmental conditions. This illustration shows how the initial library of n decapeptides may contain some compounds endowed with catalytic activity (indicated by an asterisk), and how then the ideal mutual condensation of these n decapeptides gives rise ideally to n2 20-mers, of which only m are capable of "surviving", being soluble in H2O under the given conditions. These, in turn, give rise to m2 40-residues-long peptides, of which a large number are insoluble under the given environmental conditions, and so on.

Thus, we arrive at another key assumption of our working program: The idea is that the selection is governed by the contingency of the environmental conditions, such as pH, solubility, temperature, salinity, etc. Contingently upon these conditions, the largest majority of the library structures may be eliminated (e.g., by lack of solubility, or due to aggregation), and only a few chain products may "survive" in solution, undergoing then further elongation in solution. Thus, the selection criteria conceived in our work is one that is assumed to simulate the natural chemical evolution – in particular a kind of survival of the best fit as governed by the interplay of contingent conditions (the actual pH or salinity or temperature operating at that moment of growth) and the actual physical properties of the candidate chains. Figure 3, taken from [3], gives an illustration of this process.

Is it then realistic to expect that, by this method, a sizable concentration of a given long co-oligopeptide would be synthesized? The answer appears to be positive on the basis of the procedure described in our previous work (14) which reports the fragment condensation of a 44-residues-long de novo protein – although not based on peptide catalysts, but preliminarily only on peptide synthesis.

First, two parent 40-residue peptides, P1 and P2 , were designed randomly by computer but with the constraint that the relative abundance of the 20 amino acids used in their construction maintained a 1 : 1 :1... relationship.

A matrix, A·B, of 16 20-residue peptides was constructed experimentally by the systematic combination of two small libraries A and B each comprising four ten-residue peptide sequences. The 16 20-residue sequences arrived at in this way were synthesized by the solid-phase method.

The peptide products were subjected to selection on the basis of their solubility in H_2O under well-defined conditions.

It was found thatA1B2, A2B2 , and A3B2 were completely soluble in aqueous buffer in the pH range of 5.2– 8.6; A1B3 and A3B3 were insoluble, whereas A2B3 was totally soluble, in contrast to prediction. The subsets (A·B)s that fulfilled the mentioned criterion of being soluble in H2O were then subjected to chain elongation by combination with a further small set of 20-residue sequences, C, giving rise to the new library C· (A·B)s consisting of 16 peptides which are 40-residues long.

None of the latter were soluble in aqueous buffer, but two of them, A1B2C1 and A2B2C1, turned out to be soluble in 6m guanidinium chloride (GuCl). The addition of a polar N-terminal extension to them (DDEE) resulted in the 44-residue sequences DDEE-A1B2C1 and DDEE-A2B2C1. Of these two samples, only the latter was soluble in H2O. This was further characterized and studied. Details of this work will not be given here, the interested reader is referred to ref. 14,3 and 1.

It is however very interesting at this point to mention that the far UV-CD spectrum of this de novo protein showed a high proportion of ordered structure, in particular, the presence of 49% a-helix, 12% b-sheet, and 39% aperiodic structure. Thermal denaturation experiments were performed over the 0 – 998 temperature range.

In conclusion, the 44-residues-long polypeptide sequence is to be seen as a de novo protein, and one that does not have any significant homologies with known sequences in the data bank for proteins of similar length. In addition, it displays a stable folding, and, in this sense, the 44-mer represents indeed the product of a model evolutionary design. Of course, mutatis mutandis, all what it has been stated for polypeptides can be extended to nucleic acids; the principles do not change. It should also be added that, in principle, there is no problem to obtain a few mg of such a chain with this procedure, which corresponds to an extreme large number of identical copies of such chain,

Aside from that, the approach proposed here can be conceptually generalized to a primordial mechanism that appears capable to produce a specific macromolecular sequence from an initial oligopeptide, by a step-by-step elongation which is determined by the contingency of the environmental pressure – be pH, temperature, salinity, solubility, aggregation, or other physical factors. This may well be a reasonable conceptual framework to conceive the etiology of specific macromolecular sequences, both in the case of polypeptides as in the case of nucleic acids.

Again, the synthetic procedure is not prebiotic, as the Merrifield method cannot be considered as such. As already mentioned, it is possible, however, to foresee the corresponding prebiotic synthetic scheme, based on the catalytic action of proteolitic peptides, a project that is now under scrutiny in our laboratories.

3. The Minimal Cell Project

The first two projects deal with the synthesis of macromolecular sequences. The one to be described now deals with the construction of synthetic – or better semi-synthetic –minimal living cell. The term semi-synthetic is meant to indicate that part of the material which is utilized, as well as the assembly procedure, is synthetic, while other parts (nucleic acid and enzymes) are of natural origin.

To introduce the problem, let us remind, as summarized in recent reviews [15-17], that even the simplest unicellular organisms on Earth display a staggering complexity. Escherichia coli K-12 has a genome size of ca. 4.64 Mio (check) base pairs, and Bacillus subtilis of 4.2 Mio (check) base pairs, to give examples of well-known Gram-negative and Gram-positive eubacteria, respectively. The simplest known prokaryotic cell, the obligate cellular wall-less parasite Mycoplasma genitalium, contains 517 genes with only 470 predicted coding regions [18]. The nucleomorph chromosomes from the cryptomonad Guillardia has only a 551 kb genome, and, according to Moya and co-workers [18], Buchnera species have even smaller genomes that can be reduced down to 450 kb.

The question is whether such complexity is necessary for cellular life, or whether, instead, cellular life could, in principle, also be possible with a much lower number of molecular components. This proposition is relevant also for the field of the origin of life, as it does not appear reasonable to assume that life started with cells containing thousand of genes. In fact, in the field, it is generally accepted that the extant cellular complexity is the outcome of a lengthy process of evolution, starting from primordial cells that, living in a much more permissive environment, should have been genetically much simpler. How simple would a minimal cell look like, i.e., a cell that contains the minimal and sufficient number of components to perform the basic functions of cellular life? Such a cell that contains the minimal and sufficient number of components to be defined as alive constitutes the notion of "minimal cell".

All these preliminary considerations make already clear the point, that the "minimal cell" is not a single structure, the term rather defines a family of constructs at different degrees of sophistication and complexity.

Experimental Approaches to the Minimal Cell

Having clarified, to some extent, the nature of the minimal genome, one might try to have it inserted into a cell, to see whether it works. But it is not easy to prepare the genome of Buchnera or any other micro-organism with any desired number of genes.

The alternative approach which has been considered in my and other groups is illustrated schematically in figure 4. The idea is to construct a minimal cell by inserting in a compartment a calibrated ensemble of genes and/or enzymes, increasing step by step the complexity of this added ensemble, until the construct begins to display forms of cellular life. In my group, this work is carried out by Yutetsu Kuruma, Giovanni Murtas, and Pasquale Stano.

Liposomes have been chosen as membrane compartments, since they, with their lipid bilayer, are considered the best models for the shell of biological membranes, and the procedure to insert biopolymers inside liposomes is already well-established.

Another good reason to use vesicles or liposomes is due to the fact that conditions have been described under which vesicles are capable of self-reproduction [19-20], namely, of increasing auto-catalytically their population number, which may model the behavior of living cells.

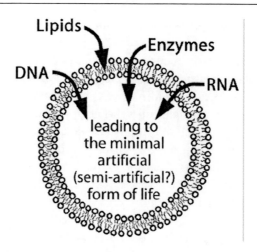

Figure 4. the approach to the semi-synthetic minimal cell, showing the encapsulation of the minimal and sufficient number of macromolecular components into a liposome to yield the minimal living cell-like system.

To arrive, in this way, at a minimal cellular life is a complex enterprise, and it is useful to divide up the "road map" to the minimal cell in different milestones with increasing complexity.

The first one, which is already under control in several laboratories, is to carry out and optimize complex enzymatic reactions in the interior of liposomes, such as the polymerase chain reaction, the biosynthesis of RNA and DNA, the condensation of amino acids, etc.

Most probably, the very first attempt to carry out biological reactions inside liposomes with the aim of creating a minimal cell is the work by Schmidli et al. [21]. The idea here was to enzymatically synthesize lecithin inside lecithin-liposomes: in this way, there would be a self-reproduction caused by an internal reaction, in keeping also with the basic ideas of autopoiesis [22-23].

The other and only other example that I like to mention here is one based on the above mentioned self-reproduction of oleate vesicles. A suggestive example of core and shell reproduction was in fact provided in 1995 by Oberhozer et al. with the use of Qbeta replicase [24]. In this experiment, while the enzyme was replicating RNA inside the vesicles, the oleate vesicles were multiplying by their own accord. At first sight, this appears already a good approximation of the living cell: there is a simple metabolism inside it, the system is replicating, and potentially capable of evolution, since there is a copying machinery of RNA that can give rise to mistakes/mutations. However, the enzyme and the RNA molecules are not reproduced from inside the system, and, after a few generations, most of the new vesicles will not be capable of further reproduction: in fact, for statistical reasons, they will not contain all original system6s components, most of them will be empty or containing only one macromolecular component. The system will undergo what we call "death by dilution" [3].

The next step in the road map to the minimal cell is the encapsulation, in the water pool of vesicles, of all components which are necessary to express proteins. Mostly, the green fluorescence protein (GFP) has been expressed until now, as it is easier to detect it. Among the research groups which are active in this field, one should mention those one by Yomo and co-workers [25], as well as Nomura et al. [26] in Japan, Noireaux and Libchaber in the States [27], our group first in Zurich and now in Rome [28-30].

In all these cases, the entire ribosomal machinery has been incorporated into the liposomes. Generally, commercial kits for protein expression have been utilized, for which the composition and the relative concentrations of components are not known.

We are then dealing with "black boxes", which contain most probably a few hundreds of enzymes.

One significant progress in the field is the description by Ueda and co-workers [31] of the so-called PURE SYSTEM. This is a system consisting of 37 enzymes (plus the ribosomes and tRNAs-a total of over 80 macromolecular components), which is capable of expressing proteins in vitro.

Protein expression is only part of the life of a cell. To have a satisfactorily minimal cell, one should reach the point at which the minimal cell is also able to self-reproduce; and we are working on that. The idea is to enrich the 37 components of the PURE SYSTEM with the minimal number of additional enzyme which permit the synthesis of the ribosomes themselves. In another direction of work, we will try to simplify the structure of the ribosomes, in order to eliminate most of the proteins.

4. Concluding Remarks

We have presented three projects that can be classified in the field of chemical synthetic biology, where the characterization of the single chemical constituents is still the major or one of the major features. In the NBPs project, the synthetic-biology products are single proteins that do not exist in nature, and, actually, the same holds for the second project presented here, where the synthesis, however, obeys a more classical organic-synthesis pattern. The project on the minimal cell is certainly the most biological of the three; however, the procedure is based on the preparation and physico-chemical characterization of vesicles of given dimensions, and the insertion of macromolecular species of known composition and concentration – a typical chemistry approach. Of these three projects, the first and the third one can be considered outcomes of modern techniques in molecular biology – in the sense that they were not technically possible ten or twenty years ago. By contrast, the second one, dealing with the prebiotic synthesis of specific macromolecular sequences, does not require any advanced modern technical skill, and one may wonder why it has not been attempted or implemented long ago. Interestingly, the minimal cell project can be seen as a concrete example of bridging systems and synthetic biology, being focused on a constructive approach of a cellular system.

It is important to mention that this experimental work has a philosophical counterpart, in the sense that it bears with fundamental questions in the field of the origin of life. Thus, the NBP project is germane to the question of the selection of our extant proteins, and, therefore, connects to the controversy between determinism and contingency in the things of nature; and so is for the second project. The third one, on the minimal cell, has directly to do with questions such as "what is life" and with the question, whether life is an emergent property arising from non-living components.

This interface between chemistry and philosophy is arising in a special way when chemistry moves towards biology, and, of course, synthetic biology is the most proper medium for this merging.

References

[1]   Luisi, P. L. (2007). Chemical synthetic biology, *Chemistry and Biodiv.,* Vol. 4, 607.
[2]   de Duve, C. (2002). *5Life Evolving*: *Molecules, Mind and Meaning6,* Oxford University Press, New York,.
[3]   Luisi, P. L. (2006). *5The Emergence of Life: From Chemical Origins to Synthetic Biology* 6, Cambridge University Press, Cambridge,.
[4]   Gould, S. J. (1989). *Wonderful Life*, Penguin Books, London,.
[5]   Monod, J. (1971). *Chance and Necessity,* Knopf, New York,.
[6]   Chiarabelli, C., Vrijbloed, J. W., Thomas, R. M. & Luisi, P. L. (2006). *Chem. Biodiv.,* **3**, 827.
[7]   Chiarabelli, C., Vrijbloed, J. W., De Lucrezia, D., Thomas, R. M., Stano, P., Polticelli, F., Ottone, T., Papa, E. & Luisi, P. L. (2006). *Chem. Biodiv.,* **3**, 840.
[8]   De Lucrezia, D., Franchi, M., Chiarabelli, C., Gallori, E. & Luisi, P. L. (2006). *Chem. Biodiv.,* **3**, 860;
[9]   De Lucrezia, D., Franchi, M., Chiarabelli, C., Gallori, E. & Luisi, P. L. (2006). *Chem. Biodiv.,* **3**, 869.
[10] Commeyras, A., Boiteau, L., Vandenabeele-Trambouze, O. & Selsis, F. (2004). in *Lectures in Astrobiology,* Vol. 1, Part 2, Eds. M. Gargaud, B. Barbier, H. Martin, and J. Reisse, Springer-Verlag, Berlin, 517-542.
[11] Taillades, J., Cottet, H., Garrel, L., Beuzelin, I., Boiteau, L., Choukroun, H. & Commeyras, A. (1999). *J. Mol.Evol.,* **48**, 638.
[12] Li, Y., Zhao, Y., Hatfield, S., Wan, R., Zhu, Q., Li, X., McMills, M., Ma, Y., Li, J., Brown, K. L., He, C., Liu, F. & Chen, X. (2000). *Bioorg. Med. Chem.,* **8**, 2675.
[13] Plankensteiner, K., Righi, A. & Rode, B. M. (2002). *Orig. Life Evol. Biosphere.,* **32**, 225.
[14] Chessari, S., Thomas, R., Polticelli, F. & Luisi, P. L. (2006). *Chem. Biodiv.,* **3**, 1202.
[15] Luisi, P. L., Oberholzer, T. & Lazcano, A. (2007). *Helv. Chim. Acta.* 2002, 85, 1759. *620 CHEMISTRY and BIODIVERSITY* – Vol. 4.
[16] Gil, R., Sabater-Munoz, B., Latorre, A., Silva, F. J. & Moya, A. (2002). *Proc. Natl. Acad. Sci., U.S.A.,* **99**,4454.
[17] Koonin, E. V. (2000). *Nat. Rev. Microbiol.* 2003, 1, 127; E. V. Koonin, *Annu. Rev. Genomics Human Genet.,* **1**, 99.
[18] Islas, S., Becerra, A., Luisi, P. L. & Lazcano, A. (2004). *Orig. Life Evol. Biosphere.,* **34**, 243.
[19] Bachmann, P. A., Luisi, P. L. & Lang, J. (1992). *Nature.,* **357**, 57.
[20] Wick, R., Walde, P. & Luisi, P. L. (1995). *J. Am. Chem. Soc.,* **117**, 1435.
[21] Schmidli, P. K., Schurtenberger, P. & Luisi, P. L. (1991). *J. Am. Chem. Soc.,* **113**, 8127.
[22] Varela, F., Maturana, H. R. & Uribe, R. B. (1974). *Biosystems.,* **5**, 187.
[23] Varela, F. & Maturana, H. (1998). *The Tree of Knowledge*, Shambala, Boston,.
[24] Oberholzer, T., Wick, R., Luisi, P. L. & Biebricher, C. K. (1995). *Biochem. Biophys. Res. Commun.,* **207**, 250.
[25] Ishikawa, K., Sato, K., Shima, Y., Urabe, I. & Yomo, T. (2004). *FEBS Letters,* **576**, 387.
[26] Yu, W., Sato, K., Wakabayashi, M., Nakatshi, T., Ko-Mitamura, E. P., Shima, Y., Urabe, I. & Yomo, T. (2001). *J. Biosci. Bioeng.,* **92**, 590.

[27] Sunami, T., Sato, K., Matsuura, T., Tsukada, K., Urabe, I., Yomo, T. (2006). *Anal. Biochem.*, **357**, 128.

[28] Nomura, S. M., Tsumoto, K., Hamada, T., Akiyoshi, K., Nakatani, Y. & Yoshikawa, K. (2003). *Chem. Bio. Chem.*, **4**, 1172.

[29] Noireaux, V. & Libchaber, A. (2004). *Proc. Natl. Acad. Sci. U.S.A.*, **101**, 17669.

[30] Pietrini, A. V. & Luisi, P. L. (2004). *Chem. Bio. Chem.*, **5**, 1055

[31] Murtas, G., Kuruma, Y., Luisi, P. L. (2007). *Biochem. Biophys. Res. Commun.*, **363**(1), 12-7

[32] Fiordimondo, D. & Stano, P. (2007). *Chembiochem.*, **8**(16), 1965-73.

[33] Shimizu, Y., Inoue, A., Tomari, Y., Suzuki, T., Yokogawa, T., Nishikawa, K. & Ueda, T. (2001). *Nat. Biotechnol.*, **19**, 751.

INDEX

D

E

F

K-12, 209
keratin, 53, 54
keratinocytes, 49
kidney, viii, 41, 47, 48, 49, 50, 58, 59, 90
kidneys, 42, 48, 78
kinase, 172
kinetic parameters, 163
kinetics, 74, 160, 168, 170, 185

L

labeling, 22, 48, 49, 50, 54
laboratory, 182, 183
lactic acid, 159, 160, 188, 195
lakes, 120
laminated, 161
lamination, 162
land, 42, 49, 54
landscape, ix, 7, 20, 21, 27, 33, 36, 38, 115, 123, 129, 136
Langerhans cells, 24
laser, 164
leaching, 161, 162, 163, 170
lead, 160, 169, 177
lecithin, 210
leishmaniasis, 134
lens, 44, 57, 59
leukemia, 20
LFA, 91
life cycle, 85, 86, 106, 115
life sciences, x, 123, 124, 131, 136, 149
lifestyle, 42
ligament, 181
ligand, 6, 11, 14, 16, 22, 23, 64, 73, 91, 169
limitation, 128, 131, 164
line, 18, 80, 94, 97, 99, 113, 132, 177
linear systems, 109, 117
linkage, 7
links, ix, 3, 105, 106, 118, 135
lipid, 209
liposome, 210
liposomes, x, 199, 209, 210, 211
liquid chromatography, 126, 127
liquid phase, 162, 188
Listeria monocytogenes, 22, 28
literature, 173, 178, 191
lithography, 164
liver, 24, 47, 90, 145
liver cancer, 145
liver cells, 90
L-lactide, 159, 192
localization, 49, 50
location, 151

luciferase, 129
lumen, 51, 52
luminescence, 62, 63, 73
lung, 154
lyme disease, 33
lymph node, 147
lymphatic system, 47
lymphocytes, 20
lymphoid, 153
lysis, 81, 85
lysozyme, 206

M

machinery, xi, 199, 200, 203, 210, 211
macromolecules, 157, 191, 206
macrophages, 153
magnetic resonance, 196
maintenance, 50, 115, 175
majority, 142, 151, 207
mammalian cells, 169
manipulation, viii, 6, 20, 23, 61, 77, 201
manufacturing, 23, 161
mapping, 17, 26, 28, 33
marine environment, 42
marrow, 153, 154, 156, 165, 167, 173, 181, 184, 185, 186, 195, 196, 197
mass spectrometry, 126, 127, 128
mast cells, 141
material surface, 168, 183
matrix, ix, 18, 84, 105, 107, 109, 110, 112, 114, 117, 126, 134, 142, 150, 155, 157, 158, 161, 166, 169, 171, 172, 173, 175, 180, 181, 188, 191, 193, 197, 207
maturation, 2, 18, 19, 32, 36, 39, 173
maxillofacial area, 152
measurement, 127
measures, 127
mechanical properties, 157, 162
mechanical stress, 157, 197
media, 65, 69, 70, 80, 85, 161, 176
mediation, 56
medicine, 150, 152, 183, 184, 197
melanoma, 27
melting, 159, 160, 161, 162, 163
melting temperature, 159
membranes, x, 80, 81, 199, 209
memory, 7, 38, 120, 168
meridian, 141, 148
mesenchymal progenitor cells, 184, 185
mesenchymal stem cells, 148, 153, 154, 155, 165, 172, 184, 185, 186, 187
mesenchyme, 82

N

Q

R

T

U

V